Indigenous Public Health

EDITED BY **LINDA BURHANSSTIPANOV** AND **KATHRYN L. BRAUN**

INDIGENOUS PUBLIC
HEALTH

Improvement through Community-Engaged Interventions

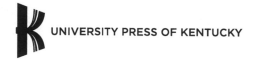

UNIVERSITY PRESS OF KENTUCKY

Copyright © 2022 by The University Press of Kentucky

Scholarly publisher for the Commonwealth,
serving Bellarmine University, Berea College, Centre
College of Kentucky, Eastern Kentucky University,
The Filson Historical Society, Georgetown College,
Kentucky Historical Society, Kentucky State University,
Morehead State University, Murray State University,
Northern Kentucky University, Spalding University,
Transylvania University, University of Kentucky,
University of Louisville, University of Pikeville, and
Western Kentucky University.
All rights reserved.

Editorial and Sales Offices: The University Press of Kentucky
663 South Limestone Street, Lexington, Kentucky 40508-4008
www.kentuckypress.com

Cataloging-in-Publication data is available from the Library
of Congress.

ISBN 978-0-8131-9584-1 (hardcover : alk. paper)
ISBN 978-0-8131-9587-2 (epub)
ISBN 978-0-8131-9586-5 (pdf)

This book is printed on acid-free paper meeting
the requirements of the American National Standard
for Permanence in Paper for Printed Library Materials.

Manufactured in the United States of America.

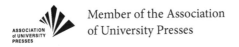

Member of the Association
of University Presses

Contents

1

Introduction

Stories of Success

Linda Burhansstipanov, Kathryn L. Braun, and
Keilyn Leina'ala Kawakami

Goal and Overview of the Book

The goal of this book, *Improving Indigenous Public Health Through Community-Engaged Interventions: Stories of Success,* is to highlight how effective community-engaged interventions, strategies, programs, and resources within Indigenous communities result in diverse, successful public health programs. The Indigenous Peoples highlighted in this book are the original peoples of the contiguous 48 states of the United States (US), Alaska, Hawai'i, and the US-Affiliated Pacific Island (USAPI) jurisdictions of American Samoa, the Commonwealth of Northern Mariana Islands (CNMI), Guam, the Federated States of Micronesia (FSM), the Republic of the Marshall Islands, and the Republic of Palau.

The US Census allows individuals of Indigenous ancestry to identify themselves as American Indian (AI), Alaska Native (AN), Native Hawaiian (NH), and/or other Pacific Islander (PI) group—for example, Chamorro, Samoan, and Marshallese.[1,2] US Census Bureau data from 2019 suggest that only 2.9% (9.7 million) of the US population were AI/AN (alone or in combination with one or more races), and the states with the highest numbers of AI/ANs were Arizona, California, Oklahoma, New Mexico, Texas, North Carolina, Alaska, Washington, South Dakota, and New York.[3]

Data from 2019 also suggest that only 0.4% (1.4 million) of the US population identified as NH/PI.[4] The states with the highest numbers of NH/PI were Hawai'i, California, Washington, Texas, Utah, Florida, Nevada, Oregon, New York, and Arizona.[4] However, other states, such as Arkansas, have large populations of PI. The 2020 United Nations estimates for populations of PI in the US-Affiliated Pacific were 55,000 in American Samoa, 169,000 in Guam, 58,000 in the Commonwealth of the Northern Mariana Islands, 115,000 in the Federated States of Micronesia, 59,000 in the Republic of the Marshall Islands, and 18,000 in the Republic of Palau.[4]

Thus, the numbers of these individuals in the US are small compared to the total population. The numbers that are included in nationally sponsored surveillance systems also are small. As a result, health data for AI, AN, NH, and PI groups are often not included in federal reports. Federal reports that include statistics on Indigenous Peoples often aggregate American Indians with Alaska Natives (AI/AN) and Native Hawaiians with other Pacific Islanders (NH/PI).[5] Although discouraged by federal law, some federal reports aggregate NH/PI peoples with Asian Americans, which masks known disparities between these groups. In this book, efforts were made to present data on AI, AN, NH, and PI health from other sources. For example, data from Hawaiʻi were used to describe the prevalence of health conditions among NH and other PI, and regionally collected data were used to describe the prevalence of health conditions among AI, AN, and PI in the USAPI jurisdictions. Also, Indigenous Peoples may have intersectional identities with other races and ethnicities, and modern-day political borders create false separations for populations, communities, and cultural groups. For example, the Pascua Yaqui have family members based in the US and Mexico, although the US is only concerned with those living in the US, and Samoans have family members living in Samoa, an independent country, as well as in American Samoa (just 140 miles from Samoa).[6]

The AI, AN, NH, and PI communities featured in this book have unique relationships with the US federal government. However, they share a history of colonization by Europeans and Americans. Colonization is defined as "the act of taking control of an area or a country that is not your own, especially using force, and sending people from your own country to live there."[7] Because of colonization, these groups experienced loss of land and power in their homelands through occupation, forced relocation, and/or mandated boarding schools. They experienced efforts to eliminate cultural strengths and resources. Most have effectively lost their right to self-determination, regardless of treaty status and agreements with the US government. As a result, the majority of Indigenous communities discussed in this book live with disparities and inequities. These include higher levels of poverty and poor health outcomes than non-Hispanic Whites.

Many government organizations (federal, state, territorial) berate Indigenous Peoples for their differences from the dominant US population and highlight their disparities. The implications are that Indigenous communities do not know how to take care of themselves or are inept at doing so, or they need the "Great White Father" to tell them what to do. These are inaccurate perspectives. When able to obtain resources and regain what was stolen, Indigenous communities are quite capable of creating, implementing, and evaluating culturally respectful interventions and programs.

Chapter 1 provides explanations or definitions for words used throughout the book and includes maps showing the areas where these populations live. It also summarizes key take-home messages from all of the chapters, and these reflect the editors' and authors' collective experiences and work with Indigenous populations. The book includes an emphasis on cancer because the majority of work completed by the editors has been focused on cancer.

Chapter 2 briefly summarizes the history and contemporary health issues of AI, AN, NH, and PI in the US. Chapter 3 explores racism and its negative impact on health status. Chapters 4 and 5 suggest principles or strategies for working more respectfully with Indigenous partners and populations, specifically strategies grounded in culture and community (Chapter 4) and in capacity building and quality improvement (Chapter 5). Chapters 6 through 10 focus on specific health issues, including sexual health (Chapter 6), cancer (Chapter 7), cancer patient navigation (Chapter 8), diabetes (Chapter 9), and heart disease (Chapter 10). Starting with Chapter 3, examples of successful, Indigenous, community-engaged interventions and strategies are highlighted. More examples are included from AI communities, as the number of AI is much bigger than of the other three groups, and AI communities have had a longer history of interactions with the US governmental policies and funding sources than the other three groups.

Indigenous Geography

US Census estimates that about 22% of AI/ANs live on reservations or other trust lands and 60% live in urban areas.[3] There are 574 federally recognized tribes,[3] and several hundred more tribes are recognized by local states. The Indian Health Service (IHS) groups AI/AN into geographic regions, referred to as Purchased Referred Care Delivery Areas (PRCDA),[8] shown in Figure 1.1.

Healthcare is delivered to AN through the 12 Alaska Native Health Corporations within the state of Alaska. The landmass of Alaska is about 570,300 square miles,[9] and distance is a key issue in healthcare delivery in Alaska. A flight from Ketchikan in the south to Barrow in the north covers 1,300 miles, and a flight from the tip of Aleutian Islands (Attu Island) to Ketchikan border covers 1,800 miles. Additionally, most regions within Alaska have no roads or only are accessible by boat and airplane. Maps of Alaska frequently show how the state is relatively small and to the lower left of the US contiguous states. However, Figure 1.2 shows the size of Alaska by overlaying it on the US map and identifies regions within the state.

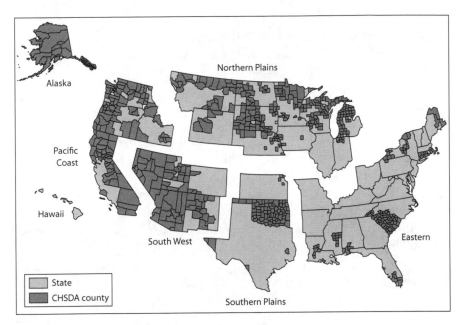

Fig 1.1. States and Contract Health Service Delivery Area (CHSDA) counties by Indian Health Service Regions, 1999–2009, *American Journal of Public Health,* 2014. Indian Health Service. These areas have since been designated as Purchased/Referred Care Delivery Areas (PRCDAs).

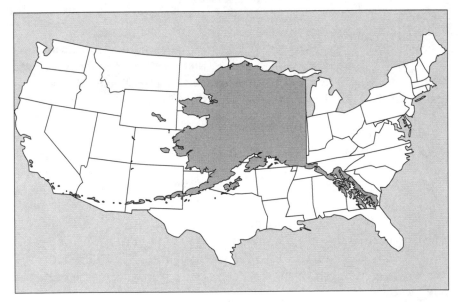

Fig 1.2a. Size of Alaska compared to the lower contiguous US states. Wikimedia.

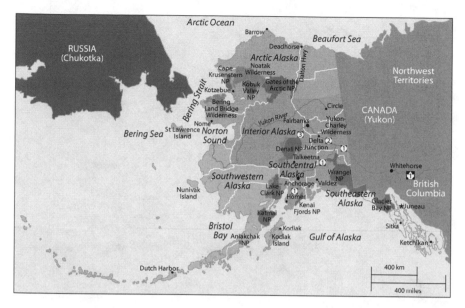

Fig 1.2b. Alaska state map with regions. Wikimedia. Original map created by Peter Fitzgerald. Redrawn for clarity and converted to black and white. https://creativecommons.org/licenses/by/3.0/deed.en.

Although the landmass of Alaska is large, the Indigenous home for NH/PI affiliated with the United States spans millions of square miles of Pacific Ocean (Figure 1.3). Native Hawaiians are the Indigenous people of the Hawaiian archipelago, which is 2,500 miles west of California, about 5 hours away by air. It takes 12 hours to fly from Hawai'i, on the eastern edge of the region, to Palau on the western edge. Each jurisdiction has its distinct language(s) and culture(s), including unique social structures.

The USAPI region includes more than 2,100 small islands and atolls within 4 million square miles of ocean. About half a million people live in a USAPI, with a collective landmass smaller than the US state of Rhode Island. The USAPI jurisdictions include American Samoa, which is in an area of the Pacific populated by Polynesians, and six jurisdictions in the area of the Pacific populated by Micronesians, including the CNMI, Guam, the FSM, the Republic of the Marshall Islands, and the Republic of Palau. The region crosses four time zones, and air travel from American Samoa to Palau can take several days, as passengers must first fly 2,500 miles north to Honolulu, then 3,800 miles west to Guam, and then 800 miles south to Palau. Health services

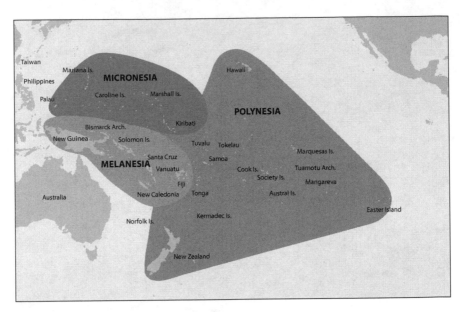

Fig 1.3. Pacific Islands map. Wikimedia.

throughout the USAPI are limited, and many individuals from the USAPI access health services in Hawai'i or the Philippines.

Terminology

Several terms and abbreviations are used throughout the book. Major terms are defined here, and Table 1.1. lists common abbreviations and acronyms.

The World Health Organization (WHO) defines "health intervention" as "an act performed for, with, or on behalf of a person or population whose purpose is to assess, improve, maintain, promote or modify health, functioning, or health conditions."[10] Interventions consist of "strategies" and may result in a "program" and/or "resource." Interventions include multiple components, each of which can be evaluated, documented, and tracked. Strategies, programs, and resources also are evaluated, but interventions are more formal and need to be validated for effectiveness, efficiency, and dissemination to others.

The phrase "social determinants of health" was first used by the WHO in 2003.[11,12] The WHO defined social determinants of health as "the conditions in which people are born, grow, live, work and age" and "the fundamental drivers of these conditions." The US Centers for Disease Control and Prevention (CDC) categorizes social determinants of health into five domains: (1) economic

Table 1.1. Abbreviations, Acronyms, and Translations Used in This Book

AAC&U	Association of American Colleges and Universities
ACE	Adverse Childhood Experience(s)
ACF	Administration for Children and Families
ACS	American Cancer Society
AI	American Indian(s)
AI/AN	American Indians and Alaska Natives
AIANNH	American Indians, Alaska Natives, and Native Hawaiians
AIDS	Acquired Immune Deficiency Syndrome
AIM	American Indian Movement
ALL	acute lymphoblastic leukemia
AN	Alaska Native(s)
ANCSA	Alaska Native Claims Settlement Act
ANILCA	Alaska National Interest Lands Conservation Act
ANMC	Alaska Native Medical Center
ANTHC	Alaska Native Tribal Health Consortium
AONN+	Academy of Oncology Nurse and Patient Navigators
APHA	American Public Health Association
APMs	alternative payment models
ARS	audience response system
ASCO	American Society of Clinical Oncology
ASU	Arizona State University
AYA	adolescents and young adults
BIA	Bureau of Indian Affairs
BIE	Bureau of Indian Education
BMI	Body Mass Index
BRFSS	Behavioral Risk Factor Surveillance System
BRTHC	Bad River Tribal Health Clinic
CAB	Community Advisory Board
CAC	Community Advisory Committee
CAIR	Center for American Indian Resilience
CBPA	community-based participatory approach
CBPR	community-based participatory research
CDC	Centers for Disease Control and Prevention
CHL	Children's Healthy Living
CHR	Community Health Representative(s)
CHSDA	Contract Health Service Delivery Areas
CLAS	Culturally and Linguistically Appropriate Services
CMS	Centers for Medicare and Medicaid Services
CNMI	Commonwealth of the Northern Mariana Islands
CNS	central nervous system
CoC	Commission of Cancer

(continued)

Table 1.1. (*continued*)

COFA	Compacts of Free Association
CPN	Cancer Patient Navigator(s)
CRC	colorectal cancer
CWC	Chuuk Women's Council
DHHS	Department of Health and Human Services
DPP	Diabetes Prevention Program
DSME	Diabetes Self-Management Education Program
EARTH	Education and Research Towards Health Study
EHR	electronic health record
FOBT	fecal occult blood test
FSM	Federated States of Micronesia
GAO	Government Accountability Office
GHWIC	Good Health and Wellness in Indian Country
GPTCHB	Great Plains Tribal Chairmen's Health Board
GLW	Guardians of the Living Water
HbA1c	hemoglobin A1c test
HDL	high-density lipoprotein
HIA	health impact assessments
HIV	human immunodeficiency virus
HOPI	Hopi Office of Prevention and Intervention
HPV	human papillomavirus
HRSA	Health Resources and Services Administration
HYSN	Hawai'i Youth Services Network
IAIA	Institute of American Indian Art
IAT	implicit association test
ICCC	International Classification of Childhood Cancer
IGRA	Indian Gaming Regulatory Act
IHCIA	Indian Health Care Improvement Act
IHS	Indian Health Service
INSPIRE	INdigenous Samoan Partnership to Initiate Research Excellence
INTERSALT	International Cooperative Study on Salt, Other Factors, and Blood Pressure
ITCM	Intertribal Council of Michigan
IRB	institutional review board
ITCA	Intertribal Council of Arizona
JTW	Journey Towards Wellness
LAC	local advisory committee
MAPP	Mobilizing for Action through Planning and Partnerships
MBSG	Mind-Body Skills Group
MFH	Messengers for Health
MGH	Moloka'i General Hospital

MHRCH	Monument Health Rapid City Hospital
MBIRI	Missouri Breaks Industries Research, Incorporated
MPHI	Michigan Public Health Institute
NACES	Native American Cancer Education for Survivors
NACP	Native American Cancer Prevention
NAU	Northern Arizona University
NBL	neuroblastoma
NCI	National Cancer Institute
NMHEP	New Mexico Health Equity Partnership
NH	Native Hawaiian(s)
NHIH	Native Hawaiian and Indigenous Health
NHANES	National Health and Nutrition Examination Survey
NHLBI	National Heart, Lung, and Blood Institute
NHHCA	Native Hawaiian Health Care Act
NHHCS	National Hawaiian Health Care Systems
NHHHI	Native Hawaiian Heart Health Initiative
NHIH	Native Hawaiian and Indigenous Health
NHIS	National Health Interview Survey
NH/PI	Native Hawaiians and Other Pacific Islanders
NHW	non-Hispanic White
NIGMS	National Institutes of General Medical Services
NIH	National Institutes of Health
NIMHD	National Institute on Minority Health and Health Disparities
NIYG	Native It's Your Game
NNACC	Native Navigators and the Cancer Continuum
NNRT	National Navigation Roundtable
NPAIHB	Northwest Portland Area Indian Health Board
NPN	Native Patient Navigator(s)
NSF	National Science Foundation
OHSU	Oregon Health & Sciences University
OPHS	Office of Public Health Studies
PAR	Participatory Action Research
PCDC	Pacific Chronic Disease Coalition
PDEP	Pacific Diabetes Education Program
PDSA	Plan-Do-Study-Act
PDTRC	Pacific Diabetes Today Resource Center
PI	principal investigator
PI	Pacific Islander(s)
PI-DPP	Pacific Island—Diabetes Prevention Program
PID	pelvic inflammatory disease
PIG-E	pancreas, insulin, glucose, and energy
PN	patient navigator(s)

(*continued*)

Table 1.1. (*continued*)

PRC	Purchased Referred Care
PROMIS	Patient-Reported Outcomes Measurement Information System
PSA	prostate-specific antigen
PSE	policy, systems, and environmental
PTSD	posttraumatic stress disorder
QI	quality improvement
Q-TIPS	Quality Tribal Improvement Programs
QOL	quality of life
RFA	Request for Applications
RMI	Republic of the Marshall Islands
SATC	Sex Abuse Treatment Center
SEARHC	Southeast Alaska Regional Health Consortium
SEM	social-ecological model
SFIC	Santa Fe Indian Center
SOE	Spirit of EAGLES
SREP	Summer Research Enhancement Program
STI	sexually transmitted infections
T2DM	type 2 diabetes mellitus
TIHP	Toiyabe Indian Health Project
THO	Tribal Health Organization
TRC	Truth and Reconciliation Commissions
TRHT	Truth, Racial Healing and Transformation
UHM	University of Hawaiʻi at Mānoa
US	United States / United States of America
USDA-NIFA	US Department of Agriculture's National Institute for Food and Agriculture
USAPI	US-Affiliated Pacific Islands
UTHSC	University of Texas Health Science Center
WHO	World Health Organization

stability, (2) education access and quality, (3) healthcare access and quality, (4) neighborhood and built environment, and (5) social and community context (Figure 1.4).[13]

In the domain of economic stability, the CDC recognizes that health can be jeopardized by poverty, unstable employment, poor working conditions, unemployment, and the need to work multiple low-paying jobs to make ends meet. Also, the stress of living in poverty can affect children's brain development, making it harder for them to do well in school. Access to quality education is essential to health, as research shows that people with more education are able to obtain better paying jobs with health insurance, and thus have more

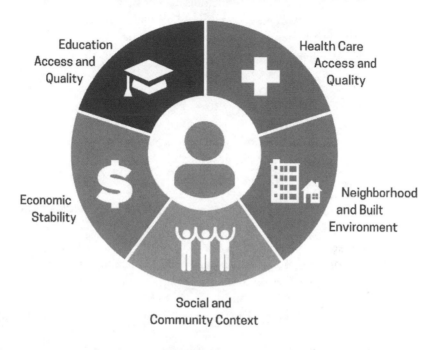

Social Determinants of Health

Education Access and Quality

Health Care Access and Quality

Economic Stability

Neighborhood and Built Environment

Social and Community Context

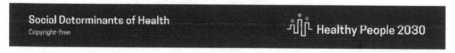

Social Determinants of Health
Copyright-free

Healthy People 2030

Fig 1.4. Social determinants of health. Courtesy of Healthy People 2030.

money to afford good housing, food, and physical activity options. Poor access to healthcare is another social determinant of health. About 1 in 10 people in the US does not have health insurance, making it difficult to see a primary care provider and to afford needed medications. Even with health insurances, some people live far from health services, and access to care also may be affected by discriminatory attitudes of providers.

One's neighborhood can be a social determinant of health, and many people in the US live in housing situations or neighborhoods that are crowded and/or have high rates of violence, unsafe air or water, noise, second-hand smoke, and other health and safety risks. Poor neighborhoods are less likely to have good options for purchasing affordable, healthy food and for safe physical activity, compared to middle-class and rich neighborhoods. The fifth category —social and community context—includes unsafe neighborhoods, discrimination, bullying, and lack of social support, all of which negatively affect health. These social determinants of health impact individual and community health, patient and family behaviors, and interactions with healthcare delivery.[14]

Healthy People 2030 defines "health disparity" as "a particular type of health difference that is closely linked with social, economic, and/or environmental disadvantage. Health disparities adversely affect groups of people who have systematically experienced greater obstacles to health based on their racial or ethnic group; religion; socioeconomic status; gender; age; mental health; cognitive, sensory, or physical disability; sexual orientation or gender identity; geographic location; or other characteristics historically linked to discrimination or exclusion."[15]

Health disparities research is devoted to advancing scientific knowledge about the influence of social (and other) determinants of health and translating this knowledge into programs and policies that can reduce health differences between groups. Because many disparities in health outcomes are rooted in disparities in social conditions, including income and living conditions, interventions for health must consider ways to reduce social disparities.[16,17]

The terms "health equity" and "health equality" are often confused with one another. Healthy People 2030 defines *health equity* as the "attainment of the highest level of health for all people."[15] As an analogy, "equality" is giving everyone a pair of shoes regardless of size (implying that one size fits all) and regardless of how many shoes they already have. But "equity" is about giving more shoes *that fit* to those who have none, while giving fewer or no shoes to those who have many. The latter implies a social justice imperative in health. Disparities and inequities begin with daily living conditions, such as being forced to live in resource-poor areas, living below the poverty level with substandard housing, having limited opportunities for education and employment, and having insufficient health insurance. "Achieving health equity requires valuing everyone equally with focused and ongoing societal efforts to address avoidable inequalities, historical and contemporary injustices, and the elimination of health and healthcare disparities."[18]

Although insufficient funding is allocated to Indigenous programs, and this impacts the potential success and/or long-term sustainability of the interventions summarized here, insufficient funding is not belabored in these chapters. Rather, the book focuses on ways community-engagement principles have been applied by and in Indigenous communities to successfully addresses disparities and work toward health equity.

"Community engagement" is a phrase used differently by different organizations. For example, the CDC defines community engagement as:

> the process of working collaboratively with and through groups of people affiliated by geographic proximity, special interest, or similar situations to address issues affecting the well-being of those people. It is a powerful vehicle for bringing about environmental and behavioral changes that will improve the health of the community and its members. It often involves partnerships and coalitions that help mobilize resources and influence systems, change relationships among partners, and serve as catalysts for changing policies, programs, and practices.[19]

Community engagement for health is integral within participatory action research (PAR). PAR requires that people affected by a health issue be involved in the identification and solving of their own problems. PAR draws on a wide range of influences, including Paulo Freire, a Brazilian educator and activist who advocated to democratize the creation of knowledge and ground it in real community needs and learning. In 1968,[20] Freire emphasized that teaching should challenge learners to examine power structures and patterns of inequality within the status quo. Community-based participatory research (CBPR) has its philosophical origins in PAR, and both stem from social justice paradigms that seeks to liberate communities from traditional, positivist forms of academic inquiry.[21] Barbara Israel and colleagues articulated nine principles of CBPR around engaging community in all aspects of research, transferring skills, and sharing power.[22]

Principles for community engagement were published by the CDC in 2011 (Table 1.2.).[19] They are organized into three sections: items to consider before beginning engagement, what is necessary for engagement to occur, and what to consider for engagement to be successful. The editors stress that community engagement does not mean "recruitment." Rather, it refers to the relationship that needs to be created between community members and collaborators to build trust to work together. Community engagement must occur before the initiation of a project.

Often when accessing needed resources for health improvement and community-engagement projects, Indigenous communities must partner with outside agencies. The external partners who collaborated on the community-engaged interventions highlighted in this book included individuals from universities, research centers, governmental bodies, healthcare organizations, and nonprofits. Extending CDC principles of community engagement, the bulleted list below summarizes some additional areas that external health

Table 1.2. CDC's Principles of Community Engagement

Before starting a community engagement effort . . .
- Be clear about the purposes or goals of the engagement effort and the populations and/or communities you want to engage.
- Focus on overall community improvement, including economic and infrastructure development, which will contribute to health.
- Ask community members to specify their health-related concerns, identify areas that need action, and become involved in planning, designing, implementing, and evaluating appropriate programs.
- Become knowledgeable about the community's culture, economic conditions, social networks, political and power structures, norms and values, demographic trends, history, and experience with efforts by outside groups to engage it in various programs. Learn about the community's perceptions of those initiating the engagement activities.

For engagement to occur, it is necessary to . . .
- Go to the community, establish relationships, build trust, work with the formal and informal leadership, and seek commitment from community organizations and leaders to create processes for mobilizing the community.
- Remember and accept that collective self-determination is the responsibility and right of all people in a community. No external entity should assume it can bestow on a community the power to act in its self-interest.

For engagement to succeed . . .
- Partnering with the community is necessary to create change and improve health.
- All aspects of community engagement must recognize and respect the diversity of the community. Awareness of the various cultures of a community and other factors affecting diversity must be paramount in planning, designing, and implementing approaches to engaging a community.
- Community engagement can only be sustained by identifying and mobilizing community assets and strengths and by developing the community's capacity and resources to make decisions and take action.
- Organizations that wish to engage a community, as well as individuals seeking to effect change, must be prepared to release control of actions or interventions to the community and be flexible enough to meet its changing needs.
- Community collaboration requires a long-term commitment by the engaging organization and its partners.

providers and researchers need to consider when working with Indigenous communities.

- The external provider or researcher must consider the Indigenous community as an autonomous and equal partner.
- Partnerships are built on trust. If trust has not yet been established between the Indigenous community and the external provider or researchers, strategies and rules of engagement to improve trust must be articulated.

- The external provider or researcher must involve the community as an expert in identifying health issues and developing interventions.
- The partnership must build public health capacity in the community.
- The external provider or researcher must be willing to learn from the community about its history, values, and respectful ways of communicating and behaving.
- Grant funding must be shared with community.
- Written protocols must be put in place for equitable decision-making and resource sharing.
- Written agreements about data ownership and management must be put in place to ensure data security, as well as appropriate and respectful dissemination of findings.

Sustainability

Many of the interventions highlighted in this book benefited from federal funding. Most of the Indigenous communities lack sufficient infrastructure to sustain public health programs beyond grant funding. In general, sustaining grant-funded interventions is difficult, and projects attempt to survive by morphing to fit new funding streams, integrating their activities into larger, more funding-secure entities, or seeking reimbursement from healthcare insurers.[23]

The second issue influencing sustainability is changing political support. For example, some AI/AN tribal nations elect new leadership (Governor, Chair, President, Principal Chief, Council) every 2 years. Newly elected officials may not want to reinforce or support the public health programs created during the previous leadership. Other times, the priorities of leadership changes, such as during the COVID-19 pandemic when some tribal nations that experienced excessive deaths voted to support only those interventions designed to address COVID-19 health issues. Other ongoing or long-term programs lost staff who were reassigned to COVID-19 prevention and control.

A third issue is staffing. Innovative interventions are often led and staffed by energetic and enthusiastic people who are able to engender support for the interventions among funders, administrators, staff, and clients. In the sustainability literature, these individuals often are referred to as champions.[24] Like all employees, champions may leave the project, for example to attend school, care for family, take a better paying job, relocate, or retire. Identifying, hiring, and training new staff and developing new champions takes time and may be difficult in rural communities. Thus, temporary funding, changing leadership, and turnover in staff are major challenges to maintaining and enhancing Indigenous public health interventions that can address inequities and reduce health disparities.

Despite the challenges of sustainability, Indigenous communities have developed many culturally appropriate and successful public health interventions. Although many Indigenous communities live in settings negatively affected by social determinants of health (Figure 1.4), with adequate resources, Indigenous communities have and can continue to implement innovative and culturally respectful public health interventions that benefit their communities. The editors are proud to be able to display their stellar work within this book.

Audiences and Authors

The book is written for several different audiences. The first audience includes public health professionals and community members working with Indigenous communities. The second audience is public health students. The third is health and social service providers who are new to Indigenous communities and need to learn more about the health issues and ways community-engagement interventions can be conducted successfully to address local health disparities. The book also may influence Indigenous policy decisions, resolutions, and ordinances.

There are other books about Indigenous health, but most provide detailed descriptions of Indigenous Peoples' disparities or focus on what Indigenous communities do wrong or how poorly people in Indigenous communities live. The editors acknowledge that Indigenous Peoples live with many disparities in comparison to other racial groups. However, a major goal of this book is to highlight ways Indigenous communities have engaged with each other and outside partners to improve their health and their communities. Much can be learned by sharing successes! Also, the editors strived to engage Indigenous Peoples in the writing of each chapter. Thus, of the 53 authors, 26 are Indigenous, and 8 are from other communities of color or under-served groups. Brief descriptions of authors are presented at the end of this book.

Key Take-Home Messages

There are seven key messages from this book:

1. Accurate Indigenous data are essential. Indigenous organizations and programs need ownership of their data, and data need to be secured within their local systems and software. This allows them to manage and control the use of data to increase the likelihood that the data are used respectfully and appropriately. Data also need to be disaggregated. For AI/AN, it is important to disaggregate data by regions defined by the IHS.[8] Data on NH/PI should never be combined with data on Asian Americans, as they differ significantly in their histories, cultures, and experiences with the US federal government.[4] Because

of the small sizes of the AI, AN, NH, and PI populations, oversampling may be required by surveillance programs.

2. Partnerships are necessary for infrastructure development, capacity building, and program sustainability. A single program cannot address every issue. Small programs must partner with other programs and communities to foster health. Organizations need to acknowledge strengths in the local Indigenous communities. Native organizations and people have the expertise to contribute to public health interventions and are willing to participate if treated as true partners. This includes being respected as decision-makers and leaders, having autonomy over their data, and both giving and receiving education. Skills to increase empowerment need to be integrated throughout public health interventions for people of all ages.

3. Trust is more likely to be developed when external providers and researchers spend time in the community. Organizations and individuals that want to work with Indigenous communities need to recognize their own implicit and explicit biases. They need to try to overcome these biases through hands-on experiences within clinical and community-based services. They need to spend time in the community to establish meaningful and trusting relationships. If trust is not established prior to receiving a grant, time for trust building needs to be scheduled within the grant cycle.

4. Interventions must be tailored to the Indigenous community of interest. There are 574 federally recognized tribes under the AI/AN label,[3] and more than 30 distinct cultural groups under the NH/PI label.[1] Each group is unique. Interventions that have proven to work in one part of the US with a certain population may not work in another part of the US or with another population. This is not to say that every intervention must be built from scratch. But an evidence-based intervention from one community must be tailored to a new community before it is implemented. Common strategies used to tailor programs to Indigenous communities involve incorporating designs and photos from the community into intervention materials, presenting evidence of the relevance of the problem to the community, using words and phrases from the community's language, drawing directly on the experience of members of the community, and reflecting the community's cultural values, beliefs, behaviors, and context.[25]

5. Traditional Indigenous cultures contribute to improved health and resiliency. Interventions need to acknowledge that most Indigenous Peoples live in

two worlds, embracing both traditional modes of living and healing and Western medicine. This is because Western medicine alone is insufficient for healing the whole self, which includes the physical, mental, emotional, social, and spiritual domains of wellness. Indigenous Peoples have been able to retain traditional cultures throughout the centuries and are very resilient. By engaging as equal partners, important elements from traditional culture can be reflected in intervention processes and products.

6. Patient navigation programs successfully address barriers to appropriate healthcare services. Indigenous Peoples are diagnosed with chronic conditions at younger ages and in more advanced stages than non-Hispanic Whites and face many barriers accessing timely and quality healthcare. Navigation programs have been shown to overcome barriers to prevention, detection, and treatment of cancer and other chronic conditions. Navigator programs help patients obtain higher quality and less costly healthcare services. Employing navigators from within the Indigenous community can help overcome trust issues and assure that local communication patterns are understood and respected. Same-group navigators also can help a patient integrate Indigenous traditional health beliefs and Western approaches to care.

7. Sustainability is a critical issue for successful public health interventions, but funding is also needed to address the social determinants of health. Sustaining successful interventions requires political support, stable funding, and program champions. The majority of Indigenous public health programs are significantly underfunded and thus jeopardized when scarce resources are reallocated to other issues, when grant funding ends, and when staff leaves. More resources need to be channeled to Indigenous communities to fund interventions and to address the social determinants of health, which often underlie health disparities. For example, addressing substandard housing on reservations and Hawaiian homesteads would reduce everyday exposure to infection and injury experienced by many Indigenous Peoples within their home settings.[26]

Summary

This chapter identified the Indigenous Peoples that are the focus of this book. Maps were included to help the reader understand where Indigenous Peoples live. Relevant terms were described, and Table 1.1. summarized the acronyms, abbreviations, and selected translations used throughout the book. Finally, the chapter presented seven key take-home messages from the book.

References

1. US Census. *The Native Hawaiian and other Pacific Islander population: 2010.* Accessed September 26, 2020. https://www.census.gov/prod/cen2010/briefs/c2010br-12.pdf.

2. US Census. *The American Indian and Alaska Native population: 2010.* Accessed September 26, 2020. https://www.census.gov/history/pdf/c2010br-10.pdf.

3. US Office of Minority Health. Profile: American Indian/Alaska Native. Accessed February 6, 2022. https://minorityhealth.hhs.gov/omh/browse.aspx?lvl=3&lvlid=62#:~:text=As%20of%202019%2C%20there%20were,of%20the%20total%20U.S.%20population.

4. US Office of Minority Health. Profile: Native Hawaiians/Pacific Islanders. Accessed February 6, 2022. https://minorityhealth.hhs.gov/omh/browse.aspx?lvl=3&lvlid=65.

5. US Office of Management and Budget. *Revisions to the standards for the classification of federal data on race and ethnicity, 2017.* Accessed September 26, 2020. https://www.whitehouse.gov/wp-content/uploads/2017/11/Revisions-to-the-Standards-for-the-Classification-of-Federal-Data-on-Race-and-Ethnicity-October30-1997.pdf.

6. Cassel KD. Using the social-ecological model as a research and intervention framework to understand and mitigate obesogenic factors in Samoan populations. *Ethn Health.* 2010;15(4):397–416.

7. Oxford Learner's Dictionaries. Colonization. Accessed September 26, 2020. https://www.oxfordlearnersdictionaries.com/us/definition/english/ colonization?q=colonization.

8. US Indian Health Service. Regional offices. Accessed September 26, 2020. https://www.ihs.gov/dcps/regionaloffices/

9. Wikipedia. Geography of Alaska. Accessed March 3, 2021. https://en.wikipedia.org/wiki/Geography_of_Alaska.

10. World Health Organization. International classification of health interventions. Accessed March 3, 2021. https://www.who.int/standards/classifications/international-classification-of-health-interventions.

11. Wilkinson R, Marmot M, eds. *The social determinants of health: The solid facts, 2nd ed.* World Health Organization Europe, 2003. Accessed September 26, 2020. https://www.euro.who.int/__data/assets/pdf_file/0005/98438/e81384.pdf.

12. Commission on Social Determinants of Health. *Closing the gap in a generation: Health equity through action on the social determinants of health.* World Health Organization, 2008. Accessed September 26, 2020. https://apps.who.int/iris/bitstream/handle/10665/43943/9789241563703_eng.pdf;jsessionid=F49278A8B7A9004027B77A0CACB9C20F?sequence=1.

13. US Department of Health and Human Services. Healthy People 2030 social determinants of health. Accessed March 4, 2021. https://health.gov/healthypeople/objectives-and-data/social-determinants-health.

14. Braveman P, Gottlieb L. The social determinants of health: It's time to consider the causes of the causes. *Public Health Rep.* 2014;129(Suppl 2):19–31.

15. US Department of Health and Human Services. Healthy People 2030 questions & answers. Accessed March 3, 2021. https://health.gov/our-work/healthy-people/healthy-people-2030/questions-answers.

16. Duran DG, Pérez-Stable EJ. Novel approaches to advance minority health and health disparities research. *Am J Public Health.* 2019;109(S1):S8–S10.

17. Srinivasan S, Williams SD. Transitioning from health disparities to a health equity research agenda: The time is now. *Public Health Rep.* 2014 January–Feburary;129 Suppl 2(Suppl 2):71–76.

18. US Department of Health and Human Services. Healthy People 2030 social determinants of health. Accessed March 4, 2021. https://health.gov/healthypeople/objectives-and-data/social-determinants-health.

19. Centers for Disease Control and Prevention. *Principles of community engagement, 2nd ed*. NIH Publication No. 11-7782, 2011. Accessed September 26, 2020. https://www.atsdr.cdc.gov/communityengagement/pdf/PCE_Report_508_FINAL.pdf

20. Freire P. *Pedagogy of the oppressed*. Continuum, 2000.

21. Wallerstein N, Giatti LL, Bógus CM, *et al*. Shared participatory research principles and methodologies: Perspectives from the USA and Brazil—45 Years after Paulo Freire's "Pedagogy of the Oppressed." *Societies (Basel)*. 2017;7(2):6.

22. Israel BA, Eng E, Schulz AJ, *et al*. *Methods in community-based participatory research for health*. Jossey-Bass, 2005.

23. Schell SF, Luke DA, Schooley MW, *et al*. Public health program capacity for sustainability: A new framework. *Implement Sci*. 2013;8:15.

24. Scheirer MA. Is sustainability possible? A review and commentary on empirical studies of program sustainability. *Am J Eval*. 2005;26:320–347.

25. Kreuter MW, Lukwago SN, Bucholtz RD, *et al*. Achieving cultural appropriateness in health promotion programs: Targeted and tailored approaches. *Health Educ Behav*. 2003;30:133–146.

26. National Congress of American Indians. Housing and infrastructure. Accessed January 1, 2021. https://www.ncai.org/policy-issues/economic-development-commerce/housing-infrastructure.

2

Standing on the Shoulders of Our Ancestors

History and Contemporary Health Status of Indigenous Peoples in the United States

Jennie R. Joe, Linda Burhansstipanov, Jessica Saniguq Ullrich, and Kathryn L. Braun

Introduction

This chapter summarizes the history and current health status of the Indigenous Peoples living on the lands now occupied by the United States (US). These lands are now known as contiguous 48 US states on the North American continent, Alaska, Hawai'i, and the US-Affiliated Pacific Islands, including American Samoa, the Commonwealth of the Northern Mariana Islands, Guam, the Federated States of Micronesia, the Republic of the Marshall Islands, and the Republic of Palau.

The purpose of this book is to highlight how these community-engaged interventions, strategies, projects, and resources within Indigenous communities produce successful public health outcomes. It is important, however, to begin by providing a brief overview on the devastating history of each Indigenous population and how this history continues to affect social determinants of health and interfere with communities' successes. Within this context, this chapter also provides the background on how Indigenous populations continue to confront and overcome issues embedded in horrific historical events.

The first inhabitants of these lands had their own cultures and identities prior to colonization, and many Indigenous Peoples continue to self-identify according to their own sense of traditional ancestral history or homeland—for example, White Mountain Apache, Tlingit, Kānaka Maoli (Native Hawaiian), Marshallese, and so on. However, in most instances, these Indigenous groups are now identified by names bestowed upon them by their colonizers and lumped into generic or geographic categories such as American Indian (AI), Alaska Native (AN), Native Hawaiian (NH), and Pacific Islander (PI). The geographical landscape also is used as a way to group Indigenous Peoples in North America—that is, Arctic, Subarctic, Northwest Coast, Plateau, California,

Southwest, Plains, Great Basin, Northeast, and Southeast. But, it is not uncommon to see American Indians and Alaska Natives (AI/AN) presented or viewed as one collective group. Similarly, Native Hawaiian and other Pacific Islanders (NH/PI) are lumped together, although this group includes more than 30 different Pacific peoples with unique cultures and languages. In this book individual group names are used, or at least one of the four relevant categories of AI, AN, NH, and PI. However, much of the data available from federal sources is presented for the larger collectives of AI/AN and NH/PI.

Attention given to group identity has increasingly become more complex, partly fueled by high rates of racial admixture, as well as the confusing way countries and state agencies classify race and ethnicity within their populations. For some data sources, individuals are allowed to specify their race. For other databases, race and ethnicity may be assigned by algorithm or "guessed at" by the data recorder. These differences increase racial misclassification problems.[1,2] However, whichever racial or ethnic classification is used for or by Indigenous Peoples, the overall intent of this publication is to bring attention to diverse Indigenous Peoples' similarities and differences in response to varying political, social, and economic conditions that contribute to their persistent state of health disparities and how some of these disparities are being addressed.

All Indigenous Peoples featured in this book have been impacted by varying degrees of colonization by European, Mexican, Asian, and US populations. For example, Mexico ruled California, Nevada, Utah, Arizona, Texas and half of New Mexico when the Treaty of Guadalupe Hidalgo ended the Mexican–American War (1846–1848).[3] Prior to colonization, Indigenous communities were self-governing with established worldviews, customs, beliefs, and taboos. They honored practices to promote health, and they made extensive use of local medicinal plants and other therapeutic interventions for treating physical, mental-emotional, or spiritual health conditions. Without question, the importance of place was central to the identity of Indigenous Peoples, with the environment shaping the group's food sources, dwellings, clothing, language, and lifestyle.

The social and cultural disruptions brought by colonization changed these norms and had a crippling impact on the health and lifestyle of most Indigenous populations. Forced colonization undermined local practices, which had developed within the context of local environmental conditions and resources. As the ability to practice time-honored and environmentally appropriate practices decreased, dependence on colonial powers increased for all things needed for survival, including food, shelter, healthcare, education, and other resources.[4]

The expansion of foreign powers across Indigenous lands led to the rapid depopulation of Indigenous Peoples through warfare, as well as through exposure to reoccurring waves of communicable diseases against which most had no immunity.[5,6] Across the continental US, Alaska, and the Pacific, the common waves of infectious diseases included smallpox, measles, influenza, bubonic plague, and sexually transmitted infections, etc.[4,7] The Indigenous healers and their treatment modalities were ineffective against the new and unfamiliar causes of diseases. Among some infectious disease survivors, consequences were devastating. For example, smallpox left many survivors with disfigurements, driving some to suicide.[8,9,10]

The high death rates from war and disease greatly impacted the Indigenous communities' most fragile members, namely, the young and the elderly. Increased infant and childhood mortality dramatically slowed population growth. The high mortality rates among elders decreased the communities' pools of knowledgeable and skilled healers, and also destroyed an irreplaceable tribal resource, as community elders were repositories of Indigenous history, language, and cultural knowledge. Because there were no formal censuses during the early periods of colonization, rates of mortality due to epidemics and warfare continue to be debated.[5,11] Estimates of the total number of Indigenous Peoples prior to European contact may have reached 100 million, and these populations likely were reduced as much as 80% following foreign occupation.[12,13]

Brief History of AI/AN under US Control

Treaties, Structures, and Laws for AI Health

The peopling of the North American continent is generally traced to theories about migrations of Indigenous Peoples moving from Asia via the Bering Straits or via sea travel. Most North America's Indigenous Peoples, however, dismiss these migration theories and hold fast to creation beliefs found in their stories and legends. Although different AI and AN tribes encountered foreign powers at different times, their experiences with colonization were similar.

Unlike other racial or ethnic groups in the US, AI have treaty-based relationships with the federal government, with treaties established by a variety of congressional actions as well as Presidential Executive Orders (Table 2.1.). During the early governmental treaty-making arrangements, the federal government's trust relationship with tribes was housed in the Indian Affairs Office within the US War Department, where there was little governmental concern for the general health and welfare of AI (other than for a few tribes considered friendly to the US). The government periodically allocated funding for immunizations to the friendly tribes, but the action was mainly to protect non-AI civilians and military personnel living near or among tribal communities.[14,15,16] History notes, for example, in 1832, the government allocated funds to buy and provide smallpox vaccinations only to tribes considered friendly to the US.[15 17]

When the US Department of Interior was established, the Indian Affairs Office was transferred out of the War Department in 1824 and given a new name—the Bureau of Indian Affairs (BIA). Initially, the office was charged to negotiate treaties, oversee trade, and deliver and provide oversight of various tribal resources, including education and healthcare promised in the treaties. The BIA website today notes that its early policies were designed primarily to subjugate and assimilate "Natives," but that these have evolved over time to policies to promote AI/AN self-determination.[18] However, BIA resources for maintaining or improving the health and education of AI/AN were and have remained insufficient to meet needs. The failure to decrease the high morbidity and mortality rates among AI/AN populations forced another congressional action in the mid-1950s by moving the healthcare responsibilities from the BIA to the US Public Health Service, which formed the federal Indian Health Service (IHS). Today, the primary healthcare delivery service system for reservation-based tribes is IHS. In recent years, a small percentage of IHS funding has been earmarked to support non-profit healthcare programs to serve AI/AN living in urban areas. In 2022, approximately 41 urban-based health programs are managed by local AI/AN boards or organizations.

Today, the basis for the IHS's authority to provide healthcare to tribes is found scattered across several pieces of legislation: (1) the Indian Citizenship Act (also called the Snyder Act) of 1921, (2) the Transfer Act of 1955, (3) the Indian Education Assistance and Self Determination Act in 1975, and (4) the Indian Health Care Improvement Act in 1976. The early policy actions were not specific to healthcare. For example, the 1921 Snyder Act was a general directive for the Indian Affairs Office to "direct, supervise, and expend such moneys as Congress may from time to time appropriate for the benefit, care, and assistance of the Indians throughout the United States." The act also included provision for "relief of distress and conservation of health." However, the Snyder Act did very little to improve healthcare for tribes, according to the Meriam Report, which was issued in 1928 by the Institute for Government Research (now called the Brookings Institution).[19]

The Indian Health Care Improvement Act of 1976 brought some additional health resources to the IHS, including recognition and some resources for urban-based health resources for those living in various cities.[20] The goal of the law was to address health inequity by improving the health status of AI/AN and bringing it more in line with that of the general US population. However, from these legal changes, a patchwork system evolved that can be difficult for today's AI to navigate. The sidebar below uses a fictitious story to illustrate how an AI woman currently functions within the healthcare system.

Table 2.1. Key Points in American Indian (AI) History

1608–1830	Treaties were made between AI Tribes and the US.
1802	War Department was created to "handle" AI.
1824	Bureau of Indian Affairs (BIA) was formed.
1850–1871	Federal reservations were established.
1871–1928	The US Congress stopped making treaties because they were seen as an impediment to assimilation into White society.
1887	The General Allotment Act (also called the Dawes Act) changed communal ownership of tribal lands to individual ownership. Each Indian male over age 18 was given an allotment, and remaining tribal lands were sold to non-Indians.
1924	Indian Citizenship Act (Snyder Act) granted US citizenship to AI born in the US, but allowed states to decide whether AI could vote, and several did not.
1934	Indian Reorganization Act set up Reservation Business Councils to govern tribes, and allowed schools on reservations.
1945–1961	In an attempt at sociocultural integration, the US Government reversed its support of the Tribal self-government movement, and more than 50 tribal governments were terminated. AI lands were sold to non-AI, putting more AI into poverty. Oil-rich lands in Oklahoma were taken by the US government and private enterprises. Reservation AI were resettled into urban centers.
1950s	BIA "Relocation Program for AI" increased migration of AI from reservations. Economic incentives were offered to bring AI to work in factories and blue-collar jobs in cities.
1955	Transfer Act transferred responsibility of providing healthcare services to AI from the BIA to the Indian Health Service.
1968	The American Indian Movement (AIM) repossessed Alcatraz Island.
1975	US Congress passed the Indian Education Assistance and Self Determination Act.
1976	The Indian Health Care Improvement Act provided funding for 34 urban AI clinics or centers in 19 states.
1988	Indian Gaming Regulatory Act was established.

A Ritual to Maintain Health: Mrs. Swift Thunder's story

Vignette:

It is 6:30 in the morning and 80-year-old Mrs. Swift Thunder sits near the door of her small, two-room house, waiting for the Community Health Representative (CHR), a local community health worker. The CHR will give Mrs. Swift Thunder a ride to the federal Indian Health Service (IHS) hospital, a 45-bed facility located 30 miles away at the end of a dirt road. Today, the road is passable, free of the seasonal rain or snow that sometimes leave behind several inches of thick, sticky mud, or slippery, snow-covered ice. Waiting for transportation has become a ritual for Mrs. Swift Thunder because she needs a ride three times a week for her renal dialysis, a procedure that replaces the work once performed by her failed kidneys. Kidney failure is a complication of type 2 diabetes mellitus, which she was diagnosed with 12 years ago, eight years after her husband was diagnosed with the same condition. His death three years ago was due to a heart failure, another common complication of diabetes.

Mrs. Swift Thunder's socioeconomic and health situation is not unique. Since the mid-1950s, diabetes has become common on many tribal reservations, and patients like her have had to accept living with a disease that dominates their daily lives. Their schedules are now organized around their dialysis appointments and their other daily self-monitoring activities, such as glucose testing, which is needed to help adjust medications.

For Mrs. Swift Thunder and others in her community, living on the reservation provides a cultural comfort. However, the well-being of many tribal members on the reservation has been and continues to be impacted by persistent poverty and a resource-poor healthcare system. Mrs. Swift Thunder, like many other American Indians, does not have private health insurance and depends on a patchwork of medical coverage provided by Indian Health Service (IHS), an organization that was formed when several tribes were forced to cede millions of acres of land to the US government.

Like many agencies that provide healthcare in rural, underserved communities, the IHS combines several sources of funding to cover the cost of providing medical care for the populations that it serves. In addition to its own federal funds, IHS utilizes Medicare, Medicaid, State, and other sources to provide coverage. However, the amount of annual federal funding for the IHS varies and is allocated at the discretion of Congress; thus, IHS is chronically underfunded. In fact, the funds that IHS uses to pay for catastrophic or unexpected emergency medical care are often depleted before the end of the fiscal year.

In Mrs. Swift Thunder's case, Medicare covers the cost of most of the care related to her diabetes (including dialysis), but cost of the medications that she takes to treat her diabetes, hypertension and elevated cholesterol levels are covered by a combination of resources. IHS provides the CHR for transportation to and from her appointments. Moreover, she needed to apply to a completely separate organization (Lions Club) to get prescription eyeglasses, and she has no coverage for routine dental care or for purchasing dentures.

Various federal policies were enacted to assimilate AI populations into White America, starting with children. For example, in 1870, with federal encouragement and permission, missionaries from various organized religions opened boarding schools to educate AI/AN children. Admission to these schools was not voluntary. Native children of school age were forcibly removed from their homes and transported hundreds of miles to unfamiliar institutions where they were required to forget their language, culture, and even, to some extent, their families. The schools were created to "kill the Indian and save the man."[21] The assimilation process began immediately upon arrival at the school; the children were scrubbed clean, issued European clothing, and told to get in line to receive European-style haircuts.

The typical boarding school curriculum emphasized vocational preparations. Classes were frequently taught by lay educators with little or no training in education and little empathy for AI/AN children. Stories told by some former boarding school attendees recounted incidences of physical, sexual, or emotional abuse by some of these caretakers. Schooling also required considerable manual labor, as most boarding schools were not well financed and had to depend on the labor of its students for the day-to-day operation by assigning students to help with food production, building maintenance, cleaning, cooking, laundry, and so on. Most school buildings also were substandard and over-crowded, facilitating rapid transmission of communicable diseases. Several of these infections were deadly, especially for children who were often malnourished and already in poor health. Most school staff and school facilities were not designed to care for ill children, and schools did not have resources to transport seriously ill children back to their families. Those who died were often forgotten, and many headstones found in old boarding school graveyards were marked "unknown."

The experience was painful for most children, leading some to run away to return home. The return, however, was not always successful. Children who were caught were returned to school, and their families were punished by the local government Indian agents, who denied them food rations, blankets, tools, or other necessities.[22] To discourage a return to life on the reservation, older students often were placed with non-Native families during school break to further their farm or homemaking skills. These "outings" were supported by the school as another way to socialize the students to become more European.

Besides the early history of forced removal of AI/AN children to boarding schools, other policies supported the placement of AI/AN foster children in non-Native homes and/or the adoption of Native children without the consent of the family. Even when voluntary, many AI families who agreed to have their children placed with non-Indian families were pressured by poverty and

Indian agents acting on behalf of the federal government. Although families were promised that their children would be well cared for and enrolled in good schools, these placements were not always positive for children, especially those who were shifted from one placement family to another when the child "could not adjust." These changes were rarely shared with the child's family. The practice continued until 1978 with the passage of the Indian Child Welfare Act, a policy enacted to give priority to placing children with family or members of their respective tribes.[23]

Unethical Health Practices

As mentioned earlier, the US government supported the giving of smallpox vaccines to "friendly" tribes and withholding it from others in the 1800s. Other health-related abuses have been documented, and as recently as the 1970s, AI women who sought care at several IHS and county health facilities were sterilized without informed consent.[24] The US Government Accountability Office (GAO) investigated these events in the 1980s and estimated that 60,000 to 70,000 AI women were sterilized without their knowledge over the course of the decade.[25]

Abuse also has occurred in research conducted with AI communities. An example is the Havasupai Study (1989–2010). In this case, researchers at Arizona State University (ASU) who had established a level of trust with the Havasupai Tribe were asked by the tribe to help them study one of their community's major health problems—type 2 diabetes. The blood collected for the study was later obtained by other researchers at ASU and another university, who analyzed the sample for other unapproved purposes, including markers for schizophrenia, inbreeding, and population migration.[26] When an investigator presented results from an unapproved study at a conference, a Havasupai tribal member was in the audience and alerted the tribal council. The Havasupai Tribe reacted quickly to the unethical sharing and misuse of specimens for a study that was not approved by the tribe's Institutional Review Board (IRB) or the IHS. In 2010, the Havasupai Tribal Nation settled a class action lawsuit against the universities. But the incident continued to fuel AI/AN mistrust of researchers.

Tribal Sovereignty

Today, the US federal government recognizes tribes as "domestic dependent nations." This means that, technically, Congress has no more power over tribal nations than it does over individual states, and states do not have power over tribal nations based within their state boundaries. The earliest legal definition of the relationship between tribes and the US government is found in the US

Constitution. Article 1, Section 8 states that "Congress shall have the power to regulate commerce with foreign nations and among the several states, <u>and with the Indian tribes</u>" (emphasis added). Thus, the Constitution placed tribes alongside foreign nations in explaining the relationship that Congress should have with them. But tribal sovereignty has historically been undermined, especially with regard to land ownership and usage. For example, in 1953, six states were mandated to transfer litigation powers from federal and tribal courts to states (Public Law 280).[27]

In the 1970s, President Richard Nixon directed Congress that "the Federal government should begin to recognize and build upon the capacities and insights of the Indian people."[28] As a result of this presidential action, and after much debate with Congress, the Indian Self-Determination and Education Assistance Act[29] passed in 1975 (Table 2.1.). Besides allowing tribes to control their own schools, this law also promoted the ability of tribes to self-govern and make decisions concerning their people. It also determined that states do not have the authority to regulate commerce with the tribes or regulate tribes. Current federal policy in the US recognizes this sovereignty and emphasizes the importance of upholding a government-to-government relationship between the US Congress and tribal nations. The relationship between the US federal government and federally recognized tribes includes a "trust," meaning that the federal government has accepted that it has a legal "duty to protect" the tribes. Still, because the tribes existed prior to the US government, they have preexisting sovereignty.

Although tribal powers do not supersede those of the US government, tribes hold the power of self-government that is independent of the control of US government. For example, mechanisms for voting for tribal leadership and the structure and function of tribal governments are completely under the control of the tribal nations. However, if a murder or suspicious death occurs on Indian land, the Federal Bureau of Investigation becomes involved in the investigation, under rules that were set as part of the historical trust agreements between tribal nations and the US Congress.

The growth of the American Indian Movement (AIM) of the 1960s brought public attention to the challenges in land use between the federal government and tribal nations. For example, a group of AI occupied Alcatraz Island in California in 1968, justifying the occupation on the basis of a federal directive that called for abandoned structures on federal lands be returned to local tribes. Thus, the abandonment of Alcatraz made it eligible for AI reoccupation. However, the US government implemented a siege of the island, removing the AI occupants. Shortly thereafter, the government converted the island into a federal park.

American Indian Gaming

Another key piece of legislation that affects the relationship between the tribes and the federal government was the Indian Gaming Regulatory Act (IGRA), which Congress passed in 1988.[30] The act established a new agency, the National Indian Gaming Commission, to help regulate gaming facilities located on any Indian reservation or lands held in trust by the US for the benefit of any Indian tribe. According to the National Indian Gaming Commission, out of 574 federally recognized tribes, only 238 tribes operated 474 gaming facilities in 28 states in 2018.[31] In fiscal year 2019, tribal gaming revenues accounted for 45% of all gaming revenue in the US.[32]

There is a popular myth that tribal members receive excessively large annual allotments or payments from the gaming operations. However, many tribal members do not receive any annual allotments or profits accrued from the gambling establishments. By law, gaming net profits may be used only to (1) fund tribal government operations or programs, (2) provide for the general welfare of their members, (3) promote tribal economic development, (4) donate to charitable organizations, and (5) help fund operations of local government agencies.[33] In general, the profits have been used to improve roads and schools and to install plumbing, electricity, and phone lines. Tribes that vote to distribute gaming revenue as payments to their tribal members first must develop a "revenue allocation plan" and then gain approval of that plan from the Secretary of the US Department of the Interior.

There are some tribes that run resort-type casinos, but many tribal gaming facilities are simply trailers where bingo games are held. Although gambling facilities located close to major state highways tend to be very profitable, those on tribal lands in remote, rural areas do not fare so well. Almost all Indian gaming tribes also pay monies to the local state governments. In 2014, tribal casinos generated $96.6 billion, of which $33.2 billion was paid in wages to employees and $16.0 billion was paid in taxes and direct payments to federal, state, and local governments.[34]

Urban American Indians

The living conditions on AI reservations have long been abysmal. Until 1917, migration off reservations was limited and controlled. During World War I, thousands of AI/AN joined the military or supported the war effort in other ways, such as by buying war bonds or taking jobs in defense plants. Because of their service during the war, Congress passed the Indian Citizenship Act in 1924, granting all AI US citizenship.[35] However, some states, including Arizona and New Mexico, refused to implement the law, which meant that AI living in those states could not vote. During World War II, AI, notably the Navajo Code Talkers and Apache Code Talkers, provided significant breakthroughs in the war effort, primarily in the Pacific. But, despite their service, many Navajo Code Talkers and Apache Code Talkers were still denied the right to vote, as both tribes were based in Arizona and New Mexico.

Many of the AI/AN men and women who served in the armed forces did not return to the reservations, but instead remained in urban areas where employment and housing with indoor plumbing were more readily accessible.[36] In the mid-1940s to 1950s, the federal government initiated a major effort to address poverty and lack of employment on reservations by recruiting and relocating young AI adults to selected urban sites. Initially, the relocation process targeted those living on extremely poor reservations in the Dakotas, Utah, Colorado, and Arizona. The relocation was a one-way ticket to the cities, where relocatees were strategically scattered throughout various low-income sections of the city. The recruits were promised job training or other work-skill development opportunities. Some relocatees managed to survive and remain, while others found ways to return to the reservation when they were unable to find meaningful work and/or cope with isolation from family and friends. Voluntary migration to the urban areas continued, however, and 71% of AI/AN lived off-reservation by 2010.[37]

Throughout the 1960s, programs designed to improve the educational status of AI/AN were implemented throughout the US. The programs offered financial assistance to AI/AN college students who wished to pursue degrees in certain needed academic areas. For example, the Indians into Medicine Program offered assistance to those who desired a career in healthcare.[38] AI/AN college and university students who accepted these scholarships were typically required to work in an AI/AN community for at least 2 years after graduation. However, following this "payback" period, many elected to move to urban areas.

Many urban-dwelling AI migrate back and forth between reservations and urban areas. The urban choice often offers better employment and educational opportunities. Urban areas also provide better quality of care for complex health conditions (such as cancer), while the reservations tend to offer access to basic health care through IHS and tribal facilities. In some cases, Native people work in urban areas and send money home to the reservation.

Brief History of AN People under US Control

Alaska Native peoples resided on this land about 15,000 years ago. Today, the AN label encompasses 20 different languages and distinct tribal groups, including:

the Eyak, Tlingit, Haida, and Tsimshian peoples in the southeast; the Inupiaq and St. Lawrence Island Yupik in the north and northwest; Yup'ik and Cup'ik Alaska Natives in the southwest; the Athabascan and Denaina in the interior and south-central region; the Alutiiq (Sugpiaq) in southcentral and Aleutian Islands, and the Unangax of the Pribolof and Aleutian Islands.[39] The beautiful diversity of Alaska's first people reflects the variation of Alaska's landscape, which ranges from a vast tundra, to windswept islands, to boreal forests and rainforests. Approximately 150 Alaskan communities are considered rural and are accessible only by boat or plane.[40] Today, AN people comprise approximately 18% of the Alaska population, and about a third live in large cities, such as Anchorage and Fairbanks. Alaska has the highest proportion of AI/AN people in the nation.[41]

The first European colonizers of Alaska were Russian (Table 2.2.). In 1867, US Secretary of State William H. Seward signed a treaty with Russia for the purchase of Alaska for $7.2 million. Despite the bargain price of roughly 2 cents an acre, the Alaskan purchase was ridiculed in Congress and in the press as "Seward's folly," "Seward's icebox," and President Andrew Johnson's "polar bear garden."[42] In 1900, the capital of Alaska was moved from Sitka to Juneau. In 1918, influenza decimated the AN population, with some communities losing 60% of their people. In 1942, during World War II, Japan invaded the Aleutian Islands of Attu and Kiska, and the American military did not retake the islands until a year later. In January 1959, almost 100 years after its purchase, Alaska became the 49th US state.

Although missionary work had been occurring throughout Alaska since the latter 1800s, in 1885 Presbyterian minister Sheldon Jackson assigned specific geographic regions of the state to different religious groups.[44] Episcopalians were assigned to Point Hope, Presbyterians to Barrow, Congregationalists to Nome, Quakers to Kotzebue, and Russian Orthodox throughout the south and southwestern regions of the state. As with AI, many AN children were forced from their homes into boarding schools in Alaska or in the "lower 48" to assimilate them.[45]

Unlike AI tribes in the lower 48, there were no treaties between the US government and AN tribes, as treaty-making with tribes was terminated by Congress in 1871. AN tribes were able to obtain federal recognition in 1993 when the Indian Reorganizations Act of 1934 was extended to Alaska.[46] Alaska had 229 federally recognized tribes and represented almost 40% of the 574 federally recognized tribes.[36]

The US government's awareness of the failures of the reservation system led to the passage of the Alaska Native Claims Settlement Act (ANCSA), which President Richard Nixon signed into law in 1971. The act "implicitly extinguished the tribe's dependent Indian community status" and created regional

Table 2.2. Key Points in AN History[43]

1741	A Russian expedition led by Vitus Bering and George Steller made the first "discovery" of Alaska, landing near what today is Kayak Island.
1740s–1830s	Russians enslaved Unangan and Sugpiaq people for fur trading.
1778	Captain James Cook sailed along the central and western coast of Alaska, Bering Strait, and entered into the Arctic Ocean.
1850s–1920s	Commercial whalers nearly destroyed whale population in Arctic waters.
1867	The United States purchased Alaska for $7.2 million in gold (roughly 2 cents an acre).
1880	Sheldon Jackson divided Alaska into religious denominational service areas.
1912	The first hospital for AN people opened in Juneau and closed due to lack of funding. The 1915 US Congress funded the 25-bed Native hospital in Juneau with the oversight of the Bureau of Education.
1917–1920	Worldwide flu epidemic decimated Alaska Native villages, losing up to 75% of some communities. TB epidemic rapidly spread among communities.
1932	Wrangell Institute, a BIA boarding school, was opened in southeast Alaska. This school closed in 1975. Many children were abused.
1942	Japanese bombed Dutch Harbor and occupied Attu and Kiska Islands. Many Unangan people were relocated and did not survive.
1953	Alaska Native Service opened a 400-bed hospital with a dedicated TB wing in Anchorage, Alaska.
1955	The Territorial Legislature engaged in a constitutional convention with one AN person (Tlingit) as an elected delegate.
1955	The federal government transferred Alaska Native health care from Bureau of Indian Affairs to US Public Health Service, Division of Indian Health.
1959	Alaska became the 49th state.
1971	The Alaska Native Claims Settlement Act was passed, which resulted in the loss of aboriginal title to land and rights. This act cleared the way for the trans-Alaska pipeline and allowed the State of Alaska to claim 104 million acres from being considered "Indian Country." Only one community retained "Indian Country" status—Metlakatla.
1972–1976	A class action lawsuit was filed, the Mollie Hootch case, which ended with the discontinuation of sending students past the 8th grade from rural communities to boarding schools.
1993	Head of BIA from 1993–1997, Ada Deer, provided full recognition of tribes, allowing for Alaska's tribes to enter government to government relations with the federal government.
1997	The Alaska Native Tribal Health Consortium was established. ANTHC is owned and managed by AN tribal governments and their regional health organizations. A new Alaska Native Medical Center replaced the one built in 1953.

for-profit corporations.[47] All Alaska tribes lost their Indian Country or reservation status, except for Metlakatla, which opted out of ANCSA.

This act transferred 44 million acres to AN regional and village corporations and compensated the newly formed AN corporations $962.5 million for land lost.[48,49] Through the Alaska Federation of Natives, AN Peoples then established 12 regional Native corporations, and each region also contained numerous village corporations, about 225 in all. Native corporations are the largest private landowners in Alaska, with title to 44 million acres. Development of the resources beneath their lands offers Native corporations an opportunity to generate jobs and other economic benefits for their Native shareholders. A 13th regional corporation headquartered in Seattle was later established for AN who live outside of Alaska, although this corporation did not receive land and ultimately dissolved.

The Alaska National Interest Lands Conservation Act (ANILCA) was passed in 1980 and created the huge public lands system in Alaska. This law protected the subsistence needs of rural AN. Subsistence hunting and fishing on federal lands and waters is regulated by the federal government under a state–federal comanagement memorandum of understanding.[50] Under Alaska state law, subsistence use includes the customary and traditional uses of fish and wildlife outside of areas that are designated as nonsubsistence use, regardless of ethnicity. Marine mammals are the single exception. Under the federal Marine Mammal Protection Act, only AN who live on the coast of the North Pacific Ocean, Bering Sea, or the Arctic Ocean may harvest marine mammals (e.g., sea otters, polar bears, walrus, seals, sea lions, whales) for subsistence purposes. The ANILCA designated more than 100 million acres of land for preservation and protection throughout Alaska.

The IHS began to offer healthcare to AN in the 1950s. In 1953, the 400-bed Anchorage Medical Center of the Alaska Native Service opened in Anchorage. This facility was originally built to care for AN people suffering from tuberculosis, which affected large proportions of AN living in rural Alaska. In 1997, the Anchorage Medical Center was replaced by the Alaska Native Medical Center (ANMC), and the transition to AN ownership was completed with its transfer to the Alaska Native Tribal Health Consortium (ANTHC) and Southcentral Foundation.[51] Today, ANTHC has the responsibility for operating the majority of the programs of the IHS Alaska Area office and is the agency that embodies healthcare self-determination for AN people. The IHS has agreements with another 35 smaller, regional health corporations around the state, from the Southeast Area Regional Health Center (SEARHC) serving the communities around Juneau, to the Arctic Slope Native Association that operates the Samuel Simmonds Memorial Hospital in Barrow.[52]

Although AN have access to comprehensive healthcare resources in Anchorage and many services in Fairbanks, healthcare staff and services in rural villages and towns vary greatly. In the most rural areas, AN may rely on the availability and skills of Community Health Aide/Practitioners (CHA/Ps) and visits from physicians and registered nurses who fly in to provide care a few days a week or a few days a month. In 2004, a study of referral patterns between tribal health organizations and the ANMC in Anchorage found that AN cancer patients were referred 13 times before being transferred to Anchorage for care.[53] This illustrates insufficient infrastructure and capacity.

Demographics, Health, and Resiliency

As of 2020, there were 574 federally recognized tribes in the lower 48 states and Alaska that were eligible for funding and services from the BIA. Tribal constitutions determine the criteria for an individual's tribal enrollment. For example, many tribes require that an individual trace ancestry to someone named on the tribe's base roll, the original list of members designated in a tribal constitution, or other document specifying enrollment criteria. Other tribes require a specified blood quantum, tribal residency, or continued contact with the tribe.[54] In 2021, there were 331,893,745 people living in the US,[55] of which 9.7 million (2.9%) were AI/AN.[56] The federal government most often aggregates statistics related to AI/AN, and it is almost impossible to find demographic data presented separately for these two groups. Thus, much of the data in this section are provided for AI/AN together.

People's socioeconomic status affects where they live and work and holds substantial influence over their health, with effects accumulating over a lifetime.[57] Compared with other populations in the US, AI/AN peoples are more likely to have lower socioeconomic status and also more likely to live in poverty than non-Hispanic Whites. In the US, the indicators that researchers use most commonly to measure the effect of socioeconomic status on health are educational attainment and income. For example, in 2019, 84.4% of AI/AN had at least a high school diploma, compared to 93.3% of non-Hispanic Whites, and 20.8% of AI/AN age 25 and over had at least a bachelor's degree, compared to 36.9% of non-Hispanic Whites.[56] Although the Indian Self-Determination and Education Assistance Act of 1975 allowed AI to operate their own schools, with funding from the US government,[29] the BIA documented that many tribal schools lacked heating, plumbing, and/or up-to-date books and computers and that teaching staff were under-paid and lived in substandard housing. In Colorado, Indigenous students report high prevalence of bullying, fighting, e-cigarette use, and attempted suicide,[58] all of which contribute to high drop-out rates.

AI/AN adults are more likely to be obese, use tobacco, and have diabetes or high blood pressure than non-Hispanic Whites.[59] Frequently, AI/AN peoples are physically inactive. For example, a third of AI/AN participants in the Education and Research Towards Health (EARTH) Study did not meet current physical activity recommendations, and a high proportion were completely sedentary during leisure time.[60] In surveys conducted by researchers at the Centers for Disease Control and Prevention (CDC), 29.5% of AI/AN reported having no healthcare provider (vs. 18.9% of Whites), and 24.2% of AI/AN reported having no healthcare coverage (vs. 12.5% of Whites) in 2014.[61] AI/AN also have less access to cancer prevention and screening and other healthcare services than people with higher socioeconomic status.[62]

The health of today's AI/AN is marked by increased mortality and morbidity associated with chronic diseases, accidents, and unhealthy lifestyle choices such as substance misuse rather than by infectious diseases. However, the COVID-19 pandemic highlighted continued vulnerabilities of AI/AN communities. Data from 2020 suggested AI/AN in New Mexico accounted for 57% of the COVID-19 cases and 75% of COVID-19 deaths in that state, although they comprise only 11% of the population.[63,64] High prevalence and mortality rates can be attributed to the social determinants of health. For example, many tribal members live in multigenerational homes with large families in close quarters, making it hard to socially distance.[65] Households tend to be crowded, and housing on some reservations often lack indoor plumbing. Differences in socioeconomic factors also contributed to elevated COVID-19 mortality.[66] Such barriers include lack of private health insurance, limited access to the Internet (for information and resources), and limited transportation options. All these factors can delay access to care or result in more severe illness that is less amenable to treatment.[67]

Although AI/AN continue to struggle with health inequities, they have many strengths. AI/AN have survived hundreds of years of occupation. Their traditions include honoring and respecting their elders and families, despite historical trauma. Their communities have strong foundations and emphasize the need to be healthy and to emulate their ancestors by continuing to speak Native languages, consume traditional foods, reserve tobacco for ceremonial uses only, and participate in daily prayers, healing rituals (such as sweat lodges), and formal ceremonies as part of their organized religion. These strengths affect the spirits, minds, emotions, bodies, and social interactions of AI/AN peoples and contribute to the balance of these aspects of life to promote health and wellness.

Among the things that make AI/AN unique are tribal sovereignty and their government-to-government relationships to the US. The Indian Self-

Determination and Education Assistance Act provides that tribes may process applications for Certificate Degree of Indian Blood and Indian Preference in Employment for anyone who can provide documentation of AI/AN quantum and/or ancestry.[68] As noted, each Tribal Nation determines criteria for enrollment within the tribe, making AI/AN the only group in the US with a provision for maintaining legal documentation of ancestry.

Brief History of Native Hawaiians under US Control

According to the 2019 US Census Bureau estimate, roughly 0.4% (1.4 million) of US population are NH or PI alone or in combination with other races.[69,70] NH are the Polynesian Peoples that first inhabited the Hawaiian archipelago, a 1,500-mile island chain that spans the Tropic of Cancer in the Pacific Ocean. The seven inhabited islands are at the southeastern tip of the chain and stretch over about 350 miles. Hawai'i is approximately 2,500 miles west of California. Because of its distance from major land masses, the Hawaiian archipelago has been called the most isolated land on the planet.

When the archipelago was first visited by Europeans, they found a healthy people living in harmony with the land (Table 2.3.). Hawaiian society was organized into land units called ahupua'a, wedge-shaped pieces of land that follow valley formations, each with a pinnacle on the mountain top and a base at the sea.[71] The ahupua'a system allowed each community access to a range of resources for food, shelter, and the practice of cultural traditions. Land was not owned; rather, the ali'i (leaders) were stewards for their land areas and the people living there. A kapu (taboo) system of laws and regulations was in place to guide behaviors. For example, there were kapu to regulate the times and places people could fish to prevent overfishing and environmental degradation.

Estimates of the size of the Native Hawaiian population prior to Western contact range from 120,000 to 600,000. Despite controversy about the size of the population when colonization occurred, scholars agree that within 100 years of European contact, the population of Hawai'i had declined by more than 80%.[7] Like the AI/AN populations, Native Hawaiians contracted and died from infectious diseases (e.g., smallpox and measles), decreased fertility, high infant mortality, poor living conditions, shrinking access to land and nutritious foods, and increased access to alcohol and tobacco.[72]

After NH learned about the monarchical structure of governance from the British, they established the Kingdom of Hawai'i in 1795. The kingdom unified five of the seven independent islands under the first king, King Kamehameha. The other two inhabited islands joined the kingdom in 1810. The kingdom was recognized as a sovereign nation by the US and major European powers.[73] Missionaries, primarily from New England, translated the Bible into

Table 2.3. Key Points in Hawai'i History

1778	Captain James Cook landed on Kaui'i and named the archipelago the "Sandwich Islands."
1810	Kamehameha I united the Hawaiian Islands, and the Kamehameha dynasty reigned until 1874.
1819	Liholiho, son of Kamehameha, defied the tradition of men and women eating separately during a feast, which leads to the abolishment of the *kapu* system.
1820	The first missionaries arrived in Hawai'i.
1822	A Hawaiian alphabet book and reading primers were published and, by 1834, close to 95% of Native Hawaiians were literate in the Hawaiian language.
1835	The first sugar plantation opened, and industrial agriculture became the dominant economic force.
1830s–1848	To keep lands in Hawaiian hands, Kamehameha III divided the land into thirds—one-third to the Hawaiian crown lands, one-third to the chiefs, and one-third to the people. However, because land ownership was a new concept, few Hawaiians filed land claims and lost their lands.
1850s	As Hawaiians died of introduced diseases, the plantations began to import labor, primarily from China, Japan, Korea, the Philippines, and Portugal.
1874	King Lunalilo died leaving no heirs. David Kalakaua was elected as Lunalilo's successor and initiated the first Hawaiian Renaissance.
1887	The 1887 Constitution of the Kingdom of Hawai'i was signed, stripping King Kalakaua and therefore the Hawaiian monarchy of much of its authority.
1893	Local sugar planters, with the help of the US Marines, forced Queen Lili'uokalani to step down, and Sanford Dole was proclaimed president.
1898	Hawai'i was annexed by the US through the Newlands Resolution.
1900	The Organic Act established the Territory of Hawai'i.
1921	Congress passed the Hawaiian Homes Commission Act, setting aside lands for Native Hawaiians and requiring that people had to have 50% blood quantum to get onto the list to acquire land.
1959	Hawai'i became the 50th state.
1970s	The second Hawaiian Renaissance began.
1975	Hōkūle'a, a traditional Hawaiian voyaging canoe, took its first long-distance voyage to prove that Polynesians migrated throughout the Pacific, navigating by the stars, currents, winds, and other elements of the environment.
1978	The Hawai'i State Constitutional Convention amended the state Constitution to increase visibility and rights of Hawaiians.
1988	The US Congress passed the Native Hawaiian Health Care Improvement Act.

1993	A joint US congressional resolution acknowledged the 100th anniversary of the 1893 overthrow of the Kingdom of Hawai'i, and offered an apology to Native Hawaiians on behalf of the US for the overthrow.
1993	The US military stopped bombing the island of Kaho'olawe, a practice that had gone on for 50 years.
2013–2017	Hōkūle'a and her sister canoe the Hikianalia covered more than 60,000 nautical miles, and reached 100 ports in 27 nations on a mission to demonstrate sustainable living and to share Polynesian cultural values.

a written form of the Hawaiian language, and Native Hawaiian literacy rates soared.[74] Between 1834 and 1948, Hawai'i was home to more than 100 Hawaiian-language newspapers.[75]

The Kamehameha line ruled Hawai'i from 1795 until the death of King Lunalilo in 1874. King David Kalakaua, Lunalilo's successor, initiated the first Hawaiian Renaissance, bringing back into prominence the practice of hula, which had been suppressed by the missionaries. Kalakaua formed a palace hula troupe, and it was during his reign that hula gained the reputation of being the national symbol of Hawai'i.

However, within 50 years of their arrival in Hawai'i, US missionaries and businessmen had gained complete control of the economy. Subsistence fishing and farming were replaced by large-scale industrial agriculture (e.g., sugar and pineapple plantations) and fishing for export. To ensure that there were enough laborers to maintain the sugar and pineapple plantations, the leaders of these foreign business interests imported workers from China (50,000 starting in 1852), Portugal (10,000 starting in 1877), Japan (200,000 starting in 1885), Korea (8,000 starting in 1902), the Philippines (30,000 starting in 1905), and other countries.[76]

Queen Lili'uokalani was the ruling monarch when the US and European settlers overthrew the monarchy in 1893, with backing of the US military.[77] Despite opposition from the majority of the Hawaiian people, the islands were annexed by the US in 1898.

The subsequent US colonization and occupation of Hawai'i was a process of forced assimilation to American laws, language, culture, and religion, and included criminal consequences for those who resisted.[78] Following annexation, the Hawaiian language was entirely banned from schools and government, although some Hawaiian-language newspapers continued to publish until the middle of the twentieth century. Native Hawaiians intermarried with the descendants of the missionaries and immigrants, in some cases to hide their Hawaiian ancestry or to strengthen their bloodline against disease. Militarization accompanied colonization. In 2021, the US military owned about

21% of the land in Hawai'i and, although it offers employment opportunities for local residents, it also restricts their access to large areas of land and ocean.

Unlike AI, NH were not forced into reservations. However, European notions of land ownership were not well understood by NH, and they lost access to almost all the land to settlers. In 1921, the US Congress passed the Hawaiian Homes Commission Act to "provide for the rehabilitation of the Native Hawaiian people through a government-sponsored homesteading program."[79] Under the act, NH could be provided a 99-year homestead lease, and in 1990, the leases were extended another 100 years. Homestead leases are for residential, agricultural, or pastoral purposes and Native Hawaiians had to be at least 50% blood quantum to be eligible to receive land. However, the act is not well implemented and, in 2017, 22,000 NH were on the waiting list for housing, no new housing was built, and the agency closed out the fiscal year with $30 million in unspent federal housing funds.[80]

A self-governance movement among Native Hawaiians blossomed in the 1970s, igniting a revival of the Hawaiian language and culture.[81] Hawai'i activists supported the Hawai'i Constitutional Convention of 1978, which codified many of the demands of NH for rights and recognition. Amendments to the constitution established the Office of Hawaiian Affairs, a semi-autonomous agency that advocates for Hawaiian issues, provides scholarships to NH students, supports health and education programs, and maintains a loan program to help NH start businesses, improve homes, consolidate debt, and continue education. Amendments also guaranteed NH access to the mountains and the sea to maintain their livelihood and culture. Hawaiian became an official state language of the state.[82]

In 1993, the US government formally apologized for the overthrow of the Hawaiian monarchy 100 years earlier.[83] In a joint congressional resolution, Congress acknowledged the historical significance of this event, which resulted in the suppression of the inherent sovereignty of the NH people and the deprivation of the rights of NH to self-determination. The resolution included a hope that this acknowledgment would provide a foundation for reconciliation between the US and the NH people and urged the US president to support reconciliation efforts. Also that year, Congress returned to Hawai'i the island of Kaho'olawe (near Maui), which had been used by the US military for bombing practice for more than 50 years. A major source of pride among Hawaiians is the revival of long-distance ocean voyaging using traditional navigation by stars, currents, winds, and other elements of the environment, proving that Polynesians were the world's greatest ocean navigators.[84]

In 1988, the US Congress passed the Native Hawaiian Health Care Improvement Act.[85] This act established Papa Ola Lōkahi, the Native Hawaiian

Board of Health, as well as the Native Hawaiian Scholarship Program to support NH entering health professions and serving in Hawaiian communities. It also funded five Native Hawaiian Health Care Systems (NHHCS) to increase access to Western and traditional health services for NH. In 2020, the five NHHCS served more than 25,000 NH and their families on the seven inhabited islands of the state, working to (1) build trust in agency–client relationships, (2) provide culturally competent outreach and services, (3) ensure access to primary care services, (4) develop collaboration and partnerships among existing health service providers, and (5) focus on health promotion, disease prevention, and health education methods that incorporate traditional Hawaiian values and beliefs. Examples of NHHCS services include diabetes self-management support; hypertension self-management support and stroke prevention; transportation; oral health/dental services; asthma programs; cancer education, screening, and patient navigation; nutrition and fitness programs; cardiovascular education and screening; women's health and perinatal education programs; support for traditional Hawaiian diet and healing practices; and behavioral health services including substance abuse and tobacco cessation. In addition, four NHHCSs offer primary care services. Indigenous health systems are attractive to NH because they place culture at the center of the delivery of services. Culture is reflected in the educational materials provided to patients and in artwork and landscaping of the center. It also is seen in faces, language, and interaction style of the staff, and in the type of services provided.

Brief History of the US-Affiliated Pacific Islands

Pacific Islanders are the Indigenous Peoples of the islands and atolls in the Pacific Ocean. Most of these islands were colonized by Europeans, and some still are considered territories of other nations. For example, French Polynesia (including Tahiti) and New Caledonia remain territories of France, and Rapanui (Easter Island) is a territory of Chile. Similarly, several Pacific Island jurisdictions are territories of or have military ties to the US, including American Samoa (population 55,000), Guam (population 169,000), the Commonwealth of the Northern Mariana Islands (CNMI, population 58,000), the Federated States of Micronesia (FSM, population 115,000), the Republic of the Marshall Islands (population 59,000), and the Republic of Palau (population 18,000).[86, 87] These six groups of islands are collectively referred to as the US-Affiliated Pacific Island (USAPI) region, which is the focus of this section. The six jurisdictions in the USAPI region include 2,000 islands in an area four times the size of contiguous US, crossing four time zones.[88]

Like Hawai'i, the USAPI nations were colonized by foreign powers. For example, Guam and the CNMI were colonized by Spain. After the Spanish–American War of 1898, Guam became a territory of the US. The CNMI was sold to Germany, then controlled by Japan, and then became a US possession after World War II. Following disputes by Germany, Great Britain, and the US over who should control the Samoan Islands, the islands were divided in 1900, with Germany taking the western islands and the US taking the eastern islands. The Marshall Islands were initially under the influence of Spain, then Germany, then Japan (from 1914 to 1945), and then, following World War II, the US. The FSM and Palau also came under US rule with the expulsion of the Japanese after the war.[89] Although Indigenous oral histories and records from early European visitors to the Pacific indicate that these PI were once healthy and hardy peoples, foreign contact brought communicable diseases, discrimination, and disadvantageous social and land-tenure structures that negatively affected their health.[90,91]

World War II in the Pacific brought famine to the islands, and the US brought welcomed food and supplies. However, the foods were high in refined sugar, salt, and fat, and after the wars ended, these foods remained in the diets of USAPI residents, largely supplanting traditional foods.[92] The term coca-colonization refers to these dietary changes among peoples of the developing world, including the US territories in the Pacific Basin.[93]

The islands have different relationships with the US. American Samoa and Guam are US territories, the CNMI has commonwealth status with the US, and the FSM, the RMI, and Palau are "freely associated states" under Compacts of Free Association (COFA). All six jurisdictions provide the US military with access to their lands and waters in return for economic aid. Between 1946 and 1958, the US military used the region to detonate thermonuclear devices in the Marshall Islands, which led to devastating environmental and health consequences for PI across the region.[94]

All six jurisdictions use US currency and have US zip codes and area codes, so they generally are not considered foreign countries. Wages tend to be lower than in the continental US, Alaska, and Hawai'i. USAPI residents are not allowed to vote in US elections. American Samoa, CNMI, and Guam elect representatives to the US House of Representatives, who can participate in discussions and serve on committees, but they are not allowed to vote. Residents of all six jurisdictions can migrate freely to the US and do so in search of better education, work, and healthcare options. Many migrate to Hawai'i, which is the closest US neighbor, but Arkansas and surrounding states are home to an estimated 12,000 Marshallese, many working in poultry production.

Table 2.4. Key Points in USAPI History

1898	The US acquired Guam from Spain following the Spanish American War, and Guam was governed between 1898 and 1950 by a US Navy officer.
1898	Under the German–Spanish treaty, Germany purchased the Northern Mariana Islands, Palau, Yap, Chuuk, Pohnpei, Kosrae, and the Marshall Islands
1900	The second Samoan Civil War was resolved by the Western powers, following which Germany took control of the western islands, and the US took control of eastern islands, renaming them American Samoa.
1914	With Germany's entry into World War I, the Japanese navy took possession of Micronesia and the Northern Mariana Islands (but not Guam).
1941	Japan took control of Guam from the US and established military bases throughout the region to support Japanese expansion to the south and east.
1944	The US retook control of Guam and also took control of the Northern Mariana Islands.
1941–1945	Although attacked only once, American Samoa served as an essential communication link and sea lane between the US, Midway, Fiji, Australia, and New Zealand.
1946–1962	The US conducted 105 atmospheric and underwater nuclear tests in the Pacific. Many of the islands are still contaminated from the nuclear fallout, and islanders continue to suffer high incidence of cancer and other health problems.
1947	President Truman signed an agreement with the United Nations establishing the Trust Territory of the Pacific Islands, which included the Northern Mariana Islands, Palau, Yap, Chuuk, Pohnpei, Kosrae, and the Marshall Islands.
1950	Guam became a US territory.
1975	The Northern Mariana Islands became a US Commonwealth and was renamed the Commonwealth of the Northern Mariana Islands (CNMI), giving it the same territorial status as Guam.
1981	The Republic of Palau, including 340 small islands, was organized.
1979	The Republic of the Marshall Islands (RMI), including 5 islands and 19 atolls, was organized.
1979	The Federated States of Micronesia (FSM), including more than 600 islands in the states of Yap, Chuuk, Pohnpei, and Kosrae, was organized.
1986	The RMI and the FSM entered into Compacts of Free Association (COFA) with the US. These were renewed in 2004.
1994	Palau became independent and entered into a 50-year COFA agreement with the US.
2018	An estimated 40,000 individuals from COFA nations were living in the US, including about 12,000 in Arkansas.

This migration suggests that the US is not fulfilling its assurances of increasing the self-reliance of the region and developing needed health, education, and welfare infrastructures.[95] Despite economic aid, most jurisdictions are economically unstable, with only marginal health and educational systems. All jurisdictions may apply for grants from the CDC, the Health Resources and Services Administration (HRSA), and the National Institutes of Health (NIH), and people living in American Samoa, the CNMI, and Guam have access to Medicare and Medicaid programs. Still, health services are generally underdeveloped in the USAPI region, and all six jurisdictions have health professional shortages. Cancer care services are very limited.[96] Those who migrate to the US, however, encounter healthcare that is very different from that of their homelands. Interview research with Marshallese in Hawai'i revealed that many migrants did not seek healthcare until they perceived that they were having a health crisis. This pattern may stem from the very limited availability of health services, especially preventive health services, on their home islands.[97]

Demographics and Health of NH/PI

Traditionally, population and health data for NH/PI were aggregated with data for Asian Americans, which masked the disparities experienced by NH/PI. The separation of NH/PI data from Asian American data was mandated in 1997 revisions to Directive 15 of the Office of Management and Budget, so more NH/PI data have become available. However, some US agencies continue to combine data from NH/PI with data from Asian Americans. In contrast, the State of Hawai'i publishes data for NH separately from other PI groups, and Guam and American Samoa participate in the Behavioral Risk Factor Surveillance System (BRFSS). Thus, where possible in this section, data specific to NH and other PI groups are presented. Otherwise, data are presented for NH/PI in aggregate.

NH/PI reside in all 50 states, but the largest concentrations are in Hawai'i (29%), California (23%), Washington (6%), Texas (4%), and New York, Florida, Utah, and Nevada each with 3%.[87] NH/PI account for less than 1% of the population in most states; however, they comprise 26% of the population of Hawai'i, 57% of the population of Guam (predominantly Chamorro), and 95% of American Samoa (predominantly Samoan). In Hawai'i, a NH is legally defined as a person who has at least one ancestor native to the Hawaiian Islands prior to 1778 when Captain James Cook made landfall. However, an individual must be 50% NH to secure Hawaiian Homestead lands and 25% NH to inherit homestead land from a relative.

The NH/PI population is relatively young. Less than 6% of NH/PI in the US are ages 65 and older, compared with about 13% of the general population.

The median age of NH/PI in the US is 10 years younger than that of the US population as a whole (27.1 years vs. 37.6 years). According to data gathered during the 2012–2016 American Community Survey of the US Census, NH/PI in the US are less likely than the US population as a whole to have a college degree (21.8% vs. 30.2%) or to own a home (49.7% vs. 63.4%), and more NH/PI live in poverty (17.7% vs. 13.4%).

In Hawaiʻi, the health status of NH is poorer than that of dominant racial/ethnic groups. NH have the shortest life expectancy of Hawaiʻi's five largest ethnic groups, living about 4 years less than White residents of the state.[98] NHs also face elevated risks of cancer, diabetes, hypertension, heart disease, and stroke.[99] They have high rates of obesity and obesity-related health problems. They are more likely than other groups to use tobacco and other substances. About 12% of NH adults report being bothered by depression.[100]

Disparities in rates of obesity, diabetes, heart disease, and cancer are likely linked to social determinants of health. From a historical perspective, the disparities in diet-related disease that exist today are the result of the historical assimilation of NH to a high-fat, Western diet, as well as the disruption of the traditional NH food systems that occurred with occupation.[101] From a cultural perspective, diet-related disparities also are a consequence of the barriers to self-determination, which greatly reduced the NH's autonomy to make food choices that would resonate with their cultural values, such as focusing their choices on their relationships with the land and with their community, and nurturing a spiritual connection to their food.[102] Many NH believe that good health is a reflection of lōkahi, which is one's ability to balance responsibilities to the group, the land, and the spiritual world (including ancestors and family gods).[103]

As noted above, some NH live on Hawaiian Home Lands, which are lands that the US Congress set aside for NH, with eligibility based on Hawaiian blood quantum.[104] Available demographic and socioeconomic data on the NH who live on Hawaiian Home Lands suggest that they experience lower socioeconomic status, higher unemployment rates, lower educational levels, and higher levels of poverty compared with other NH and the general population of Hawaiʻi. This may increase the experiences of adversity by NH residing on Hawaiian Home Lands.

In 2014, a number of federal agencies collaborated to administer the National Health Interview Survey to a sample of NH/PI residents in the US. They succeeded in gathering data from 3,197 households, including 11,085 individuals in 3,212 families.[105] The survey found that NH/PI in the US were less likely to have excellent or very good health (61.4%) compared with the overall US population (67.3%). The findings also confirmed that NH/PI data should not be aggregated with data from Asian Americans, as the survey showed that rates of health conditions among NH/PI are considerably different from the rates of the same health conditions in Asian Americans. For example, NH/PI were more likely to report serious psychological distress (4.1% of NH/PI vs. 1.6% of Asian Americans), asthma (9.8% NH/PI vs. 4.9% of Asian Americans), cancer (5.7% of NH/PI vs. 3.3% of Asian Americans), and lower back pain (28.3% of NH/PI vs. 17.6% of Asian Americans).

In terms of health behaviors, NH/PI were more likely to report participating in enough leisure-time aerobic and muscle-strengthening activities to meet the 2008 federal physical activity guidelines (25.6% NH/PI vs. 17.0% of Asian Americans). But they also were more likely to smoke (16.5% of NH/PI vs. 9.5% of Asian Americans), and drink alcohol (27.8% of NH/PI vs. 13.3% of Asian Americans).

The CDC estimates the age-adjusted rate of diabetes among NH/PI adults in the US as 23.7%, compared to 7.6% for Whites.[106] In a household survey with data from 2,522 people who had migrated to Hawai'i from the FSM and the Marshall Islands, 35% of participants ages 40 and older reported having diabetes.[107] In another survey, 47% of adults in American Samoa reported that they have been diagnosed with diabetes.[108] The prevalence of overweight and obesity also is high among NH/PI adults, estimated at 61.1% in Guam, 78.5% for NH in Hawai'i, and 93% in American Samoa.[109]

With residents from the USAPI region now migrating to all 50 US states, it is important to understand that these peoples are burdened with health conditions found in both developing countries (e.g., malnutrition, filariasis, dengue fever, tuberculosis, and Hansen's disease), as well as with diseases associated with developed countries (e.g., diabetes, heart disease, and cancer). Additionally, US testing of thermonuclear devices by atmospheric explosions in the Marshall Islands has had serious health consequences. The residents of Rongelap Atoll in the Marshalls, for example, developed acute radiation sickness during the bombing and, over the next 30 years, 33% developed thyroid nodules, including 63% of children who were under age 10 at the time of exposure. The land was poisoned and remains that way. The residents of Bikini Atoll still cannot eat food grown there due to high radiation levels in the soil. Compensation by the US is limited to residents of certain of the Marshall Islands who develop certain types of cancer. However, a growing number and variety of cancers are being diagnosed in individuals from atolls and islands outside the US-defined risk area, for which the US is reluctant to acknowledge responsibility. For example, residents of Kosrae and Pohnpei States (FSM) participated in the clean-up of the nuclear detonation sites, and radioactive strontium from the weapons testing was documented to have reached the shores of Guam; yet, the US has not provided any compensation for these people.[110]

COVID-19 presented additional challenges to NH/PI. Data from 2020 suggested a case rate of 217.7 per 100,000 NHPI in California, compared to a statewide rate of 62.4 per 100,000. NH/PI also had high case rates in Washington, Oregon, and Utah. The rates of COVID-19 positive cases among NH/PI within these states was greater than those reported for African Americans and AI/AN.[111] PI communities in Hawai'i were more than twice as likely to be killed or hospitalized by the coronavirus than other racial and ethnic groups, after adjusting for age and gender.[112] Reasons included the fact that high proportions of NH/PI are employed in service-related jobs, with high people contact and low wages. Because of culture and financial constraints, they are more likely than most other racial/ethnic groups to live in larger multigenerational households and densely populated neighborhoods. Also, NH/PI are disproportionately represented in the incarcerated and homeless populations, which are very vulnerable to contracting COVID-19.

Cultural values, which are the enduring philosophies that influence the social structures of a culture, can have a significant effect on people's beliefs about health and well-being. Among Indigenous Peoples, cultural identity may serve as a coping resource by helping individuals to feel an increased sense of belonging, specifically with their identified cultural group. Cultural identity also helps Indigenous Peoples to find meaning within their cultural context, and to approach challenges based on the values and viewpoints that align with their cultural beliefs.

Most Pacific cultures place individuals within the context of a larger group, such as the family, clan, village, their church structures, and the land. In traditional Hawaiian values, aloha (sharing in the joyous hā, or breath of life) serves as a central foundation for other Hawaiian values and ethics through its emphasis on love and affection. Samoan culture (known as faaSamoa, or the Samoan way) is rooted in strong family dynamics, powerful ties to the land, a deep reverence for the church, and a respect for both reciprocity and authority.[113] As a result, Samoans may link poor health to disharmony across these domains, as well as to aitu (spirits).[114] Chamorro culture places great importance on family and community, nature, spirituality, and communal society, with some believing that illness is caused by island spirits.[115,116] In Samoan communities, elders are responsible for imparting traditional Samoan culture to the younger generation, and assisting them to traverse their American and Samoan identities.[117] Similar to other PI peoples, NH extend aloha to their 'ohana, or kin, which may include immediate and extended families who are central to social and economic endeavors.[118]

Summary

There are similarities and differences across the groups of Indigenous Peoples in the lower 48, Alaska, Hawai'i, and the USAPI jurisdictions. AI, AN, NH, and other PI peoples have all experienced loss of land and power in their homelands because of colonization. Most have effectively lost their right to self-determination, regardless of treaty status and agreements with the US government. All have been discriminated against, and some languages and communities are at risk of disappearing altogether. In general, these populations experience lower income, lower educational attainment, and lower rates of home ownership in comparison to Whites. They all have been subjected to unethical research practices, which in many ways served to further stigmatize them.

Foremost among the differences between these Indigenous groups are their official relationships with the US government. For example, AI and AN are in government-to-government relationships with the US, whereas NH have no official government-to-government agreement. In the USAPI region, two jurisdictions are territories (American Samoa and Guam) and one has commonwealth status (CNMI). The other three USAPI jurisdictions—the FSM, the Marshal Islands, and Palau—are part of COFA. Another major difference is that many AI/AN tribes experienced the forced removal of children, who were sent to boarding schools to "Americanize" them. This was not common practice in Hawai'i or the Pacific.

Despite these historical challenges and injustices, Indigenous communities continue to persevere, and many are revitalizing their cultures. For example, more NH and non-Hawaiians are engaging in Hawaiian cultural practices, especially those related to hula and canoe paddling, and the number of people who can speak the Hawaiian language is increasing. Many AI/AN tribes are returning to traditional religious practices and making efforts to preserve their languages and cultural practices. Indigenous communities are building on their cultural strengths to engage in projects to improve the health and well-being of their peoples. This book seeks to highlight and celebrate some of these efforts.

References

1. Jim MA, Arias E, Seneca DS, *et al*. Racial misclassification of American Indians and Alaska Natives by Indian health service contract health service delivery area. *Am J Public Health*. 2014;104(Suppl 3):S295–S302.

2. Houghton F. Misclassification of racial/ethnic minority deaths: The final colonization. *Am J Public Health*. 2002;92(9):1386.

3. Gray T. The treaty of Guadalupe Hidalgo. National Archives. Accessed February 3, 2022. https://www.archives.gov/education/lessons/guadalupe-hidalgo#:~:text=The%20Treaty

%20of%20Guadalupe%20Hidalgo%2C%20that%20brought%20an%20official%20 end,the%20advance%20of%20U.S.%20forces.

4. Braun KL, LaCounte C. The historic and ongoing issue of health disparities among native elders. *Generations*. 2015;38:60–69.

5. Crosby AW. *The Columbian exchange: Biological and cultural consequences of 1492*. Greenwood Publishing, 1972.

6. Cook SF. The significance of disease in the extinction of the New England Indians. *Hum Biol*. 1973;45:485–505.

7. Fuchs LH. *Hawai'i pono: A social history*. Harcourt Brace Jovanovich, 1961.

8. Stearn EW, Stearn AE. *The effect of smallpox in the destiny of Amerindian*. Bruce Humphries, 1945.

9. Fortuine R. Traditional surgery of the Alaska Natives. *Alaska Med*. 1951;26(1):22–25.

10. Duffy J. Smallpox and the Indians in American colonies. *Bull Hist Med*. 1951;25:324–341.

11. Fuchs LH. *Hawai'i pono: A social history*. Harcourt Brace Jovanovich, 1961.

12. Dobyns HF. Estimating Aboriginal American population: An appraisal of techniques with a New Hemispheric estimate. *Curr Anthropol*. 1966;7:395–416.

13. Thornton R. *American Indian holocaust and survival: A population history since 1492*. University of Oklahoma Press, 1990.

14. Cohen FS. *Handbook of federal Indian law*. Michie Co., 1982.

15. Bergman AB, Grossman DC, Erdrich A, *et al*. A political history of the Indian Health Service. *Milbank Q*. 1999;77(4):571–604.

16. Pearson JD. Medical diplomacy and the American Indian. *Wíčazo Ša Rev*. 2004;19(1):105–130.

17. Patterson KB, Runge T. Smallpox and the Native American. *Am J Med Sci*. 2002 Apr;323(4):216–22. doi: 10.1097/00000441-200204000-00009. PMID: 12003378.

18. US Department of the Interior. Bureau of Indian Affairs. Accessed May 10, 2021. https://www.bia.gov/bia.

19. Meriam L. The problem of Indian administration: 1928. Accessed May 10, 2021. https://files.eric.ed.gov/fulltext/ED087573.pdf.

20. Indian Health Care Improvement Act. 1997. P.L. 94-437. Accessed May 10, 2021. https://www.ihs.gov/sites/ihcia/themes/responsive2017/display_objects/documents /home/USCode_Title25_Chapter%2018.pdf.

21. Victoriana Magazine. Native American tribes and US government. Accessed May 10, 2021. http://www.victoriana.com/history/nativeamericans.html.

22. Davis J. American Indian boarding school experiences: Recent studies from Native perspectives. *OAH Mag Hist*. Winter, 2001;15(2):20–22.

23. National Indian Child Welfare Association. About ICWA. Accessed May 10, 2021. https://www.nicwa.org/about-icwa/.

24. Burhansstipanov L, Bemis LT, Petereit DG. Native American communities: Perspective and genetics. In: Monsen R, ed. *Genetics and ethics in nursing: New questions in the age of genomic health*. American Nurses Publishing, 2007:197–199.

25. US Congress, Office of Technology Assessment. *Indian Health Care*, OTA-H-290 US. Government Printing Office, April 1986.

26. Petereit DG, Burhansstipanov L. Establishing trusting partnerships for successful recruitment of American Indians to clinical trials. *Cancer Control*. 2008;15(3):260–268.

27. Goldberg C. Unraveling Public Law 280: Better late than never. American Bar Association, 2017. Accessed February 6, 2022. https://www.americanbar.org/groups/crsj /publications/human_rights_magazine_home/vol--43/vol--43--no--1/unraveling-public -law-280--better-late-than-never/

28. Landry, A. Richard M. Nixon: "Self-determination without termination." *Indian Country Today*, 2018. Accessed February 6, 2022. https://indiancountrytoday.com/archive /richard-m-nixon-self-determination-without-termination.

29. Indian Self-Determination and Education Assistance Act. 1975. P.L. 93-638. Accessed May 10, 2021. https://www.bie.edu/sites/default/files/documents/idc2-087684.pdf.

30. To regulate gaming on Indian land. Public Law 100-497 100th Congress, 1988. Accessed May 10, 2021. https://www.nigc.gov/images/uploads/IGRA%20PL%20100-497.pdf.

31. Robertson DL. The myth of Indian casino riches. *Indian Country Today*, September 18, 2018. Accessed March 6, 2021. https://indiancountrytoday.com/archive/the-myth-of -indian-casino-riches?redir=1.

32. American Gaming Association. AGA commercial revenue gaming tracker. Accessed May 10, 2021. https://www.americangaming.org/research/.

33. National Indian Gaming Commission. Frequently asked questions. Accessed May 10, 2021. https://www.nigc.gov/commission/faqs.

34. Meister A. The economic impact of tribal gaming: A state-by-state analysis. Accessed May 10, 2021. https://www.americangaming.org/sites/default/files/Economic%20 Impact%20of%20Indian%20Gaming%20in%20the%20U.S.%20September%202017.pdf.

35. Urban Indian Health Commission. *Invisible tribes: Urban Indians and their health in a changing world*. Urban Indian Health Commission, 2007.

36. Burhansstipanov L. Urban Native American health issues. *Cancer.* 2000;88(5):987–993.

37. US Census Bureau. Census 2010 American Indian and Alaska Native Summary File; Table: PCT2; Urban and rural; Universe Total Population; Population group name: American Indian and Alaska Native alone or in combination with one or more races. US Census Bureau, 2010.

38. Klein BT. *Reference encyclopedia of the American Indian*. 6th edition. Todd Publications, 1993.

39. Alaska Federation of Natives. Alaska Native peoples. Accessed May 10, 2021. https://www.nativefederation.org/alaska-native-peoples/.

40. Goldsmith S. Understanding Alaska's remote rural economy. *Understanding Alaska.* 2008;10:1–12. Accessed May 10, 2021. https://iseralaska.org/static/legacy_publication_ links/researchsumm/UA_RS10.pdf.

41. National Congress of American Indian. Demographics. Accessed May 10, 2021. http://www.ncai.org/about-tribes/demographics.

42. History. US purchase of Alaska ridiculed as "Seward's folly." Accessed May 10, 2021. https://www.history.com/this-day-in-history/sewards-folly.

43. Alaska Native Tribal Health Consortium. National Indian Health Board awards Alaska Blanket Exercise workshop at ANTHC. Accessed May 24, 2021. https://anthc.org /news/national-indian-health-board-awards-alaska-blanket-exercise-workshop-at-anthc/.

44. National Library of Medicine. Native voices. 1885: Alaska regions assigned to religious denominations. Accessed May 10, 2021. https://www.nlm.nih.gov/Nativevoices /timeline/366.html.

45. Alaska State Archives. Boarding schools in Alaska. Accessed May 10, 2021. https://archives.alaska.gov/education/boarding.html.

46. Ford MJW, Rude R. ANCSA: Sovereignty and a just settlement of land claims or an act of deception. *Touro Law Rev.*1999;15(2):479–495.

47. Kendall-Miller H. ANCSA and sovereignty litigation. *J Land Use Environ Law.* 2004;24:465–613.

48. ANCSA Regional Association. About the Alaska Native Claims Settlement Act. Accessed May 10, 2021. https://ancsaregional.com/about-ancsa/.

49. Resource Development Council. Alaska Native Corporations. Accessed May 10, 2021. https://www.akrdc.org/alaska-Native-corporations.

50. Alaska Department of Fish and Game. Subsistence in Alaska. Accessed May 10, 2021. http://www.adfg.alaska.gov/index.cfm?adfg=subsistence.faqs#QA4.

51. Alaska Native Medical Center. History. Accessed May 10, 2021. https://anmc.org /history/.

52. Indian Health Service. Alaska area. Accessed May 10, 2021. https://www.ihs.gov /alaska/.

53. Personal communication, Tim Gilbert.

54. US Department of the Interior. Tribal enrollment process. Accessed May 10, 2021. https://www.doi.gov/tribes/enrollment

55. US Census. New vintage 2021 population estimates available for the nation, states and Puerto Rico. Accessed February 6, 2022. https://www.census.gov/newsroom/press-releases/2021/2021-population-estimates.html.

56. US Office of Minority Health. Profile: American Indian/Alaska Native. Accessed February 6, 2022. https://minorityhealth.hhs.gov/omh/browse.aspx?lvl=3&lvlid=62.

57. CDC. CDC health disparities and inequalities report—United States, 2013. *MMWR Suppl.* 2013;62(3):1–187. Accessed May 10, 2021. http://www.cdc.gov/MMWR/pdf/other /su6203.pdf

58. Colorado Department of Education. *Healthy Kids Colorado Survey 2013.* Accessed March 6, 2021. https://www.colorado.gov/pacific/sites/default/files/PF_Youth_HKCS_ Executive-Summary.pdf.

59. Yurgalevitch SM, Kriska AM, Welty TK, *et al.* Physical activity and lipids and lipo-proteins in American Indians ages 45–74. *Med Sci Sports Exerc.* 1998;30(4):543–549.

60. Duncan GE, Goldberg J, Buchwald D, *et al.* Epidemiology of physical activity in American Indians in the Education and Research Towards Health cohort. *Am J Prev Med.* 2009;37(6):488–494.

61. Cobb N, Espey D, King J. Health behaviors and risk factors among American Indi-ans and Alaska Natives, 2000–2010. *Am J Public Health.* 2014;e1–e9.

62. Kaur JS, Burhansstipanov L, Krebs LU. Understanding the true burden of cancer in American Indian and Alaska Native communities. In: Jackson T, Evans KA, eds. *Health disparities.* Nova Science Publishers, 2013.

63. Haynie D. Native Americans in Minnesota keep COVID-19 at bay. *US News and World Report,* October 7, 2020.

64. Shah A, Seervai S, Paxton I, *et al.* The challenge of COVID-19 and American Indian health. To the Point (blog), Commonwealth Fund, August 12, 2020. https://doi.org/10.26099 /m5ww-xa13.

65. McPhillips D. COVID-19's tragic effect on American Indians: A state-by-state analysis. US News and World. Accessed May 10, 2021. https://www.usnews.com/news /healthiest-communities/articles/2020-10-07/a-state-by-state-analysis-of-the-impact-of-covid-19-on-native-americans#:~:text=According%20to%20the%20Centers%20for,any% 20racial%20or%20ethnic%20group.

66. Mamelund SE, Shelley-Egan C, Rogeberg O. The association between socioeconomic status and pandemic influenza: Protocol for a systematic review and meta-analysis. *Syst Rev.* 2019;8:5.

67. Arrazola J, Masiello MM, Joshi S, *et al.* COVID-19 mortality among American Indian and Alaska Native persons—14 states, January–June 2020. *MMWR Morb Mortal Wkly Rep.* 2020;69:1853–1856.

68. US Department of the Interior. Indian Affairs. Our mission. Accessed May 10, 2021. https://www.bia.gov/bia/ois/tgs.

69. Jones N, Marks R, Ramirez R, Ríos-Vargas M. 2020 Census illuminates racial and ethnic composition of the country. Accessed February 6, 2022. https://www.census.gov/library/stories/2021/08/improved-race-ethnicity-measures-reveal-united-states-population-much-more-multiracial.html.

70. US Office of Minority Health. Profile: Native Hawaiians/Pacific Islanders. Accessed February 6, 2022. https://minorityhealth.hhs.gov/omh/browse.aspx?lvl=3&lvlid=65.

71. Mueller-Dombois D. The Hawaiian ahupua`a land use system: Its biological resource zones and the challenge for silvicultural restoration biology of Hawaiian streams and estuaries. In: Evenhuis NL, Fitzsimons JM, eds. *Bishop Museum Bull Cultur Environ Stud.* 2007;3:23–33.

72. Merry SE. *Colonizing Hawai'i: The cultural power of law.* Princeton University Press, 2000.

73. Hawaiian Kingdom.org. International treaties. Recognition of Hawaiian independence. Accessed May 10, 2021. https://www.hawaiiankingdom.org/treaties.shtml.

74. Ka Mo'olelo Hawai'i. The literacy revolution. Accessed May 10, 2021. http://www.abstracthawaii.com/journal/literary-revolution.

75. Lorenzo-Elarco JH. He Hō`ili`ili Hawai`i: A brief history of Hawaiian language newspapers. Accessed May 19, 2021. https://www.amdigital.co.uk/about/blog/item/hawaiian-language-newspapers.

76. Center for Labor Education and Research. University of Hawai'i West O'ahu. History of labor in Hawai'i. Accessed May 10, 2021. https://www.hawaii.edu/uhwo/clear/home/HawaiiLaborHistory.html.

77. Hawaiian Kingdom.org. The US occupation. Accessed May 10, 2021. https://www.hawaiiankingdom.org/us-occupation.shtml.

78. Goodyear-Ka'opua N, Hussey I, Wright EK. *A nation rising: Hawaiian movements for life, land, and sovereignty:* Duke University Press, 2014.

79. Hawai'i Department of Hawaiian Home Lands. Hawaiian Home Commissions Act. Accessed February 7, 2022. https://dhhl.hawaii.gov/hhc/laws-and-rules/.

80. Kalani N. With thousands waiting and millions unspent, Hawai'i fails to build a single home. *Governing,* October 4, 2017. Accessed May 10, 2021. https://www.governing.com/archive/tns-hawaii-homes-agency.html.

81. Marsella AJ, Oliveira JM, Plummer CM, *et al.* Native Hawaiian culture, mind and well-being. In: McCubbin HI, Thompson EA, Thompson AI, Fromer JE, eds. Resiliency in ethnic minority families. University of Wisconsin,1995: 93–113.

82. Hofschneider A. "Fragile Aloha": Why Hawaii's last constitutional convention was important. *Civil Beat,* September 13, 2018. Accessed May 10, 2021. https://www.civilbeat.org/2018/09/fragile-aloha-why-hawaiis-last-constitutional-convention-was-important/.

83. The Apology Resolution. US Public Law 103–150. Accessed May 10, 2021. https://www.govinfo.gov/content/pkg/STATUTE-107/pdf/STATUTE-107-Pg1510.pdf.

84. Thompson C. *Sea people: The puzzle of Polynesia*. HarperCollins, 2019.

85. Native Hawaiian Health Care Improvement Act. Accessed May 10, 2021. https://uscode.house.gov/view.xhtml?path=/prelim@title42/chapter122&edition=prelim.

86. US Office of Minority Health. Profile: Native Hawaiians/Pacific Islanders. Accessed February 6, 2022. https://minorityhealth.hhs.gov/omh/browse.aspx?lvl=3&lvlid=65.https://minorityhealth.hhs.gov/omh/browse.aspx?lvl=3&lvlid=65).

87. US Census. *The Native Hawaiian and other Pacific Islander population: 2010*. Accessed May 10, 2021. https://www.census.gov/prod/cen2010/briefs/c2010br-12.pdf.

88. Central Intelligence Agency. The world fact book. Accessed September 19, 2020. https://www.cia.gov/library/publications/the-world-factbook.

89. Pacific Island Health Officer Association. USAPI region. Accessed May 10, 2021. https://www.pihoa.org/usapi-region/.

90. Osorio JKK. Dismembering lahui: A history of the Hawaiian nation to 1887. University of Hawai'i Press, 2002.

91. Hezel F. Disease in Micronesia: A historical survey. *Pac Health Dialog*. 2010;16(1):11–26.

92. Cassel KD. Using the Social-Ecological Model as a research and intervention framework to understand and mitigate obesogenic factors in Samoan populations. *Ethn Health*. 2010;15(4): 397–416.

93. Omran AR. The epidemiologic transition. A theory of the epidemiology of population change. *Milbank Mem Fund Q*. 1971;49(4):509–538.

94. Yamada S. Cancer, reproductive abnormalities, and diabetes in Micronesia: The effect of nuclear testing. *Pac Health Dialog*. 2004;11(2):216–221.

95. Yamada S, Pobutsky A. Micronesian migrant health issues in Hawai'i: Part 1: Background, home island data, and clinical evidence. *Calif J Health Promot*. 2009;7(2):16–31.

96. Tsark J, Braun KL. Reducing cancer health disparities in the US-associated Pacific. *J Public Health Manag Pract*. 2007;13(1):49–58.

97. Choi JY. Seeking healthcare: Marshallese migrants in Hawai'i. *Ethn Health*. 2008;13(1):73–92.

98. Wu YY, Braun KL, Horiuchi BY, *et al*. Life expectancies in Hawai'i: A multi-ethnic analysis of 2010 life tables. *Hawai'i J Med Public Health*. 2017;76(1):9–14.

99. Office of Hawaiian Affairs. Native Hawaiian data book. Accessed May 10, 2021. http://www.ohadatabook.com/.

100. Look MA, Trask-Batti MK, Agres R, *et al*. *Assessment and priorities for health & well-being in Native Hawaiians and other Pacific peoples*. University of Hawai'i, 2013.

101. Fujita R., Braun KL, Hughes CK. The traditional Hawaiian diet: A review of the literature. *Pac Health Dialog*. 2004;11(2):250–259.

102. Oneha MF, Dodgson JE, DeCambra MH, *et al*. Connecting culturally and spiritually to healthy eating: A community assessment with Native Hawaiians. *Asian Pac Isl Nurs J*. 2016;1(3):116–126.

103. Braun KL, Kim BJ, Ka'opua LS, *et al*. Native Hawaiian and Pacific Islander elders: What gerontologists should know. *Gerontologist*. 2015;55:912–919.

104. State of Hawai'i, Department of Hawaiian Home Lands. Accessed May 10, 2021. http://dhhl.hawaii.gov/.

105. Galinsky AM, Zelaya CE, Simile C, *et al*. Health conditions and behaviors of Native Hawaiian and Pacific Islander persons in the United States, 2014. National Center for Health Statistics. *Vital Health Stat*. 2017;3(40).

106. Schiller JS, Lucas JW, Ward BW, *et al.* Summary health statistics for US adults: National Health Interview Survey, 2010. National Center for Health Statistics. *Vital Health Stat 10.* 2012.

107. Pobutsky AM, Krupitsky D, Yamada S. Micronesian migrant health issues in Hawaii: Part 2: An assessment of health, language and key social determinants of health. *Calif J Health Promot.* 2010;7(2):32–55.

108. Ichiho HM, Roby FT, Ponausuia ES, *et al.* An assessment of non-communicable diseases, diabetes, and related risk factors in the territory of American Samoa: A systems perspective. *Hawai'i J Med Public Health.* 2013;72(5 Suppl 1):10–18.

109. Aitaoto N, Ichiho HM. Assessing the health care system of services for non-communicable diseases in the US-affiliated Pacific Islands: A Pacific regional perspective. *Hawai'i J Med Public Health.* 2013;72(5):106–114.

110. Palafox NA, Tsark JT. Cancer in the US-Associated Pacific Islands (UASPI): History and participatory development. *Pac Health Dialog.* 2004;11(2):8–13.

111. Kaholokula JK, Samoa RA, Miyamoto RES, *et al.* COVID-19 hits Native Hawaiian and Pacific Islander communities the hardest. *Hawaii J Health Soc Welf.* 2020;79(5):144–146.

112. Hofschneider A. Hawai'i Pacific Islanders are twice as likely to be hospitalized for COVID-19. *Civil Beat,* November 20, 2020. Accessed May 10, 2021. https://www.civilbeat.org/2020/11/hawaii-pacific-islanders-are-twice-as-likely-to-be-hospitalized-for-covid-19/.

113. Aitaoto N, Braun KL, Dang K, *et al.* Cultural considerations in developing church-based programs to reduce cancer health disparities among Samoans. *Ethn Health.* 2007;12:381–400.

114. Hubbell FA, Luce PH, McMullin JM. Exploring beliefs about cancer among American Samoans: Focus group findings. *Cancer Detect Prev.* 2005;29(2):109–115.

115. De Frutos DA, De la Ros AC. Death rituals and identity in contemporary Guam. *J Pac Hist.* 2012;47(4):459–473.

116. Balajadia RG, Wenzel L, Huh J, *et al.* Cancer-related knowledge, attitudes, and behaviors among Chamorros on Guam. *Cancer Detect Prev.* 2008;32(1):4–15.

117. Vakalahi H. Cultural context of health and well-being among Samoan and Tongan American elders. *Indian J Gerontol.* 2012;26(1):75–93.

118. Handy ES, Pukui MK. *The Polynesian family system.* Mutual Publishing, 1999.

3

Addressing Racism in Indigenous Health

Kathryn L. Braun, Lisa D. Harjo, Linda Burhansstipanov,
Keilyn Leinaʻala Kawakami, Donna-Marie Palakiko,
Pearl A. McElfish, May Rose I. Dela Cruz,
Mapuana C. K. Antonio, Priscilla R. Sanderson,
Mark C. Bauer, and Nicolette I. Teufel-Shone

Introduction

Racism is experienced by many Indigenous Peoples, and it negatively affects all aspects of their lives. This chapter presents important definitions in the discussion of racism, followed by a summary of the negative effects of racism on health. Examples are shared of interventions that aim to address racism, including programs that expand the number of Indigenous healthcare providers, increase the cultural sensitivity of healthcare providers, and support self-determination, healing, and resilience in Indigenous Peoples. This chapter concludes with recommendations for future practice, policy, and research around racism.

Types of Racism

Racism is defined as "a [false] belief that race is the primary determinant of human traits and capacities and that racial differences produce an inherent superiority of a particular race."[1] As outlined by Jones, racism manifests in at least three ways: (1) institutionally, (2) interpersonally, and (3) internally.[2]

Institutional Racism

Institutional racism is reflected in policies and societal norms that privilege one group over another and effectively limit access to power, education, good jobs, and safe housing by nonprivileged groups. This type of racism also is called structural racism or systemic racism. Examples of institutional racism include United States (US) governmental policies that supported the confiscation and privatization of Indigenous Peoples' lands, forced resettlement of Indigenous Peoples to less desirable lands, forced removal of American Indian (AI) and Alaska Native (AN) children to boarding schools, and laws that discouraged or prohibited the use of Indigenous languages and healing traditions.[3] Other examples include the US governmental policy in the 1830s to provide smallpox vaccine only to AI tribes considered friendly to US expansion, and the US governmental policies in the 1970s to sterilize AI women without informed consent.[4,5] Institutional racism is supposed to have been eliminated via federal nondiscrimination laws. However, most US policies and institutions are embedded in the Western paradigm of individualism, capitalism, and control, so continue to privilege White Americans.

Interpersonal Racism

Interpersonal racism includes prejudice and discrimination. Prejudice refers to judging a person's worth based on preconceived notions of the intellect, attitudes, and behaviors of a specific group. Prejudice, also known as bias, can be explicit, meaning that the biased person is aware of and obvious about their feelings toward the nonprivileged group. Bias also can be implicit, meaning that the bias operates on the subconscious level.[6]

Discrimination refers to the actions that result from prejudice. For a person experiencing discrimination, this could range from being treated rudely or disrespectfully by service providers and coworkers, to being refused services or employment altogether, and to being treated with suspicion and blamed for criminal and socially unacceptable behaviors without proof.

Explicit Bias

Explicit bias includes outright violence and hate speech. These are examples of macroaggressions, which are obvious hurtful behaviors toward a specific group. While unacceptable and shocking, they are easily visible expressions of one race's feelings of superiority over another.

In contrast, microaggressions are everyday comments that more subtly communicate feelings of superiority. For example, when someone says "you are pretty smart for a Hawaiian" or "you dress well for an Indian," the underlying message is that Native Hawaiians (NH) are not expected to be smart and AI are not expected to dress well. Being ignored or served last at a store or in a waiting room also may be a form of microaggression. Unlike macroaggressions, perpetrators of microaggression may be unaware that their behavior or speech is racist.[7]

Implicit Bias

Unconscious bias also is called implicit bias.[8] These include the feelings that exist outside of an individual's conscious awareness. In a healthcare context, White providers may not consciously realize that they systematically spend less time with patients of color than with White patients. Perhaps they feel less comfortable with people unlike themselves based on subconscious feelings or prejudices about them, or they feel more comfortable with patients like themselves. These implicit biases are difficult to explore and change because of their subconscious nature.[8] This type of bias is best gauged using an Implicit Association Test (IAT).[8] IATs have been constructed to assess implicit bias against Blacks, Arab-Muslims, Asians, older adults, individuals with disabilities, individuals who are obese, nonheterosexuals, and other groups.[9]

Internalized Racism

Internalized racism occurs when nonprivileged racial group members accept the negative characterization of their race. This may be reflected as a lack of respect for other people of their own race and low expectations of themselves and their abilities to succeed.[2] An example of internalized racism includes feeling not "good enough" or "smart enough" to go to college based on one's race. Internalized racism also may also be at work when someone believes they are destined to develop diabetes or cancer because of their race and therefore do not practice healthy behaviors or participate in cancer screening. This concept is also relevant to the notion of fatalism.

Privilege

In the context of racism, privilege refers to the "invisible package of unearned assets" that people of the dominant culture take for granted and can rely on to get them through life.[10] In the US, the dominant population is the non-Hispanic White population. "Dominant" does not mean majority population, but that their racial group is privileged and favored by the political, social, education, and economic systems of the US. White people in the US are generally accepted by others without having to constantly prove their intelligence or integrity or to justify their right to live and work in spaces established and populated primarily by Whites. In other words, there is great protection and privilege in never looking "out of place."[11] In the US, White privilege goes hand in hand with White power, meaning that White people set rules and punishments based on White values and traditions.[12] Few White Americans examine White privilege or have thought about how it influences their behaviors. Being unconscious of one's "invisible package of unearned assets" is associated with prejudice toward and discrimination against those who do not live up to White standards.

This difference in perspective is inherent in the relationship between cultures and privilege. The concept of "White privilege" is illustrated by thinking of life in terms of dichotomies, or in terms of "us" versus "them." The worldview of White culture is often based on control of the environment and the struggle between "us" and "them." It is as if an imaginary line divides the world. Someone is either on the top or the bottom. For instance, a teacher might be on top, while the student is below. Humans are on top, while nature is below. Good may be on top and bad below. Man atop would mean woman is below. White on the top leads to Black below.

In the Indigenous worldview, however, a circle or triangle, rather than a line, would more readily demonstrate the relationship among individuals. A circle or triangle includes and equalizes all positions on the continuum, leaving no one out and giving no one an edge over another. The worldview of many Indigenous cultures is to live in harmony with and connectedness to the environment. This difference in perspective is inherent in the relationships between culture and privilege.

An example of privilege is when White adults are rightfully proud of how they overcame challenges in youth to become well-educated, secure a high-paying job, and live in a nice neighborhood. This is something to be proud of, but because of White privilege, it is easier for a White person to access these successes because more doors are open to them. Indigenous Peoples do not have comparable privileges. They must overcome not only individual challenges but also structural racism and cultural prejudice. White people are not acknowledging how White privilege eased their way to success when they say, "I overcame my challenges to be a success, why can't your people" or "your people just don't work hard enough to overcome hardship."

Privilege begins with the color of one's skin and then extends to ones' gender.[11] Traditionally in the US, White men were privileged, even over White women. Women's suffrage and women's liberation movements, led by White women, drew attention to and challenged White male privilege. Today, women (especially White women) have more control over their lives because of these earlier struggles. However, White privilege still exists and needs to be recognized and confronted to truly address racism in the US.[11]

Relationships between Colonization, Historical Trauma, and Racism

The Indigenous Peoples of colonized lands invariably fall into a nonprivileged racial category. Vulnerable communities, such as Indigenous communities, have been oppressed and marginalized for over 400 years due to their lack of privilege.[11] In this book, the focus is on the experiences of AI, AN, NH, and PI populations, whose lands were confiscated and/or controlled by Europeans through colonization. For all these groups, colonization brought exposure to foreign disease, loss of land, restrictions on speaking the Native language and practicing Native traditions, and the supplanting of Indigenous religions by Christianity. Many Indigenous groups also experienced armed conflict, often with genocidal intent, forced relocation, and separation of families, with children sent to distant boarding schools.[5]

Indigenous Peoples can view colonization as traumatic because it was sudden, shocking, comprehensive, and imposed from outside.[12] Historical trauma theory links colonization to an array of problems for generations of Indigenous Peoples.[13,14,15] The colonized generation is the direct recipient of subjugation and loss, dying from genocide, armed conflict, and disease, or watching the destruction of their people and way of life and subsequently experiencing depression, self-destructive behaviors, hostility, and chronic bereavement.

Succeeding generations are affected by the original trauma in several ways. Colonizers, now the dominant culture, impose their social and political structures, into which their own progeny fit but which marginalize Native Peoples (institutionalized racism). The resulting social and economic disadvantages imposed on Indigenous Peoples may reduce Native families' capacity to provide for their progeny.[16] Parents and grandparents may transmit beliefs about the status of their ethnic group, including notions of racial inferiority and fatalism (internalized racism). Active and passive forms of discrimination (interpersonal racism) promote continued marginalization, keeping Indigenous Peoples at or near the bottom of economic and social hierarchies.

Recent research also suggests that powerfully stressful environmental conditions (for example, relocation to nonsustaining lands, disease, and starvation) can impact the body on the genetic level.[17] Life course theorists have presented evidence that gene expression is modified by stressors in the environment. For example, inadequate prenatal maternal nutrition and lack of adequate nutrition in infancy can influence the expression of DNA and the timing of developmental milestones throughout one's life.[18] Changes in DNA that originated from an Indigenous population living through extreme starvation may be present in their progeny or descendants seven or more generations later. Additionally, exposure to extreme environmental hazards can cue parts of the DNA to open or close proteins linked to survival (some events directly identified through epigenetic research). Thus, historical trauma has biological as well as social and cultural consequences for Indigenous Peoples at the individual and population level.

The Impact of Racism on Health

Globally, the health status and social indicators of Indigenous Peoples are worse than those of the dominant cultures of the lands on which they live.[19] Most of the health disparities experienced by Indigenous Peoples can be linked to social determinants of health, defined as "the conditions in which people are born, grow, live, work, and age, [which are] shaped by the [unequal] distribution of money, power, and resources at global, national, and local levels."[20] Race is a social construct, as is the social assignment of racial groups along a hierarchy. In the US, the idea that one racial group is better than another was made up and agreed upon by the people in power. Thus, racism is considered a social determinant of health.[21]

Racism can impact health in several ways. For example, research suggests that patients who experience racism have poorer mental health (including depression, anxiety, and psychological stress), poorer physical health, and poorer general health than patients not experiencing racism.[22] The greater the experience of everyday and lifetime discrimination, the higher the prevalence of chronic pain.[23] People who internalize racist beliefs are more likely to be overweight, to have high blood pressure and fasting glucose levels, to have high alcohol consumption, and to feel psychologically distressed.[22,24] Indigenous patients that perceived dismissive attitudes from healthcare providers are more likely to disengage from care and to self-medicate.[25]

Almost all studies that have measured implicit bias among healthcare providers suggest it is common and that, in general, providers have unconscious positive attitudes toward Whites and unconscious negative attitudes toward people of color. Implicit bias on the part of providers toward non-Whites has been linked to poor patient–provider interactions, unequal treatment decisions, and poorer health outcomes for people of color.[8]

Racism is so prevalent in the US that individuals who are classified by other people as non-White, regardless of how they self-identify, have poorer self-rated health than those seen by others as White.[26] These findings emerged from an analysis of data from US states that added a question about the social assignment of race (i.e., How do other people usually classify you in this country?) to their Behavioral Risk Factor Surveillance System in 2004. Of the 321 individuals who self-identified as AI, 48% of them felt that others saw them as White. Controlling for age and education, 53% of AI who were perceived by others as White reported excellent or very good health, compared to only 32% of AI who were perceived by others as AI.[26]

Thus, there is ample evidence of racism's pervasiveness in the US and among healthcare providers. Fortunately, there also is growing literature about strategies to increase awareness of racism as a social determinant of health and about programs to address and overcome racism. For example, Susan Puumala, a public health researcher, has been analyzing the experiences of AI children in hospital emergency departments.[27] Puumala's work brings to light how discrimination, racism, and stereotyping from healthcare providers decrease trust in the healthcare system, therefore contributing to more health disparities and lower utilization. Based on her research, she has provided tips on how to educate providers and break down barriers for AI children, so they have better access to healthcare resources.

There are a number of efforts underway to address racism in healthcare. These include (1) training and supporting Indigenous providers, (2) following CLAS standards, (3) training staff in cultural responsiveness, (4) supporting truth and reconciliation efforts, and (5) promoting Indigenous culture and resilience.[28] The next section provides examples of work in these five areas.

Overcoming Racism in Healthcare: Training and Supporting Indigenous Providers

Historically, Indigenous Peoples have been woefully underrepresented in the health professions. For example, in 2015, more than 18,000 individuals graduated from US medical schools, and only 20 (0.1%) were AI/AN.[29] In 2010, only 3% of Hawai'i's physician workforce was NH, while NH made up 26% of the population.[30] Two programs are featured that aim to increase the number of Indigenous Peoples working in the health professions and to support their professional development.

The American Indian, Alaska Native and Native Hawaiian (AIANNH) Caucus of the American Public Health Association

Description

The caucus was created in 1980 through the inspiration and dedication of Margo Kerrigan (White Earth Band of the Minnesota Chippewa) to increase the visibility and involvement of AI/AN in the American Public Health Association (APHA), a public health professional society with more than 40,000 members. The caucus was expanded to welcome and include NH in 2001. The goals of the caucus are to (1) provide a focal point within the APHA for persons having a particular interest in AI, AN, and NH health issues, (2) help APHA link to other organizations having interests in AI, AN, and NH health issues, (3) strengthen professional development of members, (4) support research that has implications for AI, AN, and NH health, (5) advocate for quality public healthcare, policies, and programs in AI/AN and NH communities, (6) provide consultation on AI, AN, and NH health matters, and (7) develop standards for professional preparation and practice for AI, AN, and NH practitioners.

Intervention

Since 1990, the caucus has sponsored 10 or more breakout sessions at each annual APHA conference that feature presentations on AI, AN, NH, and PI health. Also, caucus leaders participate in the governance of APHA as members of the APHA Executive Board, Governing Council, Equal Health Opportunity Committee, Policy and Resolutions Committee, and Program Planning Committees. Michael E. Bird, Santo-Domingo/Kewa Pueblo, served as president of APHA in 2001.

Over the years, the caucus has applied for and obtained small grants from multiple foundations to support conference registration and travel costs for AI, AN, and NH students, young or reentering professionals, and traditional elders. Professional mentors assist new members both in understanding the complexities of the annual APHA meeting and the importance of participating in the caucus' social events for networking, support, and fun. Through the dynamic caucus program, projects from both small and large public health systems serving AI, AN, NH, and PI are highlighted and cosponsored by other groups within APHA. Also, every year, a special health and traditional values session is held to honor Indigenous elders and leaders. Although this is a break-out session, it has sometimes been attended by more than 400 people. Fund-raising efforts, such as silent auctions of Indigenous crafts and artwork, are conducted during the annual caucus social event.

Community Engagement

Caucus members are from diverse geographic regions of the US, including community-based AI, AN, and NH organizations and academic, research, state, and federal agencies. Many members, but especially the elected officials of the caucus, volunteer their time to attract Indigenous public health staff and community members to the annual meetings.

Outcomes

When the caucus began, there were 40 members. Since then, membership has fluctuated from a low of 40 to over 300. Both Natives and non-Natives who work to support AI, AN, and NH public health programs are welcomed to join. The caucus obtained its 501(c)(3) nonprofit status in 2003, which made it eligible to apply for funding. Grant funds have been used to support the APHA registration fee and partial or full travel scholarships for 3 to 25 students, young professionals, community members, and traditional elders to attend the annual meeting. Caucus members have provided both support and culturally relevant advice to public health students, helping them to complete bachelor and graduate degrees as well as obtain public health jobs. There are several examples of mentoring relationships initiated during the annual meetings that have continued for years.

Lessons Learned

The caucus provides a safe and culturally respectful setting for AI, AN, and NH members of APHA and makes sure that members can learn about successful AI, AN, and NH public health interventions. Because of the work of the caucus, APHA members have gained knowledge about Indigenous health issues and strengths.

The Native Hawaiian Health Scholarship Program

Description

The Native Hawaiian Health Scholarship Program was established by public law in 1988 as part of the Native Hawaiian Health Care Improvement Act. The goal is to recruit NH into healthcare and to support them in obtaining health degrees to serve NH communities.

Intervention

Similar to the National Health Service Corps, the program provides scholarships, trains scholars in providing culturally appropriate healthcare, and places scholars in underserved communities. Scholarship recipients must "pay back" each year of financial support with a year of employment in a priority community. The program is funded primarily by the U.S. Department of Health and Human Services Health Resources Services Administration. It has been administered by Papa Ola Lōkahi, the Native Hawaiian Board of Health in Hawai'i, since FY 2002. Activities include lectures and field trips to understand the healthcare needs and preferences of the NH communities within which the graduates are expected to work. Scholars also receive assistance with posttraining placement in NH communities and postplacement check-ins and guidance.

Community Engagement

The program operates within Papa Ola Lōkahi. The mission of Papa Ola Lōkahi is to improve the health status and well-being of NH and others by advocating for, initiating, and maintaining culturally appropriate strategic actions aimed at improving the physical, mental, and spiritual health of NH and their 'ohana (families) and empowering them to determine their own destinies. Its board of directors includes representatives from government agencies, including the Hawai'i State Office of Hawaiian Affairs and Department of Health, the

University of Hawai'i, and community-based programs and health centers serving NH. More than 75% of board members are of NH ancestry. The Native Hawaiian Scholarship Program is one of several programs of Papa Ola Lōkahi.

Native Hawaiian Health Scholarship recipients and alumni engage with Papa Ola Lōkahi and the Native Hawaiian Health Scholarship Program staff throughout the year. In 2018–2019, alumni scholars began to organize themselves by island to assist with identifying workforce needs by discipline and island. In addition, alumni serve in an advisory capacity to the Native Hawaiian Health Scholarship Program.

Outcomes

Between 1991 and 2018, 292 scholarships supported the training of physicians, physician assistants, nurses, dentists, dental hygienists, clinical psychologists, social workers, marriage and family therapists, pharmacists, dieticians, and public health professionals. Nearly 80% of the scholars obtained their degrees in Hawai'i, primarily through the University of Hawai'i. As of 2018, 235 scholars had completed or were completing their service obligations in Hawai'i. Scholars have served in NH communities on six major Hawaiian islands (Kaua'i, O'ahu, Moloka'i, Maui, Lana'i, and Hawai'i Island) for approximately 68 organizations, including the five Native Hawaiian Health Care Systems and the 15 Federally Qualified Health Centers in the state. Of the 235 scholars who completed their training and service obligations in 2018, 220 (94%) remain employed in their discipline in Hawai'i and continue to serve NH communities.

Lessons Learned

To increase retention of scholars in the program and in their placements, it is important to align scholars' long-term career goals with their placement sites. Activities that help orient scholars to the NH communities in which they will serve are essential to this process. Individuals in communities that receive a NH provider note that their trust in the healthcare system is increased because they can relate to a provider from their own culture. NH patients also report that their health is positively impacted. This program also helps increase cultural responsiveness of non-Hawaiian providers who work alongside NH providers.

Overcoming Racism in Healthcare: CLAS Standards and Cultural Responsiveness Training

Healthcare facilities are important settings in which to implement strategies and interventions to overcome racism, as racism in these settings decreases trust of the system and reduces access to care. In an effort to increase access to

Table 3.1. National Standards for Culturally and Linguistically Appropriate Services in Health and Health Care (CLAS)

Principal Standard

1. Provide effective, equitable, understandable, and respectful quality care and services that are responsive to diverse cultural health beliefs and practices, preferred languages, health literacy, and other communication needs.

Governance, Leadership, and Workforce

2. Advance and sustain organizational governance and leadership that promotes CLAS and health equity through policy, practices, and allocated resources.
3. Recruit, promote, and support a culturally and linguistically diverse governance, leadership, and workforce that are responsive to the population in the service area.
4. Educate and train governance, leadership, and workforce in culturally and linguistically appropriate policies and practices on an ongoing basis.

Communication and Language Assistance

5. Offer language assistance to individuals who have limited English proficiency and/or other communication needs, at no cost to them, to facilitate timely access to all health care and services.
6. Inform all individuals of the availability of language assistance services clearly and in their preferred language, verbally and in writing.
7. Ensure the competence of individuals providing language assistance, recognizing that the use of untrained individuals and/or minors as interpreters should be avoided.
8. Provide easy-to-understand print and multimedia materials and signage in the languages commonly used by the populations in the service area.

Engagement, Continuous Improvement, and Accountability

9. Establish culturally and linguistically appropriate goals, policies, and management accountability, and infuse them throughout the organization's planning and operations.
10. Conduct ongoing assessments of the organization's CLAS-related activities and integrate CLAS-related measures into measurement and continuous quality improvement activities.
11. Collect and maintain accurate and reliable demographic data to monitor and evaluate the impact of CLAS on health equity and outcomes and to inform service delivery.
12. Conduct regular assessments of community health assets and needs and use the results to plan and implement services that respond to the cultural and linguistic diversity of populations in the service area.
13. Partner with the community to design, implement, and evaluate policies, practices, and services to ensure cultural and linguistic appropriateness.
14. Create conflict and grievance resolution processes that are culturally and linguistically appropriate to identify, prevent, and resolve conflicts or complaints.
15. Communicate the organization's progress in implementing and sustaining CLAS to all stakeholders, constituents, and the general public.

care by all US residents, the National Standards for Culturally and Linguistically Appropriate Services in Health and Health Care (CLAS) were introduced in 2001 (Table 3.1.).[31]

These standards include 15 action steps that direct healthcare practitioners to "provide effective, equitable, understandable, and respectful quality care and services that are responsive to diverse cultural health beliefs and practices, preferred languages, health literacy, and other communication needs."[32] Operationalizing these standards has led to expanded access to language translation services, materials in non-English languages, and mandatory training in cultural responsiveness and cross-cultural communication.

Training is especially important to increase providers' skills at successfully interacting with individuals from different racial and cultural groups and to overcome their implicit and explicit biases. There are several phrases used to describe this type of training, including "cultural competence" training, "cultural responsiveness" training, and "cultural humility" training. The definitions of these focused phrases are similar and overlapping. However, there is increased recognition of the difficulty of becoming completely competent in another culture. Thus, training in "cultural responsiveness" and "cultural humility" stress the importance of respectful interactions, active listening, and self-reflection to building honest and trustworthy relationships with people of different cultures.[33,34] This chapter uses the phrase "cultural responsiveness" training as an umbrella term for trainings that aim to improve intercultural communication and understanding.

As training in cultural responsiveness has become more prevalent, researchers have begun to analyze the literature to understand important elements of training and the effectiveness of such training. Research to date suggests that lecture-based cultural responsiveness education helps increase provider knowledge of other cultures and improve their attitudes toward working with them. However, there is little evidence that this increased knowledge leads to improvements in patient care, treatment outcomes, patient perceptions of providers, or organizational procedures.[28,35]

Rather, educational opportunities need to be combined with skills training to support the integration of new learning into practice. Research from Australia and Canada suggests greater success with cultural training programs that are longitudinal. Such programs are offered over the course of a week, a month, or a semester and engage Indigenous Peoples as trainers, teach about the role of colonization and White privilege in health inequities, and include structured opportunities to work with Indigenous Peoples.[36,37,38] A program that trains healthcare providers to work with Micronesian migrants in Arkansas is featured as an example.

Increasing Provider Sensitivity to Micronesian Migrants in Arkansas

Description

Arkansas is home to a large population of migrants from the Republic of the Marshall Islands (RMI). The RMI consists of 24 inhabited islands and atolls in the Pacific Ocean, about 2,300 miles west of Hawai'i. It became a US territory after World War II and, while now quasi-independent, the US maintains use of the islands for military purposes. In exchange, residents of the Marshall Islands can freely migrate throughout the US, and about 12,000 have relocated to Arkansas to work in businesses such as poultry production. In 2014–2015, the University of Arkansas for Medical Sciences developed and tested a program to increase the cultural sensitivity of providers working with Micronesian migrants, as well as the ability of students from different health specialties to work interprofessionally.[39]

Intervention

Trainers included members of the faculty as well as Marshallese clinical educators and Marshallese stakeholders. Because the course aimed to increase interprofessional skills, the 16 faculty members involved in the course received 30 hours of training on the core competencies for Interprofessional Education Collaborative.[40] Lectures on Marshallese history and culture were provided by Marshallese faculty. These lectures focused on the historical relationship of Marshallese people to the US, including US occupation of the islands at the end of World War II and the postwar use of the Marshall Islands to test US nuclear weapons. Students also learned about the Compact of Free Association (COFA), a government-to-government relationship between the RMI and the US that allows Marshallese and other Micronesians (e.g., from the Federated States of Micronesia and the Republic of Palau) to freely migrate to the US. COFA also spells out US responsibilities for the health and education of Micronesians.

Along with seminars provided by Marshallese clinical educators, students engaged in community-based service-learning opportunities to provide health screenings and health education at faith-based organizations and spent four hours per week for six months in a clinic providing services to uninsured Marshallese patients with diabetes.

Community Engagement

The free clinic and culturally sensitive training were developed in direct response to community stakeholders' requests. Marshallese stakeholders, including community leaders, community health workers, and a physician continue to be involved in the improving the design and delivery of the course.

Outcomes

Students who took part in the mixed-methods evaluation of the course were from medicine, nursing, pharmacy, and radiologic imaging science. As part of the evaluation, students completed self-assessments of their ability to work interprofessionally and their level of cultural knowledge about the Marshallese community. Questions about interprofessional practice focused on their comfort with team care, collaboration, roles, and professional identity. Questions related to working with Marshallese included "In general, how would you evaluate your comfort level in caring for clients from a culture other than your own?" and "How knowledgeable are you about the healthcare practices of the Marshallese?" Students also participated in post-course focus groups, which explored changes to their knowledge and practice. Findings suggested that students gained skills and comfort working interprofessionally, increased their knowledge about Micronesia and Marshallese people, and increased their empathy toward with Marshallese patients. Participants in the focus groups also articulated a number of changes they had made in their communication with and service delivery to Marshallese patients.

Lessons Learned

Teaching cultural responsiveness while accomplishing interprofessional education requirements allowed for more in-depth cultural training and experience. Having the didactic seminars taught by Marshallese clinical educators and stakeholders provided students with first-hand accounts of Marshallese history and culture and helped to build relationships between providers and this community. Hands-on experience through clinical service and community-based service-learning was essential to the integration of knowledge and the transformation of practice.

Overcoming Racism in Healthcare: Truth and Reconciliation Efforts

The truth and reconciliation process is a type of restorative justice that aims to bring together offenders and community to make amends and repair harms caused by past crimes. Truth and Reconciliation Commissions (TRC) represent a contrast to the retributive approach taken by the Nuremberg Trials after World War II, which included military tribunals held by foreign powers to prosecute Nazi war criminals. The reconciliatory approach differs in that it is a national or local process and includes the presentation of past crimes, compensation for victims, and opportunities for perpetrators to ask for forgiveness.[41]

The most well-known TRC was established in 1996 in South Africa at the end of apartheid. Through this TRC, a committee heard directly from the victims of abuses perpetrated under apartheid. Based on testimony and research, the committee assessed the extent of abuse experienced by each individual victim. If this abuse was linked to the state, the individual was referred to a second committee that aimed to restore the victim's dignity and to recommend policies and programs that would support healing. Funds were available to pay reparations. Another committee considered applications from perpetrators of human rights violations, provided they admitted their wrongdoing.[42] During this South African TRC process, over 7,000 individuals told their stories. Since then, the South African Department of Justice and Constitutional Development has offered tuition assistance for basic and higher education and training to TRC-identified victims of apartheid.

Another example comes from Canada. In 2008, the Indian Residential Schools Settlement Agreement required the government of Canada to establish a TRC to hear from First Nations and Aboriginal people in Canada who had been forcibly relocated to boarding schools. More than 6,700 individuals testified, predominantly those who survived the boarding school confinement. They told of being physically, mentally, and sexually abused and of the lifelong harm of being torn from their families and cultures. This TRC endeavored to enter these stories into the historical record of Canada and to hold events across Canada to celebrate and honor First Nation and Aboriginal cultures. Non-Indigenous witnesses were invited to present statements recognizing past abuses and to express their willingness to join in the reconciliation process. Working groups also produced educational materials for school children and adults so that this history will not be forgotten.[43]

In the US, the W. K. Kellogg Foundation launched its Truth, Racial Healing & Transformation (TRHT) initiative in 2016. The purpose of the TRHT initiative was to help communities address the historic and contemporary effects of racism.[44] Fourteen multisector community collaborations received funding in 2017 to implement TRHT processes to unpack community experiences of racism, acknowledge its negative impact, and be part of the narrative change around racial healing.[45] A TRHT implementation guidebook was developed for use by other communities ready to embark on the journey of racial healing by (1) bringing together stakeholders, (2) establishing a vision of the community without racism, (3) understanding privilege, different levels of racism (interpersonal, institutional, and internalized), and implicit bias, (4) hearing about and acknowledging experiences of racism, (5) facilitating opportunities for healing and building a community of healers, and (6) taking action to dismantle structures and attitudes that perpetuate racism.[46]

In 2018, the Association of American Colleges and Universities (AAC&U) began partnering with institutions of higher education to prepare the next generation of leaders and thinkers to break down racial hierarchies. Each TRHT Campus Center prioritized expansive, community-based healing activities to change collective community narratives and broaden the understanding of diverse experiences. The University of Hawai'i was among 10 colleges and universities selected as a TRHT campus center through AAC&U, and this program is highlighted here.

TRHT and Native Hawaiian and Indigenous Health Programs at the University of Hawai'i[i]

Description

The University of Hawai'i at Mānoa (UHM) TRHT program, under the Office of the President, is dedicated to helping campus citizens heal from the disconnections caused by racism and settler colonialism in Hawai'i. As specified in the UHM Strategic Plan 2015–2025, a goal of the university is to become a "Native Hawaiian place of learning" and an Indigenous-serving institution.[47] The TRHT program helps actualize this by educating students and faculty, helping administrators and faculty integrate Hawaiian history, values, and language into teaching and research, and promoting individual and collective responsibility to care for each other.

The Native Hawaiian and Indigenous Health (NHIH) Master of Public Health program is housed in the Office of Public Health Studies (OPHS). It was developed in 2012–2013 to train public health students to better address health in Indigenous communities and to eliminate health disparities that stem from multifaceted social and ecological determinants of health, including colonization and historical trauma. Courses provide advanced training in Indigenous health policy, ethics, and research.

Intervention

The UHM TRHT and NHIH programs emphasize the importance of exploring personal narratives and mo'okū'auhau (genealogies) to understand racism and to promote health and healing. The first step for NHIH's involvement in TRHT was training, attended by two Indigenous NHIH faculty members in 2019. TRHT training participants were charged with helping their departments take responsibility to address racism and settler colonialism through a lens of Hawaiian principles, including mālama (to care) and aloha 'āina (deep love for the land).

---

i Funding from W. K. Kellogg Foundation and AACU.

Following the training, the NHIH faculty reevaluated the NHIH curriculum and courses and reaffirmed its approach to explore genealogical connections to health and wellness from an Indigenous worldview while practicing being a good (future) ancestor. This approach emphasized the importance of being pono (right or righteous) and having lōkahi (balance) in physical, mental, emotional, and spiritual aspects of health. This extends to include pono relationships with other people, the environment, and the spiritual realm. The NHIH faculty then facilitated departmental discussions and activities in faculty retreats and meetings based on the teachings and learnings from TRHT. These discussions and activities helped to raise awareness of everyone's relationships with fellow faculty, students, the Mānoa community in its entirety (including the elements, place names, and the physical surrounding environment), and the 'āina, all of which helped deepen conversations around racism.

TRHT has provided various workshops, meetings, and a summit to continuously engage TRHT participants in the discussions of aloha 'āina while providing avenues to discuss current issues regarding racism and culture. It also generated resources to promote UHM as a NH place of learning. For example, the UHM Native Hawaiian Place of Learning Advancement Office sponsors activities like Aloha 'Āina Friday, which features speakers on mālama and aloha 'āina, opportunities to engage in 'āina-based activities on and near campus, and campus tours to share stories of places that support aloha 'āina. These continued conversations and resources aid in the ongoing discussions and activities within OPHS at a faculty level. They also have increased receptivity to student-led work and trainings in antiracism.

Community Engagement

The work of the UHM TRHT and NHIH programs required engagement from multiple entities, including champions of the work, organizational and community leaders, and community voices at large. A valuable teaching tool for both programs was the exploration of mo'okū'auhau and the way genealogy influences conceptualizations of being, truth, and ways of knowing. While acknowledging the various communities that have shaped and paved the way for TRHT and NHIH, the work around jettisoning racism is still in progress. It will require strengthening existing relationships and building new ones to expand the circle of people and groups dedicated to dismantling racism on campus and in Hawai'i.

Outcomes

Although the TRHT and NHIH programs are in their early stages, the outcomes thus far have demonstrated promise. For the NHIH program and the department within which it is housed, there is clearly an increased sense of place. Every meeting is begun with a collective chanting of *Welina Mānoa*, written by Keawe Lopes, to acknowledge and be welcomed by Mānoa, the valley in which the university is situated. Other outcomes have included an increased sense of connections by exploring kuleana (deep responsibility) to understand "isms" of disconnect, to care for Mānoa, and to connect with students, faculty, and Mānoa as a whole. Through active discussion and activities, faculty have become more open to hearing the cultural and ancestral stories of students, reflecting proper pronunciation of their Hawaiian names, and practicing cultural humility.

For the NHIH curriculum, the TRHT program reaffirmed its epistemological approach to health and wellness. Within OPHS, TRHT materials were shared with students in undergraduate, masters, and doctoral courses. The teachings of TRHT helped increase the number of OPHS and student-led diversity workshops and antiracism activities. The biggest outcome has been the diversification of OPHS students and faculty to include more Indigenous Peoples.

Lessons Learned

Despite the early stages of this work, several lessons have been learned. First and foremost, the success of this work requires support from leadership and upper administration. The University of Hawai'i TRHT program is housed at the top—in the Office of the President—and is supported by the campus strategic plan. Its goals also are supported by the leadership of the school and department within which NHIH is located. This top-down support demonstrated campus-wide, school-wide, and department-wide commitment to TRHT and NHIH and supported NHIH's bottom-up approaches to jettisoning racism.

Sustained efforts of this work require cultural sensitivity and humility, which take time to develop. Faculty and students must be encouraged to open themselves to new ways of viewing the world. Faculty must learn to integrate information on Hawaiian history and the negative effects of colonization into their teaching, research, and service. Leadership must set standards related to increased diversity of students and faculty, particularly representing communities that have been marginalized over time. Doing so requires critical self-evaluation of each individual's role in the structures that continue to perpetuate racism, while creating spaces that prioritize truth, racial healing, and transformation. Given the physical, mental, and emotional investment of this work, sustained efforts require continued commitment, training, and funding. This will ultimately allow for a continued paradigm shift that focuses on people from a strength-based and resilience approach rather than a problem-based approach.

Overcoming Racism in Health Research: Promoting Culture and Resilience

Resilience is defined as the ability to bounce back from hardship and to over-come stress and adversity.[48] Resilience is often thought of as an individual-level attribute; individuals are resilient if they can bounce back from adversity and stress. Individual-level interventions, including cognitive-behavioral therapy and mindfulness training, have been used to increase individual resilience, with good results.[49]

However, resilience is not simply a matter of personal strength. Resilience also is built through family, nonfamily, and community supports. Communities can be resilient, for example displaying an ability to come together to recover from a natural disaster. In this case, resilience is defined as a "collective bouncing back," and this is more likely when communities have strong social networks and shared cultural beliefs and practices to draw upon.[48] This research has led to the development of interventions that can help increase resilience in vulnerable individuals and communities.[50]

The term "cultural resilience" also has been proposed as synonymous with community resilience, with special relevance for AI communities. This term refers to a distinct community or cultural system that can cope with distur-bance and evolve in ways that adapt to change but preserve the culture's dis-tinctness. The worldview, values, and practices of the culture serve as sources of strength, and cultural stories can hold lessons that can help individuals and communities to endure and evolve in positive ways.[51]

AI research centers and service programs are now exploring ways to increase individual and community resilience, especially through the publica-tion of positive stories and the development and testing of culture-based inter-ventions. An example is the Center for American Indian Resilience (CAIR) in Arizona.

Center for American Indian Resilience[ii]

Description

The Center for American Indian Resilience (CAIR) was a collaboration between Northern Arizona University (NAU), the University of Arizona (UA), and Diné College, the Navajo Nation's first tribally controlled college, which is located on the Navajo Nation. Funded by the National Institutes of Health (NIH), the Center's mission was to partner with AI communities to promote

---

ii Funding from NIH NIMHD P20MD006872.

health and resilience. CAIR defined resilience as the "ability to move forward like a willow with renewed energy, with a positive outlook and attainable goals to achieve one's dreams and overcome negative life experiences from current and past political and historical events, with the goal to reduce health disparities among AI."[52] The specific goals of the center were to (1) examine community assets, including the role of traditional knowledge, collective memory and cultural strategies in teaching health behaviors and supporting positive health outcomes, (2) document these health strategies and positive behaviors oftentimes not collected in public health research, and (3) transfer and integrate tribal elders' wisdom, knowledge and experience into contemporary public education and health promotion interventions.

Intervention

CAIR was established with four cores. The Administrative Core provided administrative structure, coordination, evaluation and resources for resilience research and education. The Research Core engaged investigators from the regional tribal entities and universities in community-based participatory research (CBPR) with AI communities. The Research, Education, and Training Core coordinated training and education events for students and junior investigators, including a Summer Research Enhancement Program (SREP) and a conference to share findings on AI strengths and resiliencies.[53] The SREP curriculum emphasized resilience and assets-based approaches.[54] The Community Engagement and Outreach Core built local capacity in applying a resilience approach to AI health promotion programs, disseminated culturally relevant health promotion programs to AI communities, and supported students to develop community-engaged resilience activities.[55]

An example of a CAIR research that had a resilience-focused intervention component was *Documenting and Promoting Resilience in Urban AI*. In collaboration with the Tucson Indian Center and AI community members, life narratives of urban AI elders were documented. The narratives were converted into digital stories kept at the Tucson Indian Center and incorporated into a workbook for a health promotion program developed for youth, consisting of 12 bi-monthly workshops that focused on historical trauma and resilience.[56,57]

Another CAIR collaborative project involved a partnership with Ndee Bikiyaa (the People's Farm) in Whiteriver, Arizona, on the White Mountain Apache Nation. The partnership investigated the link between the traditional Apache diet, health, and resilience among White Mountain Apache citizens. The primary goal of the project was to document the nutritional value of traditional meals to ensure they met requirements for institutional settings and to determine the barriers for institutions to regularly serve traditional foods.

Findings were used to create sample menus of traditional meals that met institutional requirements, such as for a senior center, nursing home, or school.

Community Engagement

CAIR activities primarily focused on partners in the states of Arizona and New Mexico. Collaborators were AI that represented Diné (Navajo), White Mountain Apache, and urban AIs in Tucson, Flagstaff, Phoenix, and Albuquerque. CAIR projects engaged AI in identifying wellness strategies, assessing healthcare providers' perceptions of AI wellness behaviors, and suggesting strategies for enhancing provider–AI patient interactions. CAIR also received a NIH diversity supplement to build an AI community/social resilience research instrument. Through this study, the research team engaged AI accessing urban centers in New Mexico and Arizona in focus groups to identify culturally relevant AI social and community resilience themes.

Outcomes

During the funding period, CAIR expanded partnerships to include 45 additional organizations or programs. The center implemented 62 outreach/community engagement activities—for example, on digital storytelling training and development, video, curriculum presentations, and workshops—and reached more than 1,700 people over 5 years. The CAIR team shared and disseminated findings from resilience research with 3,750 tribal members. Researchers submitted 21 grant proposals, 12 of which were funded within the grant; others were funded through other sources. Twenty (95%) of the 21 projects were directly related to tribal community needs, most were community engaged, and 5 were community led.

A total of 107 students from the institutes of higher education were mentored through CAIR. Fifty-six AI/AN students completed the SREP curriculum, and 33 community-based partners participated and/or mentored students while the program was supported by CAIR. Among the trainees, 71% strongly agreed that CAIR increased their confidence in their research abilities, and almost 62% strongly agreed that CAIR helped them enjoy working in a research environment.

Lessons Learned

CAIR documented and tracked increased community leadership for local programs that integrated CBPR principles to address traditional and contemporary issues impacting resilience. Themes reinforced positive aspects of diverse AI cultures and strategies for overcoming historical trauma and current events that contributed to inequity, discrimination, and racism among tribal communities in Arizona and New Mexico. Both community members and students from all three partnering educational institutions participated in multiple programs within CAIR. For example, several students who completed SREP also took part in cultural competency, research, and grant writing training. Partner programs were able to augment their curricula to address structural racism in public health by training AI students to develop strategies to acknowledge and support collective and individual resilience. AI communities expanded their leadership roles in creating, implementing, and evaluating culturally respectful public health programs that directly benefited local AI.

Summary

Racism is pervasive in the US and associated with a plethora of negative health outcomes for Indigenous Peoples and other people of color. Communities are engaging to address the negative impact on health-related outcomes. Promising practices include (1) training more Indigenous providers in health professions, especially those with high earning power, such as medicine, nursing, pharmacy, social work, and public health, (2) operationalizing CLAS standards, especially in the provision of training in cultural responsiveness that is longitudinal, addresses Indigenous Peoples' experience with colonization and trauma, features instructors from the Indigenous group, and requires fieldwork with the Indigenous group of interest, (3) supporting organized truth and reconciliation efforts that increase awareness of past abuses, host mechanisms for social apologies, and provide monetary reparations, and (4) celebrating and building interventions grounded in cultural strengths and resiliency factors important to Indigenous Peoples. While promising, none of these approaches are addressing structural racism, which refers to inequities caused by policies and laws created by the dominant culture that privilege the dominant culture at the expense of nondominant cultures. Dismantling structural racism will require policies that explicitly address disparate outcomes based on race and provide mechanisms to reduce those disparities. For example, policies are needed that guarantee Indigenous Peoples access to good education, living wage jobs, adequate housing, and full health coverage. Policies should allow Indigenous Peoples to fully express themselves both culturally and spiritually. Finally, Indigenous Peoples should be supported to increase their civic participation and be involved in the process of developing policy to overcome centuries of being denied access to critical resources.

References

1. Merriam-Webster dictionary. Racism. Accessed September 14, 2020. https://www.merriam-webster.com/dictionary/racism.

2. Jones CP. Levels of racism: A theoretical framework and a gardener's tale. *Am J Public Health.* 2000;90:1212–1215.

3. Sotero MM. A conceptual modal of historical trauma: Implications for public health practice and research. *J Health Disparities Res Pract.* 2006;1(1):93–108.

4. Burhansstipanov L, Bemis LT, Petereit DG. Native American communities: Perspective and genetics. In: Monsen R, ed. *Genetics and ethics in nursing: New questions in the age of genomic health.* American Nurses Association, 2009:179–199.

5. Thornton R. *American Indian holocaust and survival: A population history since 1492.* University of Oklahoma Press, 1990.

6. Hall WJ, Chapman MV, Lee KM, *et al.* Implicit racial/ethnic bias among health care professionals and its influence on health care outcomes: A systematic review. *Am J Public Health.* 2015;105(12):e60–e76.

7. Sue DW, Capodilupo CM, Torino GC, *et al.* Racial microaggressions in everyday life: Implications for clinical practice. *Am Psychol.* 2007;62(4):271–286.

8. Greenwald AG, Poehlman TA, Uhlmann EL, *et al.* Understanding and using the Implicit Association Test: III. Meta-analysis of predictive validity. *J Pers Soc Psychol.* 2009;97(1):17–41.

9. Project Implicit. Accessed March 16, 2021. https://www.projectimplicit.net/.

10. McIntosh P. *White privilege: Unpacking the invisible knapsack.* Peace and Freedom, 1989. Accessed September 14, 2020. https://psychology.umbc.edu/files/2016/10/White-Privilege_McIntosh-1989.pdf.

11. Burke NS. 6 steps to de-weaponize "privilege." Accessed September 29, 2020. https://medium.com/@natalie4health/6-steps-to-de-weaponize-privilege-bab24972699d

12. Sztompka P. Cultural trauma: The other face of social change. *Eur J Soc Theory,* 2000;3(4):449–466.

13. Brave Heart MY, DeBruyn LM. The American Indian holocaust: Healing historical unresolved grief. *Am Indian Alsk Native Ment Health Res.* 1998;8(2):56–78.

14. Evans-Campbell T. Historical trauma in American Indian/Native Alaska communities: A multilevel framework for exploring impacts on individuals, families, and communities. *J Interpers Violence.* 2008;23(3):316–338.

15. Wesley-Esquimaux C, Smolewski M. *Historic trauma and aboriginal healing.* The Aboriginal Healing Foundation, 2004. Accessed September 14, 2020. https://epub.sub.uni-hamburg.de//epub/volltexte/2009/2903/pdf/historic_trauma.pdf.

16. Wilk P, Maltby A, Cooke M. Residential schools and the effects on Indigenous health and well-being in Canada a scoping review. *Public Health Rev.* 2017;38:8.

17. Walters KL, Mohammed SA, Evans-Campbell T, *et al.* Bodies don't just tell stories, they tell histories: Embodiment of historical trauma among American Indians and Alaska Natives. *Du Bois Rev.* 2011;8(1):179–189.

18. Halfon N, Larson K, Lu M, *et al.* Life course health development: Past, present and future. *Matern Child Health J.* 2014;18(2):344–365.

19. Anderson I, Robson B, Connolly M, *et al.* Indigenous and tribal peoples' health: A population study. *Lancet.* 2016;388(10040):131–157.

20. World Health Organization. Social determinants of health. Accessed September 14, 2020. www.who.int/social_determinants/sdh_definition/en/.

21. Williams DR, Mohammed SA. Discrimination and racial disparities in health: Evidence and needed research. *J Behav Med.* 2009;32(1):20–47.

22. Paradies Y, Ben J, Denson N, *et al*. Racism as a determinant of health: A systematic review and meta-analysis. *PLoS One*. 2015;10(9):e0138511.

23. Brown TT, Partanen J, Chuong L, *et al*. Discrimination hurts: The effect of discrimination on the development of chronic pain. *Soc Sci Med*. 2018;204:1–8.

24. Kelaher MA, Ferdinand AS, Paradies Y. Experiencing racism in health care: The mental health impacts for Victorian Aboriginal communities. *Med J Aust*. 2014;201(1):44–47.

25. Goodman A, Fleming K, Markwick N, *et al*. 'They treated me like crap and I know it was because I was Native:' The healthcare experiences of Aboriginal peoples living in Vancouver's inner city. *Soc Sci Med*. 2017;178:87–94.

26. Jones CP, Truman BI, Elam-Evans LD, *et al*. Using "socially assigned race" to probe White advantages in health status. *Ethn Dis*. 2008;18(4):496–504.

27. Pickner WJ, Ziegler KM, Hanson JD, *et al*. Community perspectives on emergency department use and care for American Indian children. *J Racial Ethn Health Disparities*. 2018;5(5):939–946.

28. Clifford A, McCalman J, Bainbridge R, *et al*. Interventions to improve cultural competency in health care for Indigenous peoples of Australia, New Zealand, Canada and the USA: A systematic review. *Int J Qual Health Care*. 2015;27(2):89–98.

29. Association of American Medical Colleges. Table B-4: Total U.S. Medical school graduates by race/ethnicity (alone) and sex, 2014–2015 through 2018–2019. Accessed September 14, 2020. https://www.aamc.org/download/321536/data/factstableb4.pdf.

30. Ambrose AJ, Arakawa RY, Greidanus BD, *et al*. Geographical maldistribution of Native Hawaiian and other Pacific Islander physicians in Hawai'i. *Hawai'i J Med Public Health*. 2012;71(4 Suppl 1):13–20.

31. US Department of Health and Human Services, Office of Minority Health. National standards for culturally and linguistically appropriate services in health care. Accessed March 16, 2021. https://minorityhealth.hhs.gov/omh/browse.aspx?lvl=2&lvlid=53.

32. Think Culture Health. The national CLAS standards. Accessed September 13, 2020. https://thinkculturalhealth.hhs.gov/clas#:~:text=The%20National%20CLAS%20Standards%20are,culturally%20and%20linguistically%20appropriate%20services.

33. Brach C, Fraserirector I. Can cultural competency reduce racial and ethnic health disparities? A review and conceptual model. *Med Care Res Rev*. 2000;57(1 suppl):181–217.

34. Yeager KA, Bauer-Wu S. Cultural humility: Essential foundation for clinical researchers. *Appl Nurs Res*. 2013;26(4):251–256.

35. Horvat L, Horey D, Romios P, *et al*. Cultural competence education for health professionals. *Cochrane Database Syst Rev*. 2014;(5):CD009405.

36. Beavis ASW, Hojjati A, Kassam A, *et al*. What all students in healthcare training programs should learn to increase health equity: Perspectives on postcolonialism and the health of Aboriginal Peoples in Canada. *BMC Med Educ*. 2015;15:155.

37. Bullen J, Flavell H. Measuring the gift: Epistemological and ontological differences between the academy and Indigenous Australia. *Higher Educ Res Dev*. 2017;36(3):583–596.

38. Prout S, Lin I, Nattabi B. Green C. 'I could never have learned this in a lecture': Transformative learning in rural health education. *Adv Health Sci Educ Theory Pract*. 2014;19(2):147–159.

39. McElfish PA, Moore R, Buron B, *et al*. Integrating interprofessional education and cultural competency training to address health disparities. *Teach Learn Med*. 2018;30(2):213–222.

40. Interprofessional Education Collaborative. IPEC core competencies. Accessed January 15, 2021. https://www.ipecollaborative.org/ipec-core-competencies.

41. International Justice Resource Center. Truth and reconciliation commissions. Accessed September 14, 2020. https://ijrcenter.org/cases-before-national-courts/truth-and-reconciliation-commissions/.

42. Sarkin-Hughes J. *Carrots and sticks: The TRC and the South African amnesty process.* Intersentia, 2004.

43. University of Manitoba, National Centre for Truth and Reconciliation. Teaching resources. Accessed September 14, 2020. https://education.nctr.ca/teaching-resources/.

44. Christopher G. Truth, racial healing, and transformation: Creating public sentiment. *Natl Civic Rev.* 2017;106(3):12–19.

45. W.K. Kellogg Foundation. Truth, racial healing, and transformation. Accessed September 14, 2020. https://healourcommunities.org/.

46. W.K. Kellogg Foundation. *Truth, racial healing, and transformation implementation guidebook.* Kellogg Foundation, 2016.

47. University of Hawai'i at Mānoa. UH Mānoa strategic plan. Accessed February 22, 2021. https://manoa.hawaii.edu/strategicplan/.

48. Kirmayer LJ, Tait CL, Simpson C. The mental health of Aboriginal peoples in Canada: Transformations of identity and community. In: Kirmayer LJ, Valaskakis GG, eds. *Healing traditions: The mental health of Aboriginal peoples in Canada.* UBC Press, 2009:3–35.

49. Joyce S, Shand F, Tighe J, et al. Road to resilience: A systematic review and meta-analysis of resilience training programmes and interventions. *BMJ Open.* 2018;8:e017858.

50. Luthar SS. Resilience in development: A synthesis of research across five decades. In: Cicchetti D, Cohen DJ, eds. *Developmental psychopathology: Volume Three: Risk, disorder, and adaptation, 2nd ed.* Wiley Online Library, 2015:739–795.

51. Oré CE, Teufel-Shone NI, Chico-Jarillo TM. American Indian and Alaska Native resilience along the life course and across generations: A literature review. *Am Indian Alsk Native Ment Health Res.* 2016;23(3):134–157.

52. Northern Arizona University, Center for AI Resilience. What is resilience? Accessed September 14, 2020. https://nau.edu/CAIR/What-is-Resilience/.

53. Garrison ER. Transforming biology curriculum at Navajo Community College to include Navajo and Western cultural knowledge. *J Navajo Educ.* 1994;2(1):18–22.

54. Kahn CB, Dreifuss H, Teufel-Shone NI, et al. Adapting summer education programs for Navajo students: Resilient teamwork. *Front Sociol.* 2021;6:1.

55. Darroch F, Giles A, Sanderson PR, et al. The United States does CAIR about cultural safety: Examining cultural safety within Indigenous health contexts in Canada and the United States. *J Transcult Nurs.* 2017;28(3):269–277.

56. Kahn CB, Reinschmidt K, Teufel-Shone NI, et al. American Indian Elders' resilience: Sources of strength for building a healthy future for youth. *Am Indian Alsk Native Ment Health Res.* 2016;23(3):117–133.

57. Reinschmidt KM, Attakai A, Kahn CB, et al. Shaping a stories of resilience model from urban American Indian elders' narratives of historical trauma and resilience. *Am Indian Alsk Native Ment Health Res.* 2016;23(4):63.

4

Using Community-Based Participatory Research to Address Indigenous Health

Suzanne Held, Alma Knows His Gun McCormick,
Vanessa Simonds, Kathryn L. Braun, Linda Burhansstipanov,
Emily Haozous, Valerie Rangel, Jane J. Chung-Do,
Ilima Ho-Lastimosa, Rachel Novotny, and
Marie Kainoa Fialkowski Revilla

Introduction

This chapter focuses on multiple ways to engage Indigenous communities in the creation, implementation, and continued maintenance or sustainability of interventions and programs that are grounded in the local culture and driven by the local community. Chapter 1 briefly referred to Paulo Freire's work from the mid-twentieth century that introduced the right to question outside control of knowledge.[1] This became the foundation for participatory action research (PAR), which was defined as "a cycle of engaging teams in a process of reflection and action to bring about change."[2,3] Freire's work also informed the development of frameworks and principles of community-based participatory research (CBPR).[4,5] Both PAR and CBPR acknowledge the expertise of the community and their lived experience as a valuable form of knowledge, which diverges from traditional views that scientific evidence stems solely from the observations of objective, academically trained researchers.[5]

Nine principles of CBPR were outlined by Barbara Israel and colleagues in the 1990s (Table 4.1.)[4] and were contextualized through an Indigenous lens in 2009.[6] Because these nine principles have relevance for community-engaged research, PAR, and CBPR, they are reviewed in this chapter. This review is followed by descriptions of five CBPR projects conducted with Indigenous communities. The first, Messengers for Health (MFH), is a long-running partnership that uses a CBPR approach among the Apsáalooke (Crow) Nation in Montana, and it is described in detail to illustrate the nine CBPR principles. The other four CBPR projects are described in less detail, including the 2017 Santa Fe Indian Center Health Impact Assessment, Guardians of the Living Water, the MALAMA Aquaponics Study with Native Hawaiian Families, and

Table 4.1. Principles of CBPR[4]

1. Acknowledges community as a unity of identity.
2. Builds on strengths and resources within the community.
3. Facilitates collaborative and equitable partnerships in all phases of research, involving an empowering and power-sharing process that attends to social inequalities.
4. Fosters colearning and capacity building among all partners.
5. Integrates and achieves a balance between knowledge generation and intervention for the mutual benefit of all partners.
6. Focuses on the local relevance of public health problems and on ecological perspectives that attend to the multiple determinants of health.
7. Involves systems development using a cyclical and iterative process.
8. Disseminates results to all partners and involves them in the wider dissemination of results.
9. Involves a long-term process and commitment to sustainability.

the Children's Healthy Living Project for Remote Underserved Populations in the Pacific Region.

Nine Principles of CBPR

Principle 1 is to recognize the community as a unit of identity. Communities can be centered geographically or can be defined by race, ethnicity, tribe, gender, diagnosis, profession, or something else. Community is characterized by a sense of identification and connection to other members, which usually include the sharing of values and experiences.

Principle 2 recognizes that every community has strengths and resources, and that these should be leveraged to create attractive, feasible, and effective interventions to improve community health.

Principle 3 requires researchers to facilitate collaborative partnerships with community members so they can be involved in all phases of research. This principle also confirms that community members are equal members and should share control in the identification of problems, the collection and interpretation of data, and in research resources.

Principle 4 is to promote colearning and empowerment that attends to social inequalities. This means that researchers have a responsibly to learn from community, as well as to build community capacity through training, employment opportunities, and paychecks.

Principle 5 calls on researchers to integrate knowledge and action for mutual benefit of all partners. Data should not be gathered for the sole purpose of defining problems. Rather, data need to inform actions and support advocacy that can lead to improvements in the community.

Principle 6 directs research to focus on locally relevant problems. In other words, research should address community concerns rather than researcher concerns. Research also should be conducted with an ecological perspective, considering the organizational, community, and policy causes of disparities and testing higher-level interventions.

Principle 7 involves commitment to a cyclical and iterative process in research. This means that researchers and community continue to use new learnings to refine problem statements and develop and test new actions.

Principle 8 requires that research findings are disseminated to all partners, that participants view materials prepared for publication prior to their submission, and that community members serve as coauthors and copresenters of findings.

Finally, Principle 9 relates to long-term involvement between researchers and the community, with an eye to sustaining positive changes for the community. This could include the development of new services that can be sustained in the community and the empowerment of the community to propose and win funding to do their own research and outreach projects.

Examples of Successful CBPR Projects in Indigenous Communities

Messengers for Health, a CBPR Project[i]

Description

MFH is a partnership between members of the Apsáalooke (Crow) Nation, located in southeastern Montana, and Montana State University. MFH began in 1996 from a mutual interest to address cervical cancer mortality rates among the Northern Plains Tribes that were among the highest in the United States, compared with White and American Indian/Alaska Native (AI/AN) women in other regions.[7] The team decided to first administer a women's health survey to learn about perceptions around cancer and barriers to cancer screening. These data were used to develop the MFH intervention and, in 2001 and 2005, funding was received from the American Cancer Society to study the effectiveness of utilizing community women (called Messengers) to deliver education and encourage Crow women to participate in cancer screening. Over the years, the partnership worked in multiple topic areas and has provided dozens of students experience with CBPR research.

---

i Funding from ACS RSG-01-193-05-CPPB.

Intervention

Although MFH is ongoing and has conducted many projects, this example focuses on the community engagement process of the initial MFH project on cervical cancer screening. The intervention started with a survey, which was designed in close collaboration with community partners. Then, an intervention was developed and tested through which local women were trained as Messengers to deliver cancer education and outreach to their peers.

Community Engagement

Similar to other CBPR approaches, it was important that the community expressed initial interest in working in this area and that the university partner was willing to learn the best methods that would work in this specific community (CBPR principles 1, 2, and 3). A Community Advisory Board (CAB) was established, composed of five women and two men in the community who were elders, educators, health professionals, cancer survivors, and activists for the health of the community. They provided direction and advice for the program in monthly meetings. The CAB assured that all of the work was in partnership, from providing training and developing protocols and program materials, to collecting and analyzing data, and disseminating it through papers and presentations (CBPR principles 3 and 8).

The MFH staff listened carefully to local Crow leaders about their history (CBPR principles 2, 4, and 6), which led to the development of a women's health survey interview protocol that built on community norms and capacities (CBPR principles 3 and 4). Both qualitative and quantitative interviews were implemented by program staff in a one-on-one setting as preferred by the community to hear stories from community members, and these stories helped develop community-based interventions (CBPR principle 2).

When beginning this work, project partners diligently searched for interviewer training manuals developed for Indigenous populations; however, they were not able to find any. Thus, they reviewed publications that discussed interviewer training from a majority cultural lens, which were adapted to create an interviewer training manual appropriate to the MFH project. Apsáalooke community members working with the project immediately stressed that instructions provided in guides written for the dominant US population were not appropriate for their community (CBPR principles 3, 4, and 7).

For example, MFH staff found published instructions that research interviewers should be formal, businesslike, and distant, and the interviewer should collect data quickly and efficiently. In contrast, community members felt it was more culturally appropriate to approach members of the Apsáalooke Nation with a warm greeting and to take time for casual conversation before starting to gather data (CBPR principle 2). This approach proved to set a friendly and nonthreatening tone for the whole interview and allowed interviewees to openly express themselves. Had the MFH staff followed published instructions, the person being interviewed may have felt pressured or rushed or that they were being tested on their health knowledge. They would have been less likely to share personal information or express their true thoughts.

In another example, extant interviewer guides recommended using strong persuasive tactics to recruit and enroll individuals. However, community members relayed that this behavior was inappropriate in the Apsáalooke culture. Thus, MFH was careful to thoughtfully explain the study and gave potential interviewees the choice to participate, understanding that consenting individuals would be taking time from family and community obligations to participate. MFH interviewers also made sure the interview was conducted at a time and place most convenient for participants. This was a respectful approach that acknowledged that it was an honor for MFH and community members to visit with one another to share their experiences and input (CBPR principle 6).

Another published guide noted that, often, communities do not benefit from their engagement in research. However, MFH made a commitment to community members that any data collected from them would be shared with them and would be used to their benefit to the extent possible (CBPR principles 4, 5, and 8).

Outcomes

In the partnership's first study, the team learned that women in the Apsáalooke Nation had both positive and negative experiences regarding Pap testing. Positive experiences were associated with providers with whom women had established trust and with providers that were female, polite, and personable, who offered information and reassurance, and who maintained confidentiality. Negative experiences were associated with short examinations, inconsiderate providers, male providers, and limited verbal communication with/by the provider.[6] Information was shared with Indian Health Service (IHS) to help improve provider–patient relations. They also found that there is no Crow word for cancer and that women did not talk with each other about cancer screening or diagnosis. Through the MFH program, women began talking to each other, cancer survivors started to speak out in public, and a support group was started where people publicly showed that cancer was not a death sentence. The statistically significant increase in knowledge of cervical cancer and the positive shift in attitudes regarding screening and care resulted.

An important aspect of this partnership was the involvement of Indigenous students from the Apsáalooke Nation and other Indigenous nations in the project (CBPR principle 4). Students worked with MFH through internships, paid student research positions, and as volunteers. They were involved in every aspect of MFH work, from writing grant applications to disseminating results. They were coauthors of MFH peer-reviewed published papers, and frequently presented at national conferences. Students remarked on the importance of working with the program, as it provided a family for students living away from home and helped them to be successful. As of July 2020, Messengers had two "second generation students" whose moms worked with Messengers while they were in school in the 1990s and 2000s, and now their daughters were involved as student researchers.

In the early days of MFH, research grants came into the university and the primary community partner Alma Knows His Gun McCormick and other community members were employed by the university as project staff. Although trust between the Apsáalooke Nation and the university partner was high, in thinking about project sustainability, the Apsáalooke arm of the partnership began to contemplate becoming a nonprofit organization. Assistance to become a nonprofit was provided from a number of partners, including university faculty, other nonprofit organizations, a nonprofit organizational development professional, and a local grant writer.

In 2010, the MFH partnership transitioned from a research grant into a 501(c)(3) nonprofit organization with a mission to "improve the health of individuals on the Crow Indian Reservation and outlying areas through community-based projects designed to strengthen the capacity of communities and empower them to assess and address their own unique health-related problems" (CBPR principle 9).[8] Now, grants come directly to the nonprofit, or the nonprofit can receive subcontracts from universities and other institutions. Community members have developed strong leadership skills and are seen as leaders. The group continues to partner with Montana State University on their 2017–2022 NIH Báa nnilah (advice that is received from others) program to improve chronic illness self-management within the Apsáalooke Nation.[9]

Lessons Learned

There were many lessons learned through experience about respectful behaviors that may assist non-Indigenous researchers new to partnering with Indigenous communities or Indigenous researchers partnering with an Indigenous tribe that is new to them. One of the primary lessons was the importance of understanding that everyone had expertise to share and that by listening to all partners and bringing in everyone's expertise, beneficial outcomes resulted (CBPR principle 4). It was helpful to understand that all people carried assumptions from past experiences and needed space to consider and discuss these assumptions and put them aside. When agreeing to work together in a true partnership, partners had to be willing to grow and learn from each other and to change their assumptions. This helped attain a successful result and benefited the partnership and the community.

Another lesson learned through experience was the importance of the external partner spending time in the community, willing to listen and receive (CBPR principle 9). Being present together was the most efficient and respectful way to establish relationships, which was vital to the success of partnership research. Community members felt and discerned when external partners listened carefully, honored what community members said, treated all people equally, and were sincere in their intentions. It is important for external partners to take part in social activities, to ask questions to learn about the community, and to meet and relate to community members external to the research (including children). Communities have experience with outsiders who have been present without sincerity, were judgmental, or just wanted to push their own agenda; these actions and attitudes are harmful. A true partnership happens when people worked together equally and not when someone who was "better" helped others who were "less than."

The third lesson regarding respectful behaviors was the importance of partners supporting each other and having each other's back. There were aspects of the university and of the community that were not readily apparent to those who did not live or work there. There were politics and unwritten rules and different ways of recognition and acknowledgment that existed in different settings. Over time, the partners working in the MFH project gained the ability to represent each other and the project well without the other being present. For example, the university partner could go to the community and represent the project at a community meeting, and the community partner could go to a research conference and represent the project there (CBPR principle 8). Partners depended and leaned on each other for support and talked openly about struggles that arose. There was a deep level of trust that continued to grow over time. Despite facing challenges, partners continued to maintain the focus of the project, maintain unity, and persevere.

Another lesson was to be upfront with expectations and to match words with actions (CBPR principle 5). For example, the MFH partnership surveyed women in the community at the beginning of the project. When recruiting women to complete the survey, the project staff shared that the information they provided in the survey would directly benefit community women's health. Women in the community watched the actions of the partnership over time and saw them build a program to help women receive cancer screenings. Information about the project spread and from this, more community members were involved. This was important, as the sustainability of projects was essential to positively impact the lives of community members.

The final lesson for external partners was to be ready to be personally changed by the research (CBPR principle 4). This was not the type of research where the external partner remained aloof and separate from the community. As noted by Shawn Wilson, an Indigenous educator who wrote the book *Research is Ceremony*, if you are not changed by doing research, you are not doing it correctly.[10]

2017 Santa Fe Indian Center Health Impact Assessment[ii]

Description

Santa Fe, New Mexico, has a diverse and long-established AI/AN community. Geographically located in the north-central part of New Mexico, Santa Fe is close to many of the state's Pueblo communities and is on Tesuque Pueblo's ancestral land. It also is home to the Institute of American Indian Art (IAIA), one of only three United States Congressionally chartered tribal colleges. IAIA was established in 1962 with an academic mission to study, preserve, and disseminate AI/AN arts and language.

Santa Fe County includes approximately 6,300 AI/AN, representing tribes from across the country. Santa Fe's AI/AN off-reservation community includes multigenerational families of those who left their home reservations during relocation or came to IAIA to study and stayed on after graduation. Other AI/ANs are members of nearby tribes and/or have relocated to Santa Fe for work, marriage, or its vibrant and welcoming intertribal community.

The Santa Fe Indian Center (SFIC), an urban AI/AN-serving nonprofit organization, provided resources, referrals, and hosted community events throughout the year for the local urban AI/AN community. The collaboration between Emily Haozous, a Chiricahua Fort Sill Apache and a Research Scientist with the Pacific Institute for Research and Evaluation, and the Santa Fe Indian Center (SFIC) began in 2015 when Emily attended an SFIC board meeting and offered to serve as a collaborator for any health-related research they were interested in conducting. At that meeting in 2015, the board agreed to collaborate should a grant opportunity arise that met their priorities.

Within a few months, the New Mexico Health Equity Partnership (NMHEP), an initiative at the Santa Fe Community Foundation, posted a call for applications for their Health Impact Assessments (HIA). An HIA is like a needs assessment, except an HIA is designed to focus on the impact that a

ii Funding from New Mexico Health Equity Partnership, Santa Fe Community Foundation, and W.K. Kellogg Foundation.

pending or existing policy would have on the local community. The goal of the HIA was to develop data-based policy recommendations using a tested community-oriented methodology. Through the HIA process, data-based policy recommendations were developed to mitigate health risks on a marginalized population. Emily posed the idea to the SFIC board that they could examine the policy of IHS underfunding and its impact on the local urban AI/AN community. The SFIC agreed that this would meet its priorities.

The Intervention

The HIA plan was to collect detailed survey information on the overall health, health priorities, and experiences with IHS from AI/AN who lived in Santa Fe County and had received care at the local IHS facility. Before data collection, the research team worked with a CAB to refine an existing AI/AN-centered survey to meet the specific priorities of the Santa Fe urban AI/AN community, as identified by the CAB and the SFIC. Once the survey was finalized, the HIA team submitted the research for human subjects' review. The application was approved quickly, and the team was able to begin collecting survey data at a major community event in May 2016.

The HIA team collected survey data using several strategies. They found data collection was most successful during community events such as during a city-wide Community Day. The HIA CAB and the SFIC shared a table at these events, helping each other disseminate information about the SFIC while also recruiting survey participants. This collaboration was a great opportunity for the HIA team, because it demonstrated to the community the partnership between the two groups. It also helped the SFIC show its interest in improving health of the area's AI/AN community by their investment of time in this initiative.

Participating individuals completed a paper survey with a pencil, then received a $5 gift card in recognition of their time and knowledge. Some people took only a few minutes to complete the survey; others took as long as 30 minutes to write detailed qualitative information on the forms. The survey also was available online for people to complete in private. Some community members posted a link to the survey on Facebook, making it available to local community members who were not attending events in person. Potential participants often asked the data collectors if they were employees of IHS before consenting to participate in the study. The team collected a total of 165 surveys.

They also collected qualitative interviews from a subset of participants who agreed to discuss their experiences with the IHS or other salient health concerns. Those interviews took place in people's homes, over the phone, or in other locations that were identified as most comfortable for the participants. The project team completed 17 qualitative interviews with community members.

The primary research team worked to create summaries of the key data points once data collection was completed in August 2016. Those summaries were reviewed by the CAB, which identified their priority areas of concern. The team used these priority areas to pull out details that were most related to the SFIC's priority concerns for the final report. The summary and key data findings also were presented at an open community meeting at which they received feedback from the Santa Fe AI/AN community. Researchers used this feedback to help refine the final report, identifying areas where they could dedicate more focus or investigate the existing data for additional insight. Finally, the researchers and the CAB developed a set of four policy recommendations to help guide future work. They worked closely with the NMHEP to create the final HIA report, which included a plan for dissemination, follow-up, and future work.

Community Engagement

The funding opportunity required that the project partners work collaboratively. During the grant-writing phase, the team reviewed multiple drafts of the grant, with changes made based on feedback from the SFIC board. After the grant-writing team submitted the grant application to NMHEP, more refinements were made.

The HIA CAB included several SFIC board members, but it also included other AI/AN community members who had expertise or networks in specific areas. The CAB spent the first several months of the grant building their mission as a group, deciding on the priorities of the HIA, and refining the community survey they would use in the HIA. During this early funding period, Emily hired Valerie Rangel, a community member with expertise in community organizing, as program manager for the HIA. She quickly learned how to use the data collection software so they could collect data using an online survey system, which made the overall data collection process much more streamlined.

Outcomes

The HIA report was professionally printed and distributed at a launching event in January 2017 at the SFIC. At that event, the team presented four recommendations for policy action that were supported by the data. Members of the AI/AN community, the press, and the general community attended. The event also celebrated the culmination of this long process of data collection, analysis, reporting, and collaboration. The HIA report was published on the NMHEP website, as was the PowerPoint from the January community launch meeting. The team also presented the results to the Santa Fe IHS Tribal Advisory Council, in the interest of full accountability and collaboration. The HIA report was disseminated by the local newspaper and the *Navajo Times*. The local weekly newspaper, *The Reporter*, published a long-form story about the issue of under-funding to the IHS, which drew extensively from the HIA report.

The survey data itself indicated that the Santa Fe urban AI/AN community was most concerned about diabetes, body size, mental health, heart disease, and addiction. These data also revealed that more than half (53%) of Santa Fe's AI/AN were rationing food. Thus, one of the four recommendations for IHS was to partner with the local food bank to bring food resources to the AI/AN community. Soon after the HAI report was issued with this recommendation, the IHS began a partnership with a local low-cost produce delivery service (MoGro). Subsequently, the SFIC began to collaborate with MoGro to provide discount coupons for AI/AN who wished to access the high-quality, locally grown foods available through MoGro at the Santa Fe IHS. The MoGro program ended in May 2019; however, the SFIC continues to address the food insecurity issues among Santa Fe AI/AN by partnering with Feeding Santa Fe. Every week, free bags of groceries are distributed to needy families by SFIC's Santa Fe office.

This CBPR project was ultimately a very successful collaboration between an academically based AI/AN investigator and a community-based AI/AN-serving organization. The collaboration has continued, with ongoing grants and research in related areas, with a collective goal of improving health in the urban AI/AN community in Santa Fe.

Lessons Learned

A benefit of this funding opportunity was that it included community-based training in the HIA methodology, and the team was given a coach who would meet with them to move the project forward and meet the scheduled deliverables. For Emily Haozous, who was an academic researcher, this was a difficult adjustment because she was used to making her own timelines and strategies for meeting deliverables. This level of intervention ended up uniting the team, as it provided a uniform strategy for support and accountability, and it respectfully brought in those team members who were not trained in health research.

Guardians of the Living Water[iii]

Description

In 2014, the long-standing Crow Environmental Health Steering Committee of the Apsáalooke Nation invited research partners from Montana State University to work together on water quality research. The resulting project, called

---

    iii Funding from NIGMS P20GM104417 and NSF 2006031.

Guardians of the Living Water (GLW), was a culturally grounded, water-related, environmental health literacy curriculum for youth to increase understanding of the relationship between the environment and human health. It was designed to build on the strengths inherent to the role of children in Crow families.

Intervention

The curriculum was targeted to AI/AN children in afterschool and summer programs. It focused on understanding and addressing local water quality through the integration of science, culture, and collective action. The curriculum was based on an environmental health literacy framework and included progressively more complex lessons that expanded the intervention focus each year.[11] The facilitators began with lessons about water, its importance to human health, and its significance to the Crow Peoples. Next, they focused on children sharing information with their parents. Children also shared information with the broader community through presentations at community meetings. In the 2015–2016 afterschool program, children engaged in a Photovoice project that culminated with several exhibits in local community venues and a survey of the broader community. In 2019, children partnered as coresearchers, developing their research questions and methods for educating their community about the importance of water. Children then created movies that addressed local water issues and held a film screening for the community.

Community Engagement

GLW was a CBPR project. The idea to focus on environmental health came from the community, and university researchers were invited to participate. The intervention grew out of discussions between community and academic partners regarding the central role of children in Crow culture. The program established a CAB composed of seven community members, including elementary school educators, tribal college faculty, local water quality experts, parents, and elders. The CAB met monthly to advise on all aspects of the project. The research team consisted of the local project coordinator, tribal college students, and university faculty and students; they teleconferenced weekly to plan sessions. The project coordinator ran the sessions, with tribal college interns, Montana State University team members, and teachers from the local school. After each session, research team members discussed their reflections at weekly meetings. The research team presented these reflections to the CAB each month, and together they planned future sessions. The CAB also helped identify local community members to present local water-related cultural information to students.

Outcomes

Children completed pre/posttests and qualitative interviews to measure environmental health literacy–related knowledge, skills, and attitudes. Parents completed posttests and interviews. Both children and their parents increased their knowledge of water quality issues, demonstrating a deeper understanding of the cultural significance of local water sources, bacterial contamination in local water sources, and how to protect water sources. Parents also reported that their children were sharing what they were learning with them at home.[12] Responses to the community surveys following the community and Photovoice presentations demonstrated that community members retained information shared by the children about environmental health and local water issues. The curriculum, photographs, and movies developed by the project continue to be used as resources in local schools.

Lessons Learned

It is important to develop health interventions with AI/AN communities, as this increases opportunities to incorporate culture into the intervention and to empower the community to implement the intervention.[13,14,15] As noted in other examples in this chapter, a strengths-based approach can help build trust between community and research partners and result in an intervention that is attractive and successful.[16,17] Indigenous knowledge also should be integrated throughout the research process, acknowledging that Indigenous approaches may contrast with Western ways of knowing.[18,19]

GLW is an example of culturally centered research that builds upon the knowledge inherent within Indigenous communities. For example, GLW addressed water quality, a community-identified issue, and was founded on the cultural importance of water. In the first GLW summer program, a Crow teacher identified the conflict between Western and Indigenous classifications of water as "nonliving" versus "living." The teacher explicitly discussed this conflict with youth participants, and the program continues to emphasize the importance of understanding and respecting both Indigenous and Western knowledge.

Further, appreciation of self-governance in tribal communities is integral to successful research in Indigenous communities. As tribal communities have exerted their sovereignty over research conducted with their people, Western academic culture also has begun to recognize the benefits of community engagement, including the increased likelihood that people understand the purpose and benefits of the research, which, in turn, can increase trust in research, researchers, and research institutions. The development of research guidelines and tribal research codes ensure the community's interests are at the forefront of the research agenda.

Successful research in Indigenous communities also requires a basic understanding of the social and political dimensions impacting health outcomes. For example, addressing environmental health exposures taking place on tribal lands is a complex endeavor due to overlapping and ambiguous federal, state, and tribal jurisdiction.[13] The biggest challenge the GLW project faced was identifying tangible goals that children could reasonably accomplish and that would mitigate their community's multifaceted water issues. An intervention would be remiss to neglect this as part of the context affecting environmental health outcomes in Indigenous communities.

Building relationships and trust between the community and academic research partners requires attention to the expectations and the needs of each partner.[20] Community interventions in Indigenous communities benefit from long-term partnerships, which may require more time for relationship building and less focus on academic products, which can be a challenge for academic researchers.[10] However, a respectful and responsible approach to research that honors community partners can help overcome potentially conflicting priorities.

MALAMA: Mini Ahupua`a for Lifestyle and Mea'ai (food) through Aquaponics[iv]

Description

Prior to colonization, Native Hawaiians (NH) were healthy people with a robust food system. Shaped by island geography, NH divided the land into ahupua'a, wedged areas of land running from the mountain to the sea, following the natural boundaries of the watershed. Each ahupua'a contained the resources for food, including fish, seaweed, salt, taro, vegetables, fruits, and other plants. With Western colonization came the privatization of land, mass plantations, and militarization that disrupted the traditional and sustainable food system, thereby shaping the pervasive health and socioeconomic disparities seen today.

Despite these challenges, NH communities have demonstrated resilience and strength. Starting with the Native Hawaiian Renaissance movement in the 1970s, tremendous efforts have been made to revitalize NH cultural practices, including Hawaiian language, oceanic voyaging, food cultivation, and land and

iv Funding from NIH, NIMHD, the Robert Wood Johnson Foundation, and the Detroit Community-Academic Urban Research Center.

ocean restoration. Many rural NH communities have been instrumental in retaining and promoting cultural practices, including the rural community of Waimānalo on the eastern side of the island of Oʻahu. It is home to 8,000 residents, with one-third being NH, and recognized as a medically underserved community with high levels of food insecurity and socioeconomic challenges. Waimānalo also is known for its natural resources, a history of community advocacy and organizing, and a large number of NH grassroots organizations.

Intervention

The goal of MALAMA, which stands for Mini Ahupuaʻa for Lifestyle and Meaʻai (food) through Aquaponics, was to restore the elements of NH food practices and systems by merging ancestral knowledge with modern technology of aquaponics.[21] Aquaponics combines hydroponics (raising plants in water) and aquaculture (raising fish in tanks) to create a contained, sustainable food production system that mimics the ahupuaʻa system. MALAMA was based on the grassroots community work of God's Country Waimānalo (GCW), which was founded in 2005 by Ilima Ho-Lastimosa, a Waimānalo resident and community leader. GCW aimed to promote and offer community-driven, culturally grounded programs to promote multigenerational learning by engaging keiki (children) to kūpuna (elderly) in cultural practices and food sovereignty.

Drawing on previous workshops implemented by GCW, the MALAMA program included a series of hands-on, family-based workshops that integrate NH cultural practices, such as lāʻau lapaʻau (NH traditional healing through plants and spirituality) and ʻai pono (nourishing foods). Participants learn how to build and maintain an aquaponics system, to grow, cultivate, and harvest their own herbs and plants, and to create nutritious meals and lāʻau (traditional medicine). Participants also learn about aquaponics technology, water quality, fish health, gardening, and pest control. The program culminates in a "Build Weekend," when participants collectively help each other build and install their home aquaponics systems. Aligned with Hawaiian pedagogy, the nine workshops in the curriculum emphasize collective learning.

In 2018, a feasibility MALAMA study was funded by a grant to the University of Hawaiʻi from the National Institute of Minority Health and Health Disparities (NIMHD). Ten families participated in this pilot to examine backyard aquaponics as a public health intervention. Findings demonstrated that MALAMA was feasible and culturally acceptable. This led to a 2-year randomized control trial funded by the Robert Wood Johnson Foundation. A total of 20 NH families from Waimānalo were recruited and randomly assigned to the 6-month intervention or the wait-list control group. Participants completed a health questionnaire to assess changes in their knowledge of aquaponics, eating habits, mental health, cultural identity, and sense of connectedness. Participants also were interviewed at the end of nine workshops to better understand the impacts of MALAMA. Participants received cultural gifts for their participation.

Community Engagement

The MALAMA study was initiated with the support of the Waimānalo Pono Research Hui (WPRH), a community–academic partnership to promote community-driven, culturally grounded research. WPRH was created in 2017 by Ilima Ho-Lastimosa and Jane Chung-Do through seed funding provided by the Detroit Community-Academic Urban Research Center. The mission of WPRH was to work toward a healthy Waimānalo through education, aloha ʻāina (love and stewardship of land), and the honoring and transferring ʻike (knowledge) and values of the kūpuna (elderly) to the keiki (children) through "pono" research principles. In the Hawaiian language, pono translates to righteous, goodness, uprightness, and moral qualities. The group developed protocols to ensure that research and programs proposed to the community fit the priorities of community and aligned with the mission and values of WPRH.[22] Members met monthly to discuss research findings and vet new proposals. The MALAMA research team, which includes both academic and community researchers, has provided regular updates to WPRH to obtain their feedback and continued approval.

Outcomes

Today, Hawaiʻi has one of the highest cost of living, and access to land continues to be a structural barrier for Hawaiians. These backyard aquaponics systems bring NH families together to engage in their ancestral practice of land stewardship and subsistence practices. Qualitative and quantitative data suggest that having aquaponics systems at home increases access to and consumption of healthy foods.

In addition to increased access to food, findings suggest that MALAMA restores the pilina (close relationships) that people have with their food. MALAMA also enhances pilina within families, as backyard aquaponics systems are engaging and accessible for multiple generations. MALAMA also builds pilina within the community, as families are grouped together in a cohort to collectively engage in workshops and build their aquaponics systems. Many also share their excess aquaponics produce with their neighbors and share what they learned from the workshops. In addition to improved eating and relationships, participants report that they are better equipped to care for their health through lā'au lapa'au, the practice of traditional and spiritual medicine once banned by colonizers. Participants noted that reconnecting to traditional practices that were once suppressed was powerful and transformative.[23]

Concurrently with the MALAMA project, the community founded a non-profit named Ke Kula Nui O Waimānalo with a vision to kūkulu kaiāulu (to build community).[24] The mission of this organization is to support the Waimānalo community to become self-sustainable in every way, from the mountain to the sea, with the belief that the 'āina and kai (ocean) can provide for the community as it did years ago. MALAMA is now housed within Ke Kula Nui O Waimānalo and has secured its own funding for community development and research, allowing for true community ownership and power.

Lessons Learned

As CBPR principles posit, it is important to work closely with the community so that projects are thoughtfully integrated with the community's cultural values, lived experiences, and preferences. It also is important to grow community ownership of and capacity to lead research and programs. Because MALAMA was culturally aligned with the NH worldview of health and wellness, it was successful in increasing intake of fresh vegetables, fruits, and fish, enhancing pride in traditional culture, and giving NH more control over their health.

The MALAMA study also started to shift the community's research paradigm away from conventional Western approaches to research, which have been minimally effective with Indigenous communities. Instead of focusing on problems, Waimānalo started with solutions that had already been implemented and embraced by the community, and focused on generating the evidence to prove that these community-based solutions were effective in improving health. This approach ensures community buy-in and cultural relevance, which in turn promotes program sustainability. The resulting framework, evaluation tools, and educational materials developed by the MALAMA program have the potential to assist other communities interested in developing local solutions to expanding access to healthy foods and reclaiming Indigenous food systems.

Children's Healthy Living (CHL) Project for Remote Underserved Minority Populations in the Pacific Region[v]

Description

The prevalence of childhood obesity has increased significantly over the past decades, putting children at risk for lifetime obesity, early onset of disabilities

---

v Funding from the USDA, NIFA 2011-68001-30335

and chronic diseases, and reduced life expectancy.[25,26] Children in the US-affiliated Pacific region (including Hawai'i, Alaska, American Samoa, the Commonwealth of the Northern Mariana Islands [CNMI], the Federated States of Micronesia, Guam, Palau, and the Republic of the Marshall Islands) also are affected by this problem. Findings from a meta-analysis of regional data available in 2015 estimated that children aged 2–8 years have a combined prevalence of overweight and obesity of 21% at age 2, increasing to 39% by age 8.[27]

The Children's Healthy Living (CHL) Program for Remote Underserved Minority Populations of the Pacific Region was funded for 5 years (2011–2016) by the US Department of Agriculture's National Institute for Food and Agriculture (NIFA) to develop and test an intervention to address childhood obesity in the eight US jurisdictions in the Pacific region. CHL worked with individuals based at Land Grant colleges in the region, including the University of Alaska, the University of Hawai'i, the University of Guam, Northern Marinas College, American Samoa Community College, and the College of Micronesia. The aim of this CBPR project was to work in concert with Indigenous communities and the colleges that serve them "to elevate the capacity of the region to build and sustain a healthy food and physical environment to help maintain a healthy weight and prevent obesity among young children."[28]

Intervention

Following a year of community-engaged data collection and discussion, the CHL multilevel intervention was formulated at the June 2012 annual meeting, attended by 50 individuals from across the eight Pacific jurisdictions. The intervention needed to help achieve six behavioral objectives in children, specifically to (1) decrease sugar-sweetened beverage intake, (2) increase water intake, (3) increase fruit and vegetable intake, (4) decrease recreational screen time, (5) increase physical activity, and (6) increase duration of sleep.[29]

Six interventions strategies were supported by the group: (1) introduce, enhance, and support policy for healthy eating and physical activity of young children, (2) engage young children in growing and eating local healthy foods, (3) train and support role models to promote desired behaviors, (4) increase accessibility of environments for safe play and physical activity for young children, (5) increase accessibility of good water for young children, and (6) provide other education and training related to the six CHL behavioral objectives. These strategies addressed the interpersonal (training role models, parents, and teachers), community (increasing assess to healthy foods and environments for safe play), and organizational/policy (strengthening preschool wellness policies) levels of the social-ecological model.[29]

By the end of the June 2012 meeting, these six intervention strategies were collapsed into four cross-cutting functions, signifying the four action areas of the intervention: (1) strengthen and actualize school wellness policies, (2) partner and advocate for environmental change, (3) promote the CHL message, and (4) train trainers (capacity building). Recommended activities under each cross-cutting function were provided. However, the five Land Grant institutions (in Alaska, Hawaiʻi, American Samoa, Guam, and the CNMI) were subcontracted from the grant to carry out the 2-year CHL intervention in ways that fit their community's culture, preferences, strengths, and resources.[29] For example, some communities partnered with schools to improve playgrounds, while others built school gardens, and others organized family walking events.

Community Engagement

The development of the CHL multilevel intervention was led by CHL representatives from Alaska, American Samoa, CNMI, Guam, and Hawaiʻi, who met first with communities in each jurisdiction and then weekly through teleconferencing *across seven time zones* and the international dateline. The first step in developing the CHL intervention was to engage communities to identify and prioritize preferred intervention strategies. To start, the Land Grant colleges in the jurisdictions of Alaska, American Samoa, CNMI, Guam, and Hawaiʻi invited community leaders, childhood obesity experts, childcare providers, government representatives, and others to join a Local Advisory Committee (LAC). The LAC members, in turn, helped identify role models, that is, individuals and representatives of agencies that supported healthy behaviors among children in these communities.[30] LACs hosted two rounds of community meetings to initially identify assets and potential intervention strategies and to receive feedback on and rank intervention ideas.

Across the five jurisdictions, 912 individuals participated in initial and follow-up meetings; 20% of participants were parents, 36% were from educational settings, and the remaining 44% represented health and social services, government, food suppliers, wellness professionals, church members, business leaders, and others. This helped to develop a shared vision of CHL's community involvement and guided work within the participating communities.[30]

After this year-long data-gathering period, the final CHL intervention was formulated at the weeklong June 2012 annual meeting of CHL, which was attended by representatives from all jurisdictions. At this meeting, data were shared, and meeting participants rotated through small workgroups to discuss, extend, and contextualize the proposed intervention strategies as they could influence the behaviors of children. A facilitated discussion with the entire group led to the finalization and adoption of the CHL multilevel intervention strategies.[29]

Representatives from the jurisdictions also were trained and supported in data collection and entry and were included in report and manuscript writing. Additionally, two individuals from each jurisdiction were supported financially to pursue higher education, with some relocating to the University of Hawai'i or the University of Guam and others enrolling in degree-granting distance programs.

Outcomes

The CHL intervention was tested through a cluster randomized controlled design. Before the intervention delivery, data were collected on 4,329 children ages 2 through 8 years in 27 selected communities in Hawai'i, Alaska, the CNMI, American Samoa, and Guam. Researchers and community-based individuals who underwent training collected data on anthropometry (e.g., height, weight, waist circumference) and prevalence and severity of acanthosis nigricans (darkened skin at the back of the neck, associated with diabetes or prediabetes). Children's caregivers provided a 2-day food and activity diary for their child and answered survey questions on the child's sleep, physical activity, and recreational screen time habits and about the household's income and food security level. After the 2-year intervention, the same data elements were collected from 4,042 children ages 2 through 8 years in the same 27 communities.[31]

Nine of the 27 communities received the intervention, and 18 communities served as controls (to receive an optimized intervention at a later date). Mixed models were adjusted for age and sex, community clustering, and jurisdiction strata. Intervention communities showed significant improvements compared to control communities in the following: acanthosis nigricans prevalence (-3.6%), overweight plus obesity prevalence (-4.2%), waist circumference (-1.1 cm), screen time among 6–8-year-olds (-1.1 hours/day), and in Tayside sleep disturbance score among 2–5-year-olds (+1.2) and males (+0.8).[31]

After the 5-year grant, other funds were obtained to support the CHL Center of Excellence at the University of Hawai'i, which continues to provide training, research, and outreach to maintain and extend the CHL network, examine long-term effects of the multilevel CHL intervention, and provide access to best practices in policy, systems, and environmental approaches for prevention of child obesity. Annual meetings continue to bring together representatives from across the US-affiliated Pacific region.

Lessons Learned

An evaluation of the 5-year CHL project suggests several lessons.[9] First, it is important to listen to community in developing interventions, to support community-led initiatives and organizations, and to build on current programs and community strengths. This ensures that activities will fit community needs, preferences, and resources. Second, it is essential for community-wide, multi-level interventions to establish diverse community ties. Members in a broad partnership can share assets, helping smaller organizations garner resources and expertise from outside their immediate community. Third, successful interventions must build community capacity through training, skills building, and empowerment strategies to support community voice and action. Fruitful areas of skills development within CHL ranged from assisting partners with grant writing, educating on policy-changing processes, equipping role models (champions) with leadership training, providing physical activity workshops to teachers, and sponsoring hands-on gardening and cooking workshops that affirmed Indigenous practices and cultural foods. Finally, it is important in any intervention, but especially those that are being built or tailored by the community, to factor in time for delays and required program modifications. In CHL, it took time to modify materials to fit local culture and offer needed training to empower local staff and role models. Interventions that rely on community partners also must expect organizational delays.

Summary

This chapter provided examples of successful CBPR and community-engaged programs with Indigenous communities. All five examples illustrated the operationalization of important CBPR principles. For example, all five programs were guided by an advisory group composed of local community members. Mechanisms were established to facilitate colearning across partners so that university representatives learned from community, and community members and Indigenous students built capacity in research and program delivery. All five programs built their interventions on community culture and strengths. The projects associated with the Apsáalooke (Crow) Nation, MĀLAMA, and with CHL are long term and ongoing, with partners spending considerable time in the community to establish meaningful and trusting relationships. Funds were shared equitably in multiple ways including employing community members on projects, subcontracting to community organizations, and/or by helping community organizations secure their own grant funding. By applying CBPR principles, interventions are more likely to benefit Indigenous communities and improve Indigenous health.

References

1. Freire P. *Pedagogy of the oppressed*. Continuum, 1968; reprinted 2000.

2. Wallerstein N, Giatti LL, Bógus CM, et al. Shared participatory research principles and methodologies: Perspectives from the USA and Brazil-45 years after Paulo Freire's "Pedagogy of the Oppressed." Societies (Basel). 2017;7(2):6.

3. Baum F, MacDougall C, Smith D. Participatory action research. J Epidemiol Community Health. 2006;60(10):854–857.

4. Israel BA, Eng E, Schulz AJ, et al. Methods for community-based participatory research for health, 2nd edition. Jossey-Bass Publishers, 2013.

5. Wallerstein N, Duran B. Community-based participatory research contributions to intervention research: The intersection of science and practice to improve health equity. Am J Public Health. 2010;100 (Suppl 1):S40–S46.

6. LaVeaux, D. & Christopher, S. (2009). Contextualizing CBPR: Key principles of CBPR meet the Indigenous research context. Pimatisiwin: A Journal of Aboriginal and Indigenous Community Health, 7(1), 1–25. PMID: 20150951.

7. Smith AJ, Christopher S, LaFromboise VR, et al. Apsáalooke women's experiences with Pap test screening. Cancer Control. 2008;15(2):166–173.

8. Messengers for Health: Health education and outreach for the Crow People. Accessed May 11, 2021. https://www.messengersforhealth.org/.

9. Held S, Hallett J, Schure M, et al. Improving chronic illness self-management with the Apsáalooke Nation: Development of the Báa nnilah program. Soc Sci Med. 2019;242:112583.

10. Wilson S. Research as ceremony. Columbia University Press, 2008.

11. Simonds VW, Margetts M, Rudd RE. Expanding environmental health literacy—A focus on water quality and tribal lands. J Health Commun. 2019;24(3):236–243.

12. Milakovich J, Simonds VW, Held S, et al. Children as agents of change: Parent perceptions of child-driven environmental health communication in the Crow community. J Health Disparities Res Pract. 2018;11(3):115.

13. Burhansstipanov L, Christopher S, Schumacher Sr A. Lessons learned from community-based participatory research in Indian country. Cancer Control. 2005;12 (4_suppl):70–76.

14. Christopher S. Recommendations for conducting successful research with Native Americans. J Cancer Educ. 2005;20(S1):47–51.

15. Manson SM, Garroutte E, Goins RT, et al. Access, relevance, and control in the research process. J Aging Health. 2004;16(5_suppl):58S-77S.

16. Thomas LR, Donovan DM, Sigo RLW. Identifying community needs and resources in a native community: A research partnership in the Pacific Northwest. Int J Ment Health Addict. 2010;8(2):362–373.

17. Christopher S, Watts V, McCormick AKHG, et al. Building and maintaining trust in a community-based participatory research partnership. Am J Public Health. 2008;98(8):1398–1406.

18. Simonds VW, Christopher S. Adapting Western research methods to Indigenous ways of knowing. Am J Public Health. 2013;103(12):2185–2192.

19. Braun KL, Browne CV, Ka'opua LS, et al. Research on Indigenous elders: From positivistic to decolonizing methodologies. Gerontologist. 2014;54(1):117–126.

20. Nutbeam D. The evolving concept of health literacy. Soc Sci Med. 2008;67(12):2072–2078.

21. Ho-Lastimosa I, Chung-Do JJ, Hwang PW, et al. Integrating Native Hawaiian tradition with the modern technology of aquaponics. Glob Health Promot. 2019;26(3_suppl):87–92.

22. Keaulana S, Chung-Do JJ, Ho-Lastimosa I, *et al.* Waimānalo Pono Research Hui: Establishing protocols and rules of engagement to promote community-driven and culturally grounded research with a Native Hawaiian community. *Br J Soc Work.* 2019;49(4): 1023–1040.

23. Keli'iholokai L, Keaulana S, Antonio MCK, *et al.* Reclaiming 'āina health in Waimānalo. *Int J Environ Res Public Health.* 2020;17(14):5066.

24. Ho-Lastimosa I, Keli'iholokai L, Kassebeer K, *et al.* Kōkua kaiāulu: Keeping the Native Hawaiian community in Waimānalo fed. *J Indig Soc Dev.* 2020;9(3):170–182.

25. Goran MI, Ball GDC, Cruz ML. Obesity and risk of type 2 diabetes and cardiovascular disease in children and adolescents. *J Clin Endocrinol Metab.* 2003;88:1417–1427.

26. Olshansky SJ, Passaro DJ, Hershow RC, *et al.* A potential decline in life expectancy in the United States in the 21st century. *N Engl J Med.* 2005;352(11):1138–1145.

27. Novotny R, Fialkowski MK, Li F, *et al.* Systematic review of prevalence of young child overweight and obesity in the United States-Affiliated Pacific Region compared with the 48 contiguous states: The Children's Healthy Living Program. *Am J Public Health.* 2015;105(1):e22–e35.

28. Children's Healthy Living Program for Remote Underserved Minority Populations in the US-Affiliated Pacific Region. Vision-mission-core values. Accessed April 18, 2021. https://www.chl-pacific.org/about/vision-mission-core-values/.

29. Braun KL, Nigg CR, Fialkowski MK, *et al.* Using the ANGELO model to develop the children's healthy living program multilevel intervention to promote obesity preventing behaviors for young children in the U.S.-affiliated Pacific Region. *Child Obes.* 2014;10(6): 474–481.

30. Fialkowski MK, Yamanaka A, Wilkens LR, *et al.* Recruitment Strategies and Lessons Learned from the Children's Healthy Living Program Prevalence Survey. *AIMS Public Health.* 2016;3(1):140–157.

31. Novotny R, Davis J, Butel J, *et al.* Effect of the Children's Healthy Living Program on young child overweight, obesity, and acanthosis nigricans in the US-affiliated Pacific region: A randomized clinical trial. *JAMA Netw Open.* 2018;1(6):e183896.

5

Building Infrastructure, Increasing Capacity, and Improving Quality in Indigenous Health Systems

Linda Burhansstipanov, Kathryn L. Braun,
Lisa D. Harjo, Kevin Darryl Cassel, Lana Sue I. Ka'opua,
Diana G. Redwood, Kristen Mitchell-Box,
Erin Peterson, Teshia Solomon, and
Noel L. Pingatore

Introduction

Since being recognized by the US government, Indigenous communities have been significantly underfunded, underdeveloped, and/or under-resourced. This dearth of support contributes to insufficient organizational infrastructure and capacity in several areas, creating challenges for Indigenous communities to thrive as equals with other US populations. This chapter describes areas of infrastructure that are critical to operating health programs and provides examples of several community-engaged programs to strengthen infrastructure for health in Indigenous communities.

Defining Infrastructure

In healthcare, infrastructure can refer to physical structures (buildings), equipment, personnel, care procedures and protocols, and services (such as power and electricity, water and sanitation, telecommunication), all of which are needed to provide quality care."[1] In the 2015 action plan to reduce racial and ethnic disparities, the US Department of Health and Human Services called for infrastructure strengthening through increasing the diversity of healthcare professionals and researchers and incorporating cultural and linguistic knowledge in the healthcare workforce.[2] Healthy People 2030 recognized that "a strong public health infrastructure includes a capable and qualified workforce, up-to-date data and information systems, and agencies that can assess and respond to public health needs."[3]

Quality improvement initiatives can help strengthen health infrastructure, as they entail continuous attention to improving healthcare processes and workforce capacity to increase the accessibility, affordability, appropriateness, and effectiveness of healthcare and, thus, patient outcomes. Quality improvement is referenced by several Healthy People 2030 objectives related to infrastructure, for example:

- Explore quality improvement as a way to increase efficiency and effectiveness in health departments.
- Increase the proportion of tribal communities that have developed a health improvement plan.[3]

Since 2013, the Centers for Disease Prevention and Control (CDC) has funded programs for Tribal Public Health Capacity Building and Quality Improvement. In justification of this funding initiative, the CDC recognized that the separation of tribal public health systems from the larger US public health system has limited the effectiveness of tribal public health systems, and that building tribal public health infrastructure will enhance disease prevention, health promotion, and emergency response in Indigenous communities. These funds were earmarked to improve the infrastructure and operational capacity of American Indian (AI) and Alaska Native (AN) public health systems, build data systems, strengthen workforce, and enhance tribal public health programs and services.[4]

The chapter defines infrastructure in terms of structures (e.g., buildings and equipment), workforce, and quality improvement. An overview of each area is provided, followed by examples of how Indigenous communities have improved structures, enhanced worker capacity, and attended to quality. For example, the Intertribal Council of Michigan improved cancer screening participation by extending partnerships and standardizing outreach and referral processes. The Bad River Tribe, which had minimal infrastructure for health, secured funding to hire and train staff, establish a health office, improve data collection, and provide community outreach to increase cancer screening. In an example from Alaska, health providers worked collaboratively with community to change policies and programs to improve colorectal cancer screening. The Native American Cancer Prevention (NACP) program and the INdigenous Samoan Partnership to Initiate Research Excellence (INSPIRE) focused on improving the health research workforce by training members of Indigenous communities in research and supporting research projects in their communities.

Infrastructure, Workforce Capacity, and Quality Improvement

Infrastructure as Structures and Equipment

At a minimum, health programs need dedicated workspace and equipment, like an office, desk, chair, and phone. The workplace needs to provide technology that facilitates the implementation and evaluation of activities, including computers, tablets, cell phones, data analysis software, and communications software (including webinar capacity). Security software is essential, as most public health programs store confidential community or patient data on their devices.

Unfortunately, some Indigenous public health programs do not have safe and secure workplaces. In some programs, staff may share desks, phones, and computers. Some programs provide staff with technological equipment, but the equipment may be outdated, the software may be inefficient, and computers may be blocked from accessing the Internet or email. Indigenous communities and public health programs also may be challenged by poor Internet and cellular access, especially in rural areas and on reservations, making staff dependent on landline phones and Internet dial-up services. Connection services may not exist or be limited to a single provider service that is not compatible with a staff person's phone.

Many Indigenous public health programs are responsible for people living in areas encompassing hundreds of square miles. In the lower 48, Alaska, and the Pacific, this can include reservations, villages, islands, and atolls that are hundreds of miles from diagnostic, treatment, and rehabilitation facilities. For such programs, funding must support reimbursement for ground, air, or water travel, or staff must have access to organization-owned vehicles. Similarly, staff may require overnight lodging to effectively reach and serve their designated work area. Thus, infrastructure includes providing the support and resources that allow the public health staff to conduct their jobs efficiently.

Infrastructure as Workforce Capacity

In large state or provincial public health units, most staff positions are carried out by a single employee. However, Indigenous programs frequently have one individual filling several roles, such as outreach, recruitment, education, and clerical. For small programs, this may be the only feasible approach, and it can be quite effective and efficient. For example, in small health programs, the project manager may answer the phone and coordinate schedules, communications, and event or travel logistics. But as an Indigenous public health program's funding increases and/or the program expands, additional staff support is crucial.

All staff new to a health organization serving Indigenous communities need basic training, including orientation to Indigenous organizational policies, office procedures, and cultural perspectives. Such training also is necessary for an Indigenous staff member who is from another Indigenous community, as beliefs and practices vary greatly across Indigenous groups. Staff also need training on other complementary programs within and outside the organization to avoid duplication and to encourage collaboration. Organizations with many different programs can benefit from regular meetings to introduce changes, collaborate on event, and coordinate client care. For example, several Indigenous programs encourage and support healthy eating and exercise to reduce risk of heart disease, cancer, and diabetes. Opportunities to combine efforts during community events and to reinforce healthy behavior across programs can benefit the entire community. Additionally, educational materials for one program should be reviewed internally to make sure messages do not contradict advice offered by another program. Some organizations find it useful to cross train staff so they can assist another program when needed.

Confidentiality training is particularly important, as it is critical that staff protect community members' private and personal information.[5,6,7] Violations of confidentiality affect the entire program and will reduce community trust in the program. New staff need to have opportunities to shadow comparable staff that demonstrate competencies and necessary skills on the job. Refresher training is important, and the inclusion of new topics is essential, as public health knowledge is constantly expanding.

For Indigenous programs to succeed, support is essential from administrative and other internal leadership. Without micromanaging, administrators need to receive regular reports from the people they supervise and provide summaries of decisions made by the tribal council or board meetings. A highly successful public health program can deteriorate rapidly when administrators are not active supporters.

External supporters include the local Indigenous health council, healers, elders, leaders, and community members. These individuals need to know what is going on so that they can support the organization and make sure the offered programs are attractive, culturally relevant, and meaningful to the community. These individuals also may have ideas for fundraising, outreach, publicity, and evaluation. Engaging community can decrease health disparities and address social determinants of health, while simultaneously acknowledging and respecting local sovereignty.

Some Indigenous communities have their own public health departments and colleges. But they usually benefit from collaborating with local state or city public health departments and local colleges and universities. For example, health departments and universities outside of the tribe or community can provide training on conducting needs assessment, developing policy, and developing quality assurance procedures.[8] Lack of these skills contribute to the disparities Indigenous Peoples continue to experience.[9] These partnerships also may be helpful in leveraging resources for the organization. Similarly, internal Indigenous staff can serve on advisory committees for local health departments and for research and training programs. Partnerships need to provide benefits to both organizations.

Unfortunately, there are many examples in which research collaborators are disrespectful of the local Indigenous ways or "use" the Indigenous community as "subjects" without providing training, resources, or even a summary of research findings. There are other examples of public health agencies that are resistant to respecting local cultural policies, principles, and nuances. Indigenous groups need support to develop capacity and infrastructure for health, but they also need to sustain their cultures.[10]

Among key reasons to encourage partnerships with other organizations is to collaborate during emergency situations and unpredictable threats. Such threats include the September 11th terrorist attack, the COVID-19 pandemic, and natural disasters (hurricanes, tornadoes), but also relate to daily public health issues, including low-quality housing (e.g., housing that lacks plumbing and electricity), poverty, and food insecurity.

Infrastructure as Quality Improvement

According to the American Public Health Association (APHA), quality in public health is "the degree to which policies, programs, services, and research for the population increase desired health outcomes and conditions in which the population can be healthy."[11] These processes have the purpose of improving structures and processes of care, as well as staff performance. Quality improvement (QI) focuses on improving population health by assuring that the right services are provided in the right way to the people who need them. QI also is a continuous and ongoing effort, by which the team sets and meets measurable objectives for efficiency, effectiveness, performance, accountability, outcomes, and other indicators of quality.[12]

Several models exist to guide QI initiatives. The best known is the four-step "Plan-Do-Study-Act" (PDSA) model of quality improvement.[13] In step 1, the team documents the current approach to care to identify places where things get stuck or clients fall through the cracks. Then the team proposes a strategy to improve care. In step 2, the team implements the strategy on a small scale, documents problems and successes, and collects outcome data. In step 3, the data are compared against standard care to see if an improvement was realized, and the problems are examined for ways to improve implementation of successful strategies on a larger scale. In step 4, the strategy is refined and implemented more broadly. This leads the group back to step 1, as they plan strategies to improve another aspect of care. The PDSA cycle should be repeated again and again to continuously improve the quality of care provided by the organization.[14]

Another approach is to implement initiatives to make policies, systems, and environment (PSE) more supportive of healthy behaviors. Policy changes are changes to laws and rules. Systems change usually focuses on changing structures, processes, and rewards in organizations, like schools, worksites, or health settings. Environmental changes can be actions such as adding bike lanes to city streets. The components of PSE are interrelated. For example, a policy change to make a hospital or clinic smoke-free or tobacco-free will result in an environmental change (cleaner air for patients and staff), which may lead to systems changes (more programs to help employees and patients quit tobacco). Like the PDSA model, the process is not linear. A major goal of the PSE approach is to institutionalize sustainable changes that improve the health of broad populations.[15]

Examples of Successful Communities Projects to Improve Health Infrastructure in Indigenous Communities

Intertribal Council of Michigan Q-TIPS Breast Health Project[i]

Description

The Intertribal Council of Michigan (ITCM) is a 501(c)(3) organization that represents 12 federally recognized tribes with 45,000 enrolled members in Michigan. The agency employs approximately 160 employees; 35 of these employees are based in the ITCM central office in Sault Ste. Marie, while member tribes have offices and staff on site.[16] The participating tribes operate ambulatory care clinics under the Indian Health Services (IHS), and patients are referred to local screening facilities at hospitals.

The Q-TIPS (Quality, Tribal Improvement Programs and Services) project was designed to formalize a tribal breast health quality improvement collaborative with at least four tribes participating to (1) increase breast health screening rates among the women in the targeted population ages 40 to 49 by 20%, and (2) decrease time between breast cancer screening, diagnosis, and treatment for women within the target population. State and tribal data sources

---

i Funding from CDC U38 OT000240.

revealed that screening rates were much lower for AI females (68.1%) compared to the general population at 85.3%.[17] The data found that only 37.5% of AI females having mammograms were in the 40–49 age range.

Intervention

The ITCM Breast Health Collaborative used the PDSA model to implement quality improvement projects designed to increase breast health screening services within four tribal communities in Michigan's rural Upper Peninsula. ITCM collaborated with the Michigan Public Health Institute (MPHI), with which they had a long-standing relationship. Each of the four tribes developed a team and appointed a tribal quality improvement leader. Team members organized themselves as a "learning collaborative" through which everyone agreed to keep an open mind and learn together how to improve systems of care related to breast cancer screening.[18] MPHI staff provided in-depth training on quality improvement methodology, including the PDSA model and common tools such as the team charter, aim statements, process mapping, check sheets, fishbone diagrams, affinity diagrams, and storyboards.[19] They also provided training in facilitation, group dynamics, focused conversation methods, and structured brainstorming techniques.

Community Engagement

The community was the four tribal clinics and their consumers, including clinic patients and mammography providers. The focus of the initiative was to improve the experience for the consumer by improving access to care and making services more acceptable and comfortable. In addition to clinic staff, receptionists, and representatives from referral agencies, the local quality improvement teams included community members who provided input and clarification on the processes for scheduling and receiving breast health screening from the consumer's perspective. As a part of each team, community members also provided insight into solutions and interventions to improve the process.

The first step was documenting and examining the current approach via process mapping. During this step, teams noted the actions and number of steps required by clients to obtain breast health screening. While these steps varied for each tribal site, the process typically included several cumbersome steps. For example, a screening appointment would be made, the consumer would arrive, and then the process of checking her insurance or other coverage options would take place, which required more time and paperwork. Results of the exam were delayed due to poor communication between the tribal clinic and screening facility. The team discussed ways to streamline the process so there were fewer steps for the client. The team also recommended ways to improve the timing of test reporting.

As the streamlined process was implemented at each tribal site, team leaders continued to meet and participate in additional training and technical assistance sessions. The learning collaborative model allowed teams to share lessons learned, group facilitation tips, and intervention strategies with each other. Vigorous and proactive discussions took place during each training focusing on the PDSA processes to identify feasible and effective ways to increase women's participation in mammography.

Outcomes

The learning collaborative approach to quality improvement proved to be effective for the four tribal clinics in the Breast Health Collaborative and was utilized consistently for clinic and public health programs administered by the ITCM. Tribal Health Systems staff can often feel isolated and challenged to coordinate services across multiple agencies, such as Tribal Health, IHS, local hospitals, screening facilities, and county health departments. The support from peers in the learning collaborative was beneficial in addressing these challenges.

Evaluation results of the quality improvement training were very positive, with an average rating of 3.45 on a 4.0 Likert scale among participants agreeing with the statement "*I can apply what I've learned to the PDSA cycle my team is working on.*" Ratings for other measures were similar.

Patient outcomes also were positive. For example, in a single PDSA cycle, the streamlined processes put in place resulted in a doubling of completed mammograms and a 10% increase in referrals. Sites also improved their use of Electronic Health Records (EHR) and other documentation. All sites reported the consistent use of quality improvement beyond the initial 5-year funding cycle. This indicated increased capacity, contributing to project sustainability and improved health systems change, which led to better quality and coordination of care.

Lessons Learned

Storyboards were used to communicate completed quality improvement projects to other staff, managers, tribal health boards, and community members. Teams were encouraged to celebrate the completion of each PDSA cycle and disseminate their work as well as their results. By showcasing their storyboards during staff meetings and as posters in the clinic and other common areas, the team received acknowledgment and support for further work to improve coordination and quality of care, as well as patient satisfaction.

Journey Toward Wellness[ii]

Description

The goal of the Journey Toward Wellness (JTW) project was to address excessive numbers of late-stage cancer diagnoses among the Bad River Band of the Lake Superior Tribe of Chippewa Indians by increasing cancer screening. The Bad River Band is a federally recognized tribe located on a 125,000-acre reservation in northern Wisconsin on the south shore of Lake Superior in both Ashland and Iron Counties. The tribe has 7,356 enrolled members; about 1,500 live on the reservation, and another 3,000 live in counties contiguous to the reservation and the areas served by the tribe's Health and Wellness Center. The Bad River Band is one of 11 Chippewa tribes residing and sharing the ceded territories in the states of Michigan, Wisconsin, and Minnesota.

Intervention

The intervention was provided to (1) increase early detection of cancer so people could start treatment while cancer was in the early stage, (2) provide staff education to better assist community members, and (3) improve referral services so that tribal members would come to the Bad River Tribal Health Center (BRTHC) for subsequent services. The staff of the JTW project created a stakeholder group of Bad River Tribe community members to guide the work of the project and to provide oversight to the quality improvement processes. In year 2, the JTW staff and the stakeholder group implemented a community health assessment to learn what members of the Bad River Tribe thought about their health, the BRTHC, and related topics. The results guided activities to meet the JTW goals.

Based on the needs assessment, multiple community cancer education events were developed and implemented. The events included seven women's and men's wellness events, two cancer walks, Bingo to share health awareness, a health fair, and three cancer screening educational sessions. The women's and men's wellness events included educational sessions about cancer, games, food, and health screenings for diabetes, obesity, and bone density. To improve workforce capacity, three training sessions were held on best practices in outreach and recruitment to cancer early detection screening. One session featured a local oncologist who spoke about the new cancer center and answered staff questions. Another speaker explained recommended cancer screenings for AI/AN.

---

ii Funding from CDC U38OT000248.

Community Engagement

The stakeholder group ranged from 15 to 70 community leaders who contributed greatly to engaging the tribal community in the JTW project. They shared feelings, beliefs, and actions of the tribe throughout the processes of planning and guiding activities for JTW, and they shared program information with the broader community.

A community health assessment was implemented with tribal members. The preliminary results were reviewed by JTW staff, the BRTHC, and the stakeholder group members. The results provided data to support the design of strategies to improve cancer early detection screening, staff in-services, community events, and referral services at the BRTHC. Cancer was rated as one of the top 3 concerns by community members, and this helped the BRTHC staff to shift cancer as a higher health priority. In response to the data, JTW offered the initial Women's Wellness and Men's Health tune-up events, which engaged the community in the project and built better relationships between BRTHC staff and community members. The events also increased community members' participation in cancer screenings.

Outcomes

Bad River Tribal members attended 14 cancer education events and were provided 1,089 unduplicated units of service. Attendance at Women's Wellness events increased from 41 in 2015 to 261 in 2017. All community activities included cancer screening and health education. Growing attendance demonstrated that the Bad River community was interested and committed to preventing and controlling cancer.

Many educational opportunities were created for staff-in-service trainings. Training in iCare/EHR, a cloud-based medical records system, was held to ensure staff proficiency in documenting patients' screening results and identifying patients who needed to have screenings performed. By year 3, eight staff members had been trained. During the next 2 years, a total of 16 staff members completed the trainings. The resulting success was using the iCare/EHR to start mailing reminder cards to patients for cancer screenings, resulting in over 7,500 reminder letters sent during the grant period.

Cancer education resulted in positive changes in attitudes and perceptions of cancer and cancer screening. The BRTHC implemented guidelines of screening patients for breast and colorectal cancer at the age of 45 instead of age 50, since data revealed that Northern Plains AI have a much higher risk of breast and colon cancer than non-Natives. Over the course of the project, screening for colon cancer increased from 10 individuals in 2013 to 105 in 2017, screening for cervical cancer increased from 10 individuals in 2013 to 123 in 2017, and screening for breast cancer from 30 individuals in 2013 to 78 in 2017. Screening results were uploaded into iCARE/EHR, providing a reminder for subsequent screenings. Early screening resulted in referrals to partner facilities before cancer had spread, and these facilities shared results with BRTHC to update their records.

Lessons Learned

The JTW project greatly impacted both the tribal community and the BRTHC. It promoted awareness, education, and action by tribal members to take charge of their health. Lessons learned included recognizing the value of the stakeholder group, composed of elders, community members, and JTW staff, which became the driving force behind the project and provided the insight, foresight, and hindsight to make this project successful. They continued to meet after funding ceased to keep guiding the BRTHC. Second, community engagement is essential to the success of public health interventions, as it keeps people participating and active in a project's activities and events. The JTW project also learned that maintaining staff was critical for the project. Staff turnover requires additional training and work to keep the project cohesive and responsive to the community. Finally, the JTW project learned that they can make a difference in the community by educating, screening, and building relationships with the patients they serve.

Partnership for Native American Cancer Prevention Community Grants Program[iii]

Description

The Partnership for Native American Cancer Prevention (NACP) was a joint project of the Arizona Cancer Center and Northern Arizona University, working with three tribal communities in Arizona. Initially funded by the National Cancer Institute in 2002, NACP evolved over time to include a community grants initiative. The community grants program aimed to enhance resources within AI/AN tribes and communities to increase their cancer control capacity. By providing this support, NACP was able to engage more communities at a variety of levels and provide technical assistance to improve their research and programs to address cancer disparities.

A true partnership requires a mutual benefit to all. Conducting research with community partners is a gift, not a privilege. It allows researchers to pursue their profession and bring praise and funding to the institution, while influencing the

iii Funding from the NIH NCI 2U54CA143925 and U54CA143924.

health of a population. But with that gift comes a responsibility. A way to meet that responsibility is through reciprocity. Reciprocity indicates mutual exchange that benefits both partners. This can include hiring and training community members as staff; compensating community for use of facilities, personnel, or property; providing food, supplies, and equipment; and sharing resources and gains (e.g., financial support). In this example, reciprocity occurred through shared resources and capacity building.

Intervention

The NACP Community Grants Program was modeled after the very successful Mayo Clinic Spirit of EAGLES (SOE) community grants program.[20] The NACP Outreach Core allocated $50,000 annually to fund up to five community-initiated projects in amounts between $1,000 and $10,000. Members of a sub-committee of the Outreach Core's Community Action Committee were trained on the SOE process and developed a call for proposals adapted from their materials. NACP staff promoted the opportunity to AI/AN communities in Arizona through multiple media and word-of-mouth outlets.

Capacity building came in the form of grant writing training. A multisite session was led by staff in Tucson, with virtual links with staff at four other locations between 2 and 8 hours away by car. This allowed the program to include more communities by cutting travel costs and time commitments for participants. Providing on-site staff at each location also allowed for the intimate, one-on-one technical assistance that attendees found helpful. The training covered the basics of grant writing and information specific to applying to the NACP Community Grants Program. It also included information on other community grant opportunities from the university and the community, like the Susan G. Komen Foundation. The NACP staff also provided technical assistance to applicants as part of the application process, for example answering questions and reviewing applications upon request.

Community Engagement

The community grants subcommittee and program staff established the timeline, application, and selection process, which evolved over the 4-year grant period to better serve the tribes and community organizations. Three colleagues not affiliated with NACP but familiar in working with AI/AN communities were recruited to serve on the review committee. NACP staff awarded the projects based on scores. Staff provided additional technical assistance to the communities to address weaknesses within their applications as noted by the review committee, and the NACP evaluator provided technical assistance to strengthen community evaluation skills.

Outcomes

From 2000 to 2005, the program received 39 applications and funded 18 projects that reached more than 2,500 participants. Two communities used findings gained through their community grant to apply for and receive significant funding from the CDC to enhance their cancer prevention and control initiatives. Another community was able to publish and disseminate a report on the status of cancer in their community. In another, 85% of eligible women were screened for both breast and cervical cancer. Two projects were adopted by one or more tribes and incorporated into their health department's annual budget. One was adopted and adapted for a Mexican American population in the state.

The long-term impact of these projects included using report data to begin discussions on the development of a cancer center on tribal lands and collaboration between the Arizona Cancer Center to use mobile units to improve cancer screening rates on reservations. One project was reported in the Surgeon General's report on alcohol and drugs as a model program. Another positive impact was that several of the community projects led to applications for research projects develop jointly by university and tribal partners.

Lessons Learned

The NACP Community Grants project is an example of how Indigenous knowledge can inform health research and disease prevention and control programs. It also exemplifies the important concepts of relationships, respect, responsibility, reciprocity, and relevance that are critical to successful engagement in Indigenous communities. True partnerships are built on relationships that incorporate shared resources and respect the community's knowledge about how to best address their community needs. Reciprocity includes sharing resources, as well as technical assistance and training to build community workforce capacity. The knowledge and skills associated with grant writing assist both the community and individual participants. The community organizations can develop projects and programs independent of the university, while also creating a new and marketable skillset for individual participants.

Good Health and Wellness in Indian Country, Alaska[iv]

Description

In 2014, the Alaska Native Tribal Health Consortium (ANTHC) received a 5-year CDC Good Health and Wellness in Indian Country grant to encourage healthy behaviors in AN communities through community-chosen and culturally

---

iv Funding from CDC DP005422.

adapted PSE approaches. The Good Health and Wellness in Indian Country (GHWIC) program goals were to increase access to traditional and healthy foods, increase physical activity, reduce tobacco use, improve health literacy, promote breastfeeding, and enhance community clinical linkages to reduce heart disease, diabetes, and stroke among AI/AN people. ANTHC worked with five regional Tribal Health Organizations (THO) that provided services ranging from primary and emergency care services, to behavioral and dental healthcare and health promotion and disease prevention programs. These five regional THO were responsible for providing healthcare services to 46,140 AN people (28% of the Alaska Native population) living across Alaska in over 90 communities, ranging in population size from 50 to 30,000.

Intervention

THO developed PSE change strategies and activities to make organizational improvements and increase the sustainability of program efforts after grant funding ended. Supported by ANTHC, THO staff used a systematic process to assess community needs, develop appropriate PSE changes, engage stakeholders, counter resistance, navigate the policy landscape, and work with nontraditional partners.

Community Engagement

THO staff spent the first year of the project assessing community needs using the National Association of County & City Health Officials' MAPP (Mobilizing for Action through Planning and Partnerships) strategic planning process. The MAPP process is a comprehensive approach to prioritize community public health needs, identify community assets and resources, and develop a vision statement to guide the subsequent planning process. THO staff had broad community involvement in the MAPP process and used a variety of data sources including statewide and regional data from prior assessments, community surveys, and key informant interviews and focus groups with community members and tribal leaders. This comprehensive approach resulted in a rich assessment that identified areas of need in each of the communities. THO staff selected strategies and developed activities to make progress in their identified priorities related to GHWIC program goals.

Outcomes

As of August 2018, and as a result of program efforts, a total of 30 new PSE changes were made. These included tobacco-free healthcare organization policies ($n = 3$); tobacco-free tribal resolutions ($n = 2$); tobacco-free school district policy ($n = 1$); healthy food policy and environmental changes ($n = 3$);

changes in patient–provider communication (n = 4); pre-diabetes, obesity, and/or tobacco screening and referral policies (n = 13); healthcare facility signage (n = 3); and a Baby-Friendly Hospital Initiative (BFHI) designation application to support breastfeeding (n = 1). These policies now protect the health of more than 40,000 tribal members and THO employees.

For example, a THO located in southwest Alaska completed a community health assessment indicating that residents were concerned about the high amount of tobacco use. Many people reported wanting to quit and expressed that the price of tobacco should be increased. The THO chose two strategies to improve the health of the people in the region: (1) advocating for a tobacco screening and referral policy at the THO, and (2) increasing referral options for tobacco cessation services by training at least one healthcare provider from each community as a tobacco treatment specialist. In 2016, the THO leadership passed a policy requiring all patients aged 12 and older to be screened for tobacco use, that it be documented in the EHR, and that tobacco users be provided options for evidence-based cessation treatments. A total of six staff were trained as tobacco treatment specialists. Additionally, the THO passed a tobacco-free worksite policy in 2016, which created a 100% tobacco-free environment that applied to all employees, clients, volunteers, visitors, vendors, tribal organization properties, and tribally owned or leased vehicles.

Another THO located in southeast Alaska completed a community health assessment that indicated residents were concerned about the high occurrence of diabetes. The THO chose two strategies to address this community concern: (1) expand access and availability to the Diabetes Prevention Program (DPP) and Diabetes Self-Management Education Program (DSME), and (2) implement diabetes screening and referral policies. While both DPP and DSME classes were available at the THO previously, participation in the program was modest, attrition rates were high, and many eligible patients were not appropriately referred by their healthcare providers. In May 2016, a diabetes screening and referral policy was passed by the THO's Health Board. This new policy led to changes to the EHR to create a reminder for providers to contact any patient who had declined the initial referral.

A THO located in northwestern Alaska found through their community health assessment that residents in their region were concerned about the increased prevalence of obesity. The THO chose to work on improving health literacy to help people access healthcare and the information and resources needed to maintain a healthy weight. A helpful strategy to improve patient–provider communication was to provide teach-back training to all clinicians. The teach-back method is an evidence-based strategy for healthcare clinicians to ensure the information and instructions they provide are understood by the patient. After clinicians in the region were trained in the method, they incorporated it into their discharge planning policy and procedures to make sure that patients and/or their caregivers can repeat back instructions to the provider related to recommended medications, activities, treatment, equipment, follow-up appointments, and so forth.[21]

Obesity was a concern of another THO in southeast Alaska. This THO chose to implement multiple worksite environmental change strategies to support THO employees and patients to maintain a healthy weight, including improving access to healthy foods, increasing opportunities for physical activity, and pursuing the Baby Friendly Hospital Initiative designation to support breastfeeding. Under this initiative, the hospital cafeteria developed "Mindful Meal" selections that followed recommended dietary guidelines and included nutrition information that is easy to see and understand. The hospital also developed a punch card incentive system for healthy purchases, removed soda machines in one building, reduced the number of sugar-sweetened beverages offered in the cafeteria, and supplemented other campus vending machines with small salads, fruit, jerky, and low-fat yogurts. Related to physical activity, THO staff initiated a stair climbing campaign, modeled after the CDC Stair-WELL project, and placed motivational point-of-decision signs outside the elevator and stairway doors to encourage stair use. In 2016, the THO fitness center was remodeled and expanded from 800 to 4,000 square feet, the usage policy was changed to allow access to employee family members, and a fitness consultant was available to help staff and family members set and meet fitness goals.

A THO in Interior Alaska found its community members similarly concerned about obesity. To address this issue, the staff at the THO decided to advocate for a healthy food policy at their organization. They also worked to increase access to and use of traditional and healthy foods as part of the policy. To build support for the initiative, THO staff convened a Healthy Food Policy Committee comprised of representatives from a variety of departments within the organization, and the committee distributed an opinion survey to employees and community members about the potential healthy food policy. Results indicated overwhelming support for a policy that would expand healthy options in the healthcare facility cafés, vending machines, and at THO meetings. In 2016, the THO leadership passed a healthy food policy.

Lessons Learned

PSE change within tribal communities requires a multidisciplinary team, a commitment to the process, and understanding that change takes time. Using a systematic process, including assessing community needs and developing policies with the support of community and organization stakeholders, can augment traditional public health promotion efforts and lead to more sustainable improvements in the future. These examples illustrate some of the PSE changes that were implemented to increase health and wellness in AN communities.

INdigenous Samoan Partnership to Initiate Research Excellence[v]

Description

In the Territory of American Samoa, cancer is the second leading cause of death. Colorectal cancer is the most common malignancy affecting both men and women, but only 7% of adults were up to date with colorectal cancer screening in 2013.[22] American Samoa also was challenged by lack of infrastructure to conduct research on ways to improve cancer prevention and screening behaviors. American Samoan leaders in government, health, and education indicated that many studies conducted in the territory were not reviewed by the local Institutional Review Board (IRB), which resulted in ethical concerns. In many cases, the outcomes and knowledge gleaned from these externally led studies were not shared with or used to benefit American Samoa.

To improve cancer prevention and control in American Samoa, the American Samoan Community Cancer Coalition, a diverse group of community advocates with a common goal of fighting cancer, sought assistance from long-standing research partners at the University of Hawai'i (UH). From this community-initiated partnership, the INdigenous Samoan Program to Initiate Research Excellence (INSPIRE) was proposed and funded through a 5-year grant from the National Institute on Minority Health and Health Disparities. As a community-driven project, funding was provided directly to the American Samoan Community Cancer Coalition's community-based investigators, with technical support provided by academic researchers at UH and Azusa Pacific University in California. The goal of INSPIRE was to establish a culturally grounded and durable foundation for public health research in American Samoa, with research aimed at reducing colorectal cancer-related health disparities found in the territory.[23]

Intervention

INSPIRE activities included (1) creating a community-based research facility in American Samoa, (2) providing technical assistance to the American Samoa institutional review board (IRB), charged with overseeing all research studies conducted in American Samoa, and (3) recruiting and training a cohort of

---

v Funding from NIH NIMHD U24 MD011202-01 4.

Indigenous Samoan researchers to establish a sustainable cancer control research agenda for American Samoa.

INSPIRE's office space was selected to facilitate easy access by INSPIRE research trainees, as well as by the community at large. The INSPIRE hub was outfitted with computer terminals, high-speed Internet access, software for quantitative and qualitative data collection and analyses, audiovisual capability, connection to a learning platform for blended and distance education, and other resources essential to conducting research and training. Additionally, the US coinvestigators facilitated a process whereby American Samoan investigators became associate members of the UH Cancer Center, which provided them access to online library services and external expert consultation.

To build the capacity of the existing IRB in American Samoa, technical assistance was provided to IRB members, interested healthcare providers, educators from the American Samoa Community College, and representatives of the LBJ Tropical Medical Center and the American Samoan Government (ASG). Specific training topics included an overview of research ethics, IRB procedures, human subjects' protection policies, recruiting and training of members, procedures for a rigorous review of research, and access to continuing education and consultation from other IRB.

The INSPIRE team recruited a cadre of American Samoa–based research trainees interested in advancing their research knowledge relevant to cancer health disparities. Because INSPIRE's training faculty was located in Hawai'i and California, training was primarily provided through distance technologies. Research trainees were able to interact in joint seminars and communicated via web-based conferencing and email.

Community Engagement

Guided by community-based participatory research (CBPR) principles, the INSPIRE partnership adopted a research paradigm based on fa'aSamoa (the Samoan Way), which intentionally sought to weave Western research methods with Samoan ways of knowing. Talanoga (discussion) with community partners, research trainees, and academic partners provided direction. This focus served to build on strengths and resources within the community, to facilitate collaborative partnerships, and to integrate knowledge and action that mutually benefitted all INSPIRE partners.[24]

To promote INSPIRE and its research strengthening activities, the American Samoan partners coordinated an open house reception in the first year of the project. This reception was formally opened with a traditional Samoan 'ava ceremony. 'Ava is a beverage made throughout Polynesia, and the 'ava ceremony was conducted by traditional, religious, and community leaders, orators, le taupo (chief's daughter responsible for preparation of the beverage), and 'aumaga (untitled, young men who assist le taupo and serve the beverage to honorees).[25] Subsequently, INSPIRE investigators invited community members and dignitaries to participate in informational and research training sessions.

INSPIRE faculty trainers and research trainees understood and valued the importance of open communication and mutual respect. Through open dialogue, the staff learned that the INSPIRE trainees consistently preferred learning as a group. Thus, trainings and research projects were designed to be group-based and support fa'aSamoa by working purposefully to ensure local ownership, promote effective leadership, and embed strong mentorship structures.

Outcomes

Through the project's written evaluation and group discussion, INSPIRE staff learned that INSPIRE research trainees valued collaborative learning activities and increased their commitment to health disparities research. Trainee comments included: "Discussion allowed me to compare Western culture with Samoan culture, individualism versus collectivism. I was able to understand how Samoan culture may not align with Western methods," and "Being part of INSPIRE helped me to more effectively apply Samoan traditions and values to health issues."

Several group research projects were undertaken. For example, the trainee group decided to work together to update existing population-based cancer control data resources. In another group research project, INSPIRE investigators and coinvestigators led a population-based study of 750 American Samoan adults aged 50 years and older, asking about colon cancer risk and assessing health literacy. For the latter, members of the community assisted in the adaptation of the Short Form Test of Functional Health Literacy Adults (STOFHLA) for residents of American Samoa.[26]

Lessons Learned

Consistent with tenets of CBPR, the INSPIRE partners committed to discussion and consensus agreement, with partners from American Samoa making the final decision. Treading the sensitive balance of addressing cancer disparities in American Samoa involved cultural humility, interpreted as the willingness to learn deeply and to authentically respect perceptions of "survivance" and sovereignty that differ from Western perspectives.[27] In testimony to the United Nations (2017) Tapau [Chief] Dr. Daniel Aga made the critical distinction between democratic deficiencies in relations with the US government and cultural sovereignty within the American Samoa community.[28] This sovereignty ensured the perpetuation of le gagana Samoa (the Samoan language), le fa'a matai (traditional village governance), and collectivist land tenure rights tied to kinship and village systems. US-based INSPIRE partners learned that addressing cancer disparities and the social determinants of health in American Samoa necessitated respect for diverse perceptions of cultural sovereignty and continuous examination of personal biases.

The collaboration resulted in a more comprehensive examination of the upstream or macro-level social determinants of health in American Samoa. While rich in history, cultural tradition, and social capital, American Samoa remains socioeconomically impoverished as characterized by its fragile economy, negative trade balance, relatively high levels of household poverty, and limited healthcare resources and personnel.[29,30,31] Although upstream social determinants of health are beyond the scope of INSPIRE's mission, project staff were guided by the American Public Health Association's emphasis on "health in all policies." This strategy was relevant to understanding and addressing the multiple and intersecting factors that influenced population health and health equity. Specifically recommended was multisectoral participation that involved collaboration between governmental and nonprofit entities.[32] Here the staff was reminded of the 'alagaupu (Samoan wisdom), "Ua gatasi le futia ma le umele", meaning "While the fisherman swings the rod, the others must assist him by paddling hard." In promoting health for all, diverse roles and strengths needed to be valued.

The project included partners based in American Samoa, Hawai'i, and California, and all research trainees held full-time jobs, and many had extensive family and church commitments. Web-based communications were an essential means for convening weekly team meetings across multiple time zones. Discussions were audiotaped and available to those unable to attend a meeting. The team learned that commitment to regular communications was key to advancing project aims and maintaining positive relations.

Finally, INSPIRE found great value in the strategy of weaving methodologies from fa'aSamoa and Western pedagogy. In this way, the INSPIRE team confirmed and worked to extend work of Samoan social scientists in Samoa, Aotearoa/New Zealand, and other parts of the Pacific Basin in using the metaphor of "weaving" to describe the integration of Indigenous and Western research methods to improve Indigenous self-determination, workforce capacity, and health.[33,34,35]

Summary

This chapter started with a definition of infrastructure as structures, workforce capacity, and quality improvement. Indigenous public health programs need all three to evolve and improve health equity. Five successful programs were highlighted from diverse Indigenous communities. American Samoa is a small rural community in the United States Pacific Territories with limited infrastructure. Bad River is a small rural tribe based on the Great Lakes, also with limited infrastructure. ITCM is a well-established, large tribal consortia. ANTHC coordinates and facilitates public health programs throughout Alaska, focusing on AN villages and communities. NACP primarily works in the southwest region of the U.S. Each program worked respectfully with Indigenous communities and dedicated long-term efforts to build structures, enhance workforce capacity, and improve the quality of care in communities.

References

1. Luxon L. Infrastructure—the key to healthcare improvement. *Future Hosp J.* 2015 Feb;2(1):4–7.

2. Department of Health and Human Services. HHS action plan to reduce racial and ethnic health disparities. Accessed March 16, 2021. https://minorityhealth.hhs.gov/npa/files/Plans/HHS/HHS_Plan_complete.pdf.

3. Healthy People 2030. Public health infrastructure. Accessed April 20, 2021. https://health.gov/healthypeople/objectives-and-data/browse-objectives/public-health-infrastructure.

4. Centers for Disease Prevention and Control. Tribal public health capacity building and quality improvement. Accessed April 20, 2021. https://www.cdc.gov/tribal/cooperative-agreements/tribal-capacity-building-OT18-1803.html.

5. Harjo LD, Burhansstipanov L, Lindstrom D. Rationale for "cultural" native patient navigators in Indian country. *J Cancer Educ.* 2014;29(3):414–419.

6. Petereit DG, Burhansstipanov L. Establishing trusting partnerships for successful recruitment of American Indians to clinical trials. *Cancer Control.* 2008;15(3):260–268.

7. Braun KL, Kagawa-Singer M, Holden AEC, *et al.* Cancer patient navigator tasks across the cancer care continuum. *J Health Care Poor Underserved.* 2012;23:398–413.

8. Centers for Disease Control and Prevention. Overview of CDC-RFA OT13-1302: Building capacity of the public health system to improve population health through national, nonprofit organizations. Accessed May 23, 2021. https://www.cdc.gov/publichealthgateway/docs/foa/ot13-1302_initiative overview_?pg.pdf.

9. Abbasi J. Why are American Indians dying young? *JAMA.* 2018;319(2):109–111

10. Institute of Medicine. *The future of the public's health in the 21st century.* National Academies Press, 2002.

11. American Public Health Association. Quality improvement in public health: It works! Accessed April 25, 2021. https://www.apha.org/~/media/files/pdf/factsheets/qi_in_ph_it_works.ashx.

12. Baker Jr EL, Potter MA, Jones DL, *et al.* The public health infrastructure and our nation's health. *Annu Rev Public Health.* 2005;26(1):303–318.

13. Public Health Foundation. Quality improvement accreditation preparation and support. Accessed April 25, 2021. http://www.phf.org/focusareas/Pages/Quality_Improvement_Accreditation_Preparation_and_Support.aspx.

14. Public Health Foundation. Public health quality improvement encyclopedia. Accessed April 25, 2021. http://www.phf.org/resourcestools/Pages/Public_Health_Quality_Improvement_Encyclopedia.aspx.

15. Rural Health Information Hub. Policy, systems, and environmental change. Accessed May 22, 2021. https://www.ruralhealthinfo.org/toolkits/health-promotion/2/ strategies/policy-systems-environmental.

16. Inter-Tribal Council of Michigan, Inc. Agency description. Accessed April 25, 2021. https://www.itcmi.org/about-us/agency-description/.

17. Michigan Department of Community Health and Michigan Public Health Institute. *Special cancer behavioral risk factor survey, 2008*. Accessed April 25, 2021. www.michigancancer.org/PDFs/MCCReports/SCBRFS_2008-042910.pdf.

18. Ayers LR, Beyea SC, Godfrey MM, *et al*. Quality improvement learning collaboratives. *Qual Manag Health Care*. 2005;14(4):234–247.

19. Swanwick T, Vaux E, eds. *ABC of quality improvement in healthcare*. Wiley Blackwell, 2020

20. Kaur JS, Dignan M, Burhansstipanov L, *et al*. The "Spirit of Eagles" legacy. *Cancer*. 2006;107(8 Suppl):1987–1994.

21. Yen PH, Leasure AR. Use and effectiveness of the teach-back method in patient education and health outcomes. *Fed Pract*. 2019;36(6):284–289.

22. American Samoa Community Cancer Coalition. *American Samoa comprehensive cancer control plan*, Accessed May 22, 2021. https://ftp.cdc.gov/pub/publications/CANCER/ ccc/american_samoa_ccc_plan_2012_2017.pdf

23. Tofaeono V, Ka'opua LSI, Sy A, *et al*. Research capacity strengthening in American Samoa. *Br J Soc Work*. 2020;50(2):525–547.

24. Minkler M, Wallerstein N, Oetzel J, eds. *Community based participatory research for health, 3rd ed*. Jossey-Bass, 2017.

25. Grattan F. *An introduction to Samoan custom*. R. McMillan, 1948.

26. Baker DW, Williams MV, Parker RM, *et al*. Development of a brief test to measure functional health literacy. *Patient Educ Couns*. 1999;38(1):33–42.

27. Vizenor G. *Survivance: Narratives of native presence*. University of Nebraska Press, 2008.

28. United Nations. *Report of the special committee on the situation with regard to the implementation of the declaration on the granting of independence to colonial countries and people for 2017*. United Nations, 2017.

29. US Department of the Interior. Census issues in the territories. Accessed May 22, 2021. https://www.doi.gov/ocl/hearings/110/CensusIssuesInTerritories_052108.

30. US Department of the Interior. American Samoa. Accessed May 22, 2021 https:// www.doi.gov/oia/islands/american-samoa.

31. US Department of the Interior. Economic structure of American Samoa, Commonwealth of Northern Mariana Islands, Guam, and the US Virgin Islands. Accessed May 22, 2021. https://www.doi.gov/sites/doi.gov/files/uploads/Economic_Structure_of_Territories.pdf.

32. Rudolph L, Caplan J, Ben-Moshe K, *et al*. *Health in all policies: A guide for state and local governments*. Public Health Institute and American Public Health Association, 2013.

33. Mulitalo-Lauta, P. *Faasamoa and social work within the New Zealand context*. Dunmore Press, 2000.

34. Seiuli BMS. Uputaua: A therapeutic approach to researching Samoan communities. *Aust Community Psychol*. 2012;24(1):24–37.

35. Tamasese K, Peteru C, Waldegrave C, *et al*. Ole taeao afua, the new morning: A qualitative investigation into Samoan perspectives on mental health and culturally appropriate services. *Aust N Z J Psychiatry*. 2005;39(4):300–309.

6

Addressing Sexual Health in Indigenous Communities

May Rose I. Dela Cruz, Kathryn L. Braun, Naomi R. Lee, Judith Clark, Cornelia "Connie" Jessen, Ross Shegog, Florence (Tinka) Duran, and Leah Frerichs[i]

Introduction

This chapter presents information on sexual health, beginning with a discussion of risk factors for teen pregnancy and sexually transmitted infections (STI), followed by prevalence data on teen pregnancy, chlamydia, gonorrhea, human immunodeficiency virus (HIV), syphilis, and human papillomavirus (HPV) in American Indian (AI), Alaska Native (AN), Native Hawaiian (NH), and Pacific Islander (PI) populations. The chapter then highlights four community-driven and culturally appropriate interventions aimed at reducing teen pregnancy and STI prevalence among these groups.

Risk Factors for Teen Pregnancy and STI

Risk factors for teen pregnancy and STI are overlapping. For example, early age of sexual activity, high number of sexual partners, multiple sexual partners, sexual abuse or rape, use of alcohol and drugs, and poverty are risk factors for both teen pregnancy and STI.[1,2,3] Additional risk factors for teen pregnancy include being from a single-parent home, living in foster care, having a mother who gave birth before the age of 20, living in a home with frequent family conflict, and low self-esteem.[1,2]

Limited access to private and public health insurance, primary prevention services (e.g., school-based sexual health education), and secondary prevention services (e.g., HPV vaccination and abortion) are also risk factors. Additional barriers include distance to healthcare facilities, long duration of some treatments for sexual health issues, and medical mistrust.[4,5,6] Stigmatization of sexual health education, birth control, abortion, and STI treatment may also

i Chapter preparation was supported by the NIH through the partnership for Native American Cancer Prevention (NACP) NCI - grant 2U54CA143925-11, and the Southwest Health Equity Research Collaborative, NIMHD grant 1U54MD012388-01.

present barriers, especially in small communities. Often, pregnancy and STI were portrayed as "women's health issues," making them taboo subjects and a low priority for funding in many communities.

Addressing risk factors for teen pregnancy and STI are important ways to improve sexual health in Indigenous populations. Understanding teen pregnancy and STI prevalence is a crucial first step to decreasing disease burden and designing prevention and intervention strategies. Thus, surveillance systems need to provide data for AI/AN and NH/PI groups. For programming, culturally tailored interventions are needed, keeping in mind that the cultural diversity among over 574 AI/AN tribes and over 30 different NH/PI groups does not allow for a "one size fits all" approach.

Teen Pregnancy and STI Prevalence in Indigenous Populations

Teen Pregnancy

In the United States, the teen pregnancy rate in 2013 was approximately 26.5 births per 1,000 women aged 15–19 years. In 2017, it was estimated at 18.8 per 1,000 teen women, a significant reduction.[2] However, according to 2017 data from the Centers for Disease Control and Prevention (CDC), the teen birth rate for AI/AN teens was 32.9 births per 1,000 women aged 15–19 years, and the teen birth rate for NH/PI was about 25.5 births per 1,000 women aged 15–19 years.[2]

Adolescent pregnancies can negatively affect teen parents and the growing baby. Teens girls with babies are less likely to finish high school and more likely to rely on public assistance compared to teens who delay childbearing. They also are more likely to be poor as adults, and their children are more likely to have poorer educational, behavioral, and health outcomes.[7] Teen pregnancy is highly preventable through abstinence and the use of birth control. Good education programs in late elementary school and during middle and high school can provide teens with information to help them make safe-sex choices.[2]

STI

Approximately 20 million new cases of STI are reported to the CDC every year in the US.[8] However, the burden of STI is much greater than 20 million, because only four STI—chlamydia, gonorrhea, HIV, and syphilis—are reported to the CDC, while more common viral infections, including human papillomavirus (HPV) and genital herpes, are not reported. Those four reportable STI accounted for approximately 95% of STI cases in the US in 2020, and sexually active young adults (ages 15 to 24 years) are at the highest risk, accounting for 50% of new STI cases.[8] STI are highly preventable through abstinence and the use of condoms. Most STI are treatable if caught early.[9] Of those mentioned, HIV and HPV are not currently curable, but they can be controlled by vaccination (HPV) and treatment.[10] STI usually cause discomfort, and untreated STI can lead to infertility or even death.

Chlamydia

Chlamydia is the most common *reportable* STI in the US, with approximately 1.4 million cases reported annually to the CDC.[11] In 2017, the prevalence of chlamydia in AI/AN populations was estimated at 781.2 cases per 100,000 population. This rate was 3.7 times greater than for Whites. Analysis of Indian Health Service (IHS) data suggested that, out of 12 IHS regions nationally, 10 had higher case rates for chlamydia compared to rates for all races/ethnicities.[12] For example, in 2017, the chlamydia infection rate for the Great Plains IHS region was about five times the national average rate for all races/ethnicities. In 2017, the rate of reported chlamydia cases among NH/PI was 715.4 cases per 100,000 population,[11] which was 3.4 times the rate of Whites and 5.5 times the rate of Asian Americans. Untreated infections in women can result in pelvic inflammatory disease (PID), which is a major cause of infertility, as well as ectopic pregnancy and chronic pelvic pain. Infants also can contract chlamydia from their mothers during delivery, potentially resulting in neonatal ophthalmia and pneumonia. In addition, chlamydial infections increase the risk of transmission of other STI.

Gonorrhea

In 2014, approximately 350,000 cases of gonorrhea were reported to the CDC. Throughout the 5-year period 2010–2014, AI/AN had the second-highest rate, which was 4.2 times higher than for Whites.[12] In the same period, the rate increased by 100% among AI/AN, highest among all racial/ethnic subpopulations. In a study of surveillance statistics from the IHS, 3 out of 12 IHS regions had higher case rates for gonorrhea compared to rates for all races/ethnicities.[12] For example, the Alaska IHS region had nearly a 5-fold higher annual incidence of gonorrhea than the average for all AI/AN communities, while the prevalence in the Albuquerque region was approximately 1.5-fold higher than the average for all AI/AN communities. In 2014, the gonorrhea rate among NH/PI was 102.1 cases per 100,000 population, which was 2.7 times the rate among Whites.[13] Gonorrhea infections can lead to many symptoms, including PID, septic abortions, and preterm delivery. Like chlamydia, gonorrhea can increase the transmission of other STI.[14]

HIV

HIV infections and acquired immune deficiency syndrome (AIDS) affected an estimated 1.2 million people in the United States in 2018.[15] According to the CDC, the 2016 prevalence of HIV among AI/AN (62.3 per 100,000) and NH/PI (9.9 per 100,000) was much lower than for the general US population (306.6 per 100,000).[16] The prevalence of AIDS among AI/AN (62.3 per 100,000) and NH/PI (73.7 per 100,000) also was lower than for the general population (162.5 per 100,000).[15]

Transmission of HIV occurs through three main routes. HIV is most frequently transmitted through sexual intercourse and contaminated blood products. However, in rural and impoverished communities, mother-to-child transmission is more often a route of transmission compared to communities of higher socioeconomic status. Therefore, prevention and treatment methods for at-risk populations should be implemented by elucidating prevalence and risk factors. Many tribal and urban organizations have breastfeeding promotional programs. However, for mothers infected with HIV, alternatives to breastfeeding are needed.

Syphilis

In 2017, the CDC enumerated 30,644 cases of syphilis in the US, representing a rate of 9.5 cases per 100,000 population. In 2017, the rate of reported syphilis cases among AI/AN (11.1 cases per 100,000 population) was 2.1 times the rate among Whites.[17] Out of 12 IHS Regions, 4 had higher case rates of syphilis compared to rates for all races/ethnicities.[12] In 2014, the rate of syphilis among NH/PI was 6.5 cases per 100,000 population, 1.9 times the rate for Whites.[13] The rate for NH/PI was much higher in 2017, 13.9 cases per 100,000 population, which was about 2.6 times the rate among Whites. This disparity was similar for NH/PI women (2.5 times the rate among White women) and NH/PI men (2.6 times the rate among White men).[13] Left untreated, syphilis can result in damage to the brain, nerves, eyes, or heart. It also increases one's risk of transmitting and acquiring HIV. In women, syphilis can infect the fetus and/or result in the death of the infant, even if the syphilis was acquired up to 4 years before delivery.[16]

Human Papillomavirus (HPV)

HPV is the most common STI, although it is not a reportable STI. There are more than 150 known HPV types, with 14 identified as cancer-causing types.[18] It is estimated that 50–80% of sexually active individuals will contract at least one HPV genotype in their adulthood. Among AI/AN, findings from tribe-specific HPV prevalence suggested that AI/AN women had a high prevalence of HPV.[19,20,21,22] For example, in a 2019 study among women of the Great Plains IHS, nearly 35% of AI women were positive for at least one type of HPV.[23]

Although many individuals may contract HPV, 80–90% of infected individuals will recover from HPV infections.[24] However, the remaining 10–20% will not clear the virus effectively, perhaps due to an ineffective immune response. In these cases, the disease becomes "DNA positive," resulting in a persistent infection. These persistent infections can result in genital warts (caused by low-risk HPV) or various cancers (from high-risk HPV).

High-risk HPV infections are implicated in almost all cases of cervical cancer. However, high-risk HPV also is associated with other cancers, including vulvar/vaginal, anal, penial, and oropharyngeal. Approximately 12,900 new cases of cervical cancer were diagnosed in the US in 2015.[25] While the cervical cancer mortality rate has declined, approximately 4,100 women still die from this disease every year. Data from 2009 suggested that AI women had increased cervical cancer incidence and death rate ratios (RR = 2.11 and 1.55, respectively) relative to White women.[26] In 2010 in Hawai'i, NH women had higher incidence and mortality rates of cervical cancer than White women, with an incidence of 9.6 per 100,000 (compared to 7.0 for Whites) and a mortality rate of 4.5 per 100,000 (compared to 1.8 for Whites).[27] The reasons for these disparities are not known with certainty, but they may be due to a higher prevalence of high-risk HPV genotypes and a lower prevalence of screening among these populations.[18,19] For example, in 2019 in Hawai'i only 60% of PI women and 80% of NH women reported having had a Pap smear in the past 3 years, compared to 85% of White women.[28]

HPV can be largely prevented by timely vaccination with the HPV vaccine. In 2011, the three-dose HPV vaccination was added to the Adolescent Immunization Schedule by the CDC for male and female children 11–12 years old, along with tetanus, diphtheria, and pertussis (Tdap), and meningococcal conjugate (MCV4) vaccines.[29] In 2019, CDC modified recommendations to two doses for all individuals aged 9–26 years. Since HPV causes nearly all cervical cancers, compliance with HPV vaccination would especially benefit AI/AN and NH/PI populations who have low cervical cancer screening prevalence and high mortality from cervical cancer.[30] In 2019, about 71.5% of youth aged 13–17 years had received one or more shots, and about 54.2% of youth had received the two-shot series.[31] These percentages, while having increased over the past decade, are still lower than for the age-appropriate uptake of Tdap (88.9%) and MCV4 (86.6%) on the same Adolescent Immunization Schedule as the HPV vaccine.

The next section highlights four interventions to improve sexual health in AI/AN and NH/PI communities.

Examples of Successful Indigenous Community-Engaged Interventions

HPV Is Not a Tradition: Protect the Circle

Description

The prevalence of high-risk HPV among AI women in the Great Plains IHS region was estimated at 34.8% in 2010, compared to about 20.7% in the general population[22,32] The higher prevalence of HPV likely contributed to disparities in cervical cancer incidence and mortality. Specifically, AI women in the Great Plains had approximately twice the prevalence and four times the mortality from cervical cancer compared to White women in the same region.[25] Fortunately, the HPV vaccine presented an opportunity to reduce these disparities.

Thus, when the first HPV vaccine was released in the US in 2006, the Great Plains Tribal Chairmen's Health Board (GPTCHB) recommended developing culturally appropriate strategies to facilitate vaccine uptake in the 18 Great Plains tribal nations and communities in South Dakota, North Dakota, Nebraska, and Iowa. GPTCHB was primed to take on an HPV-vaccine promotion project because of its history of developing programs and efforts through community-based participatory research (CBPR).

Intervention

The major goals of the project were to (1) determine knowledge and beliefs related to the HPV vaccine and factors that facilitate or hinder vaccination, and (2) develop an intervention with the potential to promote HPV vaccination among AI in the Great Plains region.

Community Engagement

In 2009, the GPTCHB's cancer program prioritized addressing HPV and sought to develop strategies to promote the HPV vaccine. The program team formed an advisory board consisting of a school board member, a school nurse/teacher, a community health representative, a tribal council member, a provider from IHS, an elder community member, and a cancer survivor. The advisory board met regularly to provide guidance and feedback to the project.[33] To better understand perceptions about HPV and opinions for strategies to promote the HPV vaccine, the advisory board recommended the team conduct a series of focus groups.

Ultimately, the team recruited 69 individuals who participated in four focus groups that included (1) tribal healthcare providers and community educators (n =1 0), (2) IHS clinicians (n = 7), (3) young adult women ages 19–26 (n = 20), and (4) girls aged 14–18 (n = 18) with their parents (n = 14).[33,34] Focus group discussions revealed a general awareness of HPV and the vaccine, but a lack of specific knowledge. For example, many participants indicated they had heard of the HPV vaccine but were unclear at what age one should get the vaccine. Another theme was fear and misconception that the vaccine could cause HPV or cancer. To address these issues, the participants in the focus groups emphasized a need for more culturally specific community education using a variety of channels and outlets, including health fairs, radio announcements, posters, and brochures in schools and healthcare settings.

Following the focus groups, an opportunity occurred for the cancer program to create a multimedia health education video on HPV and the vaccine.[33,34] Community members and leaders informed the development of the video that would be culturally relevant for the intended AI community. For example, the project team developed a script for the video, which was reviewed by community leaders for evaluation and feedback. The goal of the video was to provide educational content that would be engaging and relevant for AI youth. Accordingly, most of the video used clips edited together from short interviews with adolescents and young adults from representative tribes. However, feedback from community leaders indicated that more content for parents was needed. Specifically, they raised the issue that many parents were uncomfortable discussing HPV with their children, but that they often had a critical role in HPV vaccination decisions. Thus, an interview with a mother and her teenage daughter, who had just received the HPV vaccine, was added to model how to talk about the importance and benefits of the HPV vaccine. Finally, culturally relevant music, graphics, and messages were woven throughout the video, which could be viewed online. [34]

Outcomes

The GPTCHB's efforts resulted in a culturally tailored video about HPV and the vaccine. The video provided a new tool for community health educators and clinicians to use in their efforts to increase community awareness about the importance of the HPV vaccine. GPTCHB distributed the video to a diverse range of stakeholders including tribal health departments, IHS facilities, and tribal colleges. GPTCHB also provided the video to Mayo Clinic's Native CIRCLE program, a resource center that provided cancer-related materials free of charge to community and healthcare professionals involved in the education of AI/AN. Finally, GPTCHB staff used the video in their community workshops and presentations, often at the request of tribal partners. For example, it was presented at a popular annual education conference held in conjunction with a regional basketball tournament each year that brought together over 500 educators and youth from across the Great Plains region. The video was presented along with a discussion about how different communities could use the video in schools and healthcare settings. An HPV vaccine infographic was designed for community members from data after the conclusion of the Great Plains HPV study.

Lessons Learned

Using CBPR, the GPTCHB cancer program developed and disseminated a culturally relevant HPV educational video. The project began with a process to learn from the community, which helped formulate messages to address their needs and concerns. The team found that interviewing and engaging community members directly in the video, rather than using paid professional actors, had benefits, but it also took additional time and flexibility to finalize a clear and professional product. However, the locally produced video helped bring the educational content to life, featuring relatable youth from the community. Further, personal stories from individuals in the community, such as the mother talking about getting her daughter the HPV vaccine, served to potentially help other parents to have similar conversations. Overall, the video helped to address knowledge gaps in the community and engaged viewers to consider and clarify their own traditional and cultural values around health and wellness in the context of the HPV vaccine.

Native It's Your Game[ii]

Description

Native It's Your Game (NIYG) is an online sexual health curriculum for Native youth developed and tested by the Healthy Native Youth Collaborative, represented by the Alaska Native Tribal Health Consortium (ANTHC), the Inter-Tribal Council of Arizona, Inc. (ITCA), the Northwest Portland Area Indian Health Board (NPAIHB), and the University of Texas Health Science Center (UTHSC).[35,36] Together, this group served 295 tribes in three regions—Alaska, Arizona, and the Pacific Northwest. Curriculum development and testing were supported by the CDC and US Department of Health and Human Services Agency for Children and Families.

ii Funding from CDC 5U48DP001949 and DHHS ACF 2011-ACF-ACYF-AT-0157.

Surveillance data showed that AI/AN youth had higher teen birth rates and STI prevalence than White youth.[11] They also were more likely to report sexual activity before age 13 and low rates of consistent condom use.[37,38] To delay, or mitigate, the consequences of early sexual activity, effective middle school HIV, STI, and pregnancy prevention curricula were needed. However, tribal leaders felt that programs developed for dominant US cultures might not be well received and would need to be adapted for AI/AN youth.[39] Other limitations included the lack of trained educators and geographic isolation experienced by some tribes. An online curriculum offered promise to overcome these barriers. Over 76% of Pacific Northwest AI/AN youth reported experience with and comfort in searching for health information online, and Internet access in US AI/AN communities was improving.[40,41,42]

Intervention

NIYG was adapted from "It's Your Game," an evidence-based, 24-lesson, sexual health program for youth. Both "It's Your Game" and NIYG were guided by social cognitive theory, which holds that behavior is determined by the interaction of personal factors (e.g., personal values, beliefs, skills, outcome expectations, and perceived self-efficacy), social factors (role models), and environmental factors. In adapting "It's Your Game" into NIYG, members of the collaborative attended to surface structures (e.g., swapping out graphics for AI/AN photos) and deep structures (e.g., referencing cultural values and norms of AI/AN cultures).[34] For example, besides changing the name to "Native It's Your Game," adaptations involved featuring AI/AN youth, communities, music, and clothing, and changing images and names to reflect Native cultures and languages from the three different regions.

Other adaptations involved incorporating cultural, social, environmental, and psychological influences of sexual health behaviors.[34] This included the addition of videos featuring the voices of an AI/AN elder and a health education expert who reflected tribal and youth perspectives. Each region provided a video for the curriculum. For example, AI/AN elders from Arizona introduce the curriculum and sensitive lessons, such as anatomy and reproduction. The elders also reference the Native Wellness Model, an integration of physical, emotional, social, mental, and spiritual dimensions of health, and provide traditional blessings. Other video clips feature local AI/AN youth, providing heterogeneous peer perspectives on healthy friendships and protecting personal rules.

As adapted, NIYG is a stand-alone, 13-lesson, Internet-based sexual health life-skills curriculum. Each of the 13 lessons is approximately 35 minutes and covers healthy friendships, protecting personal limits, puberty and reproduction, healthy dating relationships, consequences of sex (HIV, STI, and pregnancy), refusal-skills training, testing, and condom- and contraceptive-skills training. The educational information is delivered using two-dimensional interactive activities, quizzes, animations, videos, and fact sheets.

Production elements also include video and music produced by Native artists and videos of cultural events, such as Pow Wows and Native Youth Olympics, representative of the various AI/AN Peoples in the regions. Printable fact sheets provide extended coverage of topics on pregnancy testing, menstruation, birth control, STI, HIV-testing, body art, substance use, LGBT-two spirit youth, interpersonal violence, and suicide. Parent–child homework activities are designed to facilitate dialogue on friendships, dating, and sexual behavior between parents or guardians and youth.

Community Engagement

The cultural adaptation of It's Your Game and the subsequent testing of NIYG involved AI/AN communities and stakeholders in each region.[35] Using a CBPR approach, the collaborative worked closely with key decision-makers, tribal councils, tribal health boards, and tribal health directors. This approach maximized their ownership in the development of the program and helped to assure the curriculum was responsive to the voice of regional tribes, parents, and youth. Regional communities in Alaska, Arizona, and the Pacific Northwest also were invited to participate in intervention testing. Written agreements were signed by tribal regional organization representatives outlining responsibilities for the tribe, school site, and/or regional organization and conditions of participation, and how the information would be used and disclosed.

Outcomes

The acceptability of NIYG was assessed with a total of 45 AI/AN youth, aged 11–15 years, from each region.[34] A majority agreed that NIYG met the needs of AI/AN youth. Most youths rated the lessons as credible, helpful in making healthy choices, and more fun than other school lessons, computer-based lessons, and health lessons (although not as fun as their favorite video games). Satisfaction ratings were positive for the culturally adapted learning activities, the elder's video, teen peer videos, and a private graffiti wall journaling activity. Youth rated NIYG as enjoyable, easy to use, understandable, and acceptably paced. Most indicated they would recommend NIYG to friends, but were less enthusiastic about sharing the more graphic lessons on anatomy and reproduction. Youth predominantly agreed that the program was suitable for AI/AN youth, and especially for middle school teens given the predominance of cartoons.

AI/AN adult stakeholders comprising 27 parents, health educators, health-care providers, and other community members from 13 different tribal communities participated in focus groups or advisory meetings across the three regions.[34] Although the participating stakeholders did not represent the perceptions of all communities served by the organizations in this collaborate, their input was invaluable in reviewing a cross section of adapted lessons. Stakeholders agreed all NIYG topics were important, perceiving them as helping to meet youth's sexual health needs and filling a current void in educational options. They also felt the curriculum provided a holistic approach incorporating Indigenous perspectives, values, and issues. They considered the representation of traditional values to be appropriate overall and expressed that it had achieved the aim of cultural appropriateness. Stakeholders were positive about disseminating the program, suggesting their communities would support implementation through community organizations, including health clinics, tribal councils and governments, hospitals, and schools.[34]

The effectiveness of NIYG was tested using a baseline sample through a randomized controlled trial conducted in 25 participating AI/AN sites in Alaska, Arizona, and the Pacific Northwest.[35] Sites were recruited by sending flyers to local and regional schools, tribal community centers, and after-school and summer camp programs, and by advertising on organizational websites, social media outlets, and/or newsletters. The 25 sites, comprising 13 urban and 12 rural settings, included tribal schools, tribal community health centers, tribal Boys and Girls Clubs, and after-school and summer youth programs. These sites were randomized to the treatment (NIYG) intervention ($n=14$) or the comparison intervention ($n = 11$). The comparison intervention comprised other health-related computer-based programs that addressed tobacco smoking, hearing, alcohol and drugs, and diet and physical activity.[36] These comparison programs were delivered in a standard number of sessions ($n = 13$) and duration (approximately 35 minutes) that was comparable to the NIYG learning time.

Of the 523 youth in the baseline sample, 402 (77%) youth were retained at follow-up. Of the 402, 86% were AI/AN, and the mean age was 13 years. At first follow-up, AI/AN youth exposed to NIYG reported increased knowledge about condoms and HIV/STI, increased self-efficacy to acquire condoms and use condoms, and more reasons not to have sex than youth receiving the comparison intervention.[35] The community sites had sufficient computer access and Internet connectivity to implement the online health education programs with adequate fidelity. However, variable bandwidth and technical issues led some sites to access programs via back-up modalities (e.g., uploading the programs from a USB drive).

Lessons Learned

This project demonstrated that NIYG was well accepted and effective in the communities in which it was delivered. Findings also suggest that disseminating Internet-based health promotion programs is a promising strategy to address health disparities for this underserved population. The provision of back-up modalities was recommended to address possible connectivity or technical issues.

After the NIYG trial, the collaborative between ANTHC, ITCA, NPAIHB, and UTHSC established the Healthy Native Youth portal.[43] This online resource provides a "one-stop shop" for tribal health advocates and educators to access age-appropriate curricula. Besides NIYG, the website includes many other sexual health curricula: Circle of Life, Respecting the Circle of Life, Native STAND, Native Voices, Healing of the Canoe, and Safe In The Village.[44,45,46,47,48] In addition to the Healthy Native Youth portal, the NPAIHB also hosts WeRNative,[49] a comprehensive health resource and text messaging campaign for Native youth, by Native youth, providing content and stories about the topics that matter most to them.[50] Similarly, ANTHC hosts I Know Mine,[51] a youth wellness website that provided information and resources, including access to free condoms and STI and HIV self-testing, to support Alaska Native youth and their allies.

'Imi Hale Native Hawaiian Cancer Network's HPV Vaccine Brochure[iii]

Description

Hawai'i has a diverse, multiethnic population of 1.4 million people, with 23% NH, 23% Japanese, 19% Caucasian, 15% Filipino, and 20% other ethnicities, including other Asian and PI ethnicities.[52] Because of small numbers, the National Immunization Survey-Teen database does not publish HPV vaccination prevalence for NH/PI or Asian ethnic groups. Thus, a statewide parent survey on their child's HPV vaccine uptake was conducted by 'Imi Hale Native Hawaiian Cancer Network ('Imi Hale) in 2014. Based on findings from this survey and other research, culturally grounded health education materials were developed. 'Imi Hale was a community-based program active from 2000 through 2017 based at Papa Ola Lōkahi, a nongovernmental entity that oversees the Native Hawaiian Healthcare Improvement Act, Hawaiian health policy, and healthcare. 'Imi Hale's work was guided by principles of CBPR.[53]

---

iii Funding from The Queen's Medical Center (Hawai'i), NIH NCI U54CA153459, and NIMHD U54MD007584.

Intervention

In 2014, 'Imi Hale recruited parents from across the state to complete a telephone survey to assess their knowledge of the HPV vaccine, the status of their child's HPV vaccine uptake, and barriers and motivators to uptake.[54] Parents of 11-to-18-year-old children in Hawai'i's four major ethnic groups—NH, Filipinos, Japanese, and Caucasians—were identified, and 799 parents (about 200 in each group) completed the survey. Findings suggested that about 35% of daughters and 19% of sons had received all three doses of the HPV vaccine, as recommended at the time. Vaccine uptake was associated with knowledge about the vaccine, believing in its effectiveness, and the older age of the child. Motivators for HPV vaccination were physician's recommendation and wanting to protect one's child. The primary barrier to uptake was a lack of knowledge about the vaccine, especially for NH and Filipino parents.[52] Since there was no Hawai'i-developed brochure for the HPV vaccine, 'Imi Hale decided to develop a local HPV vaccine brochure and test it locally for attractiveness, readability, and comprehension.

Community Engagement

To inform the development of the brochure, 'Imi Hale staff conducted interviews with 20 parents of 11-to-18-year-old children who were NH ($n = 5$), Filipino ($n = 4$), Japanese ($n = 5$), or White ($n = 6$).[28] They confirmed that the brochure should address knowledge and misconceptions (e.g., only girls need to be vaccinated and age 11–12 is too young to be vaccinated against HPV) and include pictures of children that reflected local faces, testimonials, vivid colors, and an immunization chart.

Based on findings from the literature and the parent interviews, 'Imi Hale staff members drafted a brochure.[55] Fifteen health educators and nine physicians reviewed the brochure to ensure the accuracy of the content, and they provided their preliminary endorsement. Next, the brochure was tested with eligible parents, which were those who had an 11-to-18-year-old child in Hawai'i and were responsible for taking the child to get vaccinated. Participants were mailed a mock-up of the HPV vaccine brochure and a survey soliciting feedback on the brochure. The latter included questions on the brochure's attractiveness, acceptability, messenger effectiveness, personal relevancy, readability, suggestions for improvement, parent demographics, and child vaccination status. Additional questions asked parents to confirm comprehension, new words they encountered, and suggestions for improvements to the brochure (Table 6.1.). In all, 52 parents provided feedback on the brochure. The brochure received a final review and endorsement from engaged physicians and community members.

Table 6.1. Material Feedback Outcomes from Parents (*n* = 52)

Measure	*n* (%)
Attractiveness	
If I saw this in a doctor's office, I would pick it up.	44 (84.6)
The messages, visuals, colors, and voices were appealing to me.	50 (96.2)
The people shown look like someone I know.	50 (96.2)
Acceptability	
I feel comfortable sharing this brochure with another parent.	52 (100)
I think other parents of adolescents would benefit from this brochure.	52 (100)
Messenger Effectiveness/Testimonies	
I found the quote from the doctor to be helpful.	51 (98.1)
I found the quote from the mother something I can relate to.	50 (96.2)
Personal Relevancy	
The messages and pictures were meaningful to me as a parent.	50 (96.2)
Readability	
I found this brochure easy to read.	52 (100)
Were there words new to you?	4 (7.7)

Other research by 'Imi Hale provided additional information on preferred delivery routes for health education materials by island.[56]

Outcomes

Nearly all (over 90%) of participating parents were positive about the brochure's appearance. They reported that the brochure was easy to read, informative, appropriate, and useful. They most appreciated the photos of local children and testimonies from a NH pediatrician and a Filipino parent. Overall, they reported that the brochure increased their knowledge of the vaccine and their intent to vaccinate their child. Parents also said they would share the brochure with their provider and with other parents.[29]

A key component of evaluating the utility of a brochure was to assess the target audience's comprehension of the brochure using open-ended questions, including "What is this brochure about?" In response, parents highlighted specific information, such as the benefits of the vaccine for cancer prevention (44%) and the need for boys and girls aged 11–18 years old to be vaccinated (40%). Having the parents report that the HPV vaccine was for both girls and boys after reading the mock-up was especially gratifying.[29]

Lessons Learned

Community participation of local providers and parents was critical for developing an HPV brochure to fit Hawai'i's context. This study fulfilled a need for

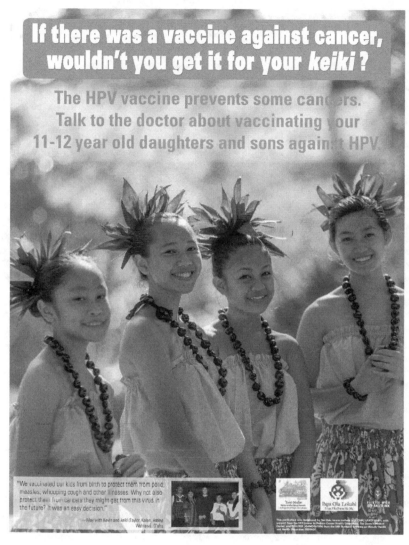

Fig 6.1. HPV vaccine poster. Used with permission by May Rose I. Dela Cruz.

a local HPV vaccine brochure for parents in Hawai'i. After receiving the endorsement from providers and community members, 40,000 brochures were printed for clinics, community health centers, the Native Hawaiian Healthcare Systems, and other health offices in the state of Hawai'i. Two large posters also were created for clinics and health offices to enhance provider and parent discussions about the HPV vaccine (Figure 6.1).

Building Capacity for Teen Pregnancy Prevention in the Northern Mariana Islands[iv]

Description

The Hawai'i Youth Services Network (HYSN) is a coalition of youth-serving organizations in Hawai'i that provides services and training in Hawai'i and the Pacific. This organization has a long history of helping service providers adopt and implement evidence-based curricula to improve the sexual health of youth. The Pacific Pregnancy Partnership is a partnership between the Public School System of the Commonwealth of the Northern Mariana Islands (CNMI) and the HYSN of Honolulu, Hawai'i.

HYSN began partnering with the CNMI Public School System in 2009 with the goal of (1) reducing the risk of unplanned pregnancy and STI and increasing the likelihood of successful transition to adulthood for youth, (2) increasing the number of adolescents that abstained from sex, delayed initiation of sex, used effective contraception if sexually active, and had fewer sexual partners, and (3) reducing the teen birth rate.

Beginning in 2012, the program was funded through the federal Personal Responsibility and Education Program with the CNMI Public School System as the grantee. The CNMI public school teachers and counselors delivered the program. HYSN provided ongoing training, technical assistance in adapting and delivering the program, and evaluation services that addressed teen pregnancy/STI prevention and healthy adolescent development.

Intervention

The program, called the Pacific Pregnancy Partnership, included three parts: (1) a classroom-based sexual health education program for grades 6 and higher, (2) parent education, and (3) an after-school/summer program for middle school youth. The sexual health education program was implemented in every middle and high school throughout CNMI. The curriculum "Making a Difference" was taught to 6th graders, the curriculum "Making Proud Choices" was taught to 7th graders, and the curriculum "Be Proud Be Responsible" was taught in the high schools. These three curricula were developed by the same curriculum developer, ETR.[57]

Early in the development of the program, the three evidence-based curricula were adapted to ensure cultural relevance for PI students. For example, HYSN developed culturally relevant sexual health and bullying prevention videos for the population, which is composed primarily of PI, Filipino, and

iv Funding from the US ACF 2001MPPREP and 90AK0037.

mixed-race youth. The youth were extensively involved in the production and editing of the videos. Two of the videos won national awards from the CDC and the US Substance Abuse and Mental Health Services Administration.

Every school conducted a parent night meeting prior to classroom instruction. Parents and family members learned the importance of talking to their children about sensitive subjects like sexual health. They were told that schools can teach knowledge and skills, but it was up to families to discuss what was right and wrong. Parents who became advocates for the program were invited to present at parent night and meetings with the CMNI Education Commissioner and administrators. The after-school/summer component of the program provided positive youth development activities and adult supervision to help prevent risky behaviors. The program provided lessons that reinforced the knowledge, attitudes, and skills learned in the classroom.

In addition to being trained to deliver the curricula, teachers and counselors also received training in ways to improve their delivery of the program. For example, HYSN offered introductory training on sexual health called "Sex Ed 101 for Educators," which covered the basics of anatomy, puberty, contraception, and STI. "Helping Our Parents Educate" focused on parent–child communication about sexual health. Workshops also were conducted on safe environments for lesbian, gay, bisexual, transgender, and queer students and on the prevention or bullying. HYSN and the program coordinator worked together to assure that teachers and schools had continuing access to technical assistance.

Community Engagement

The CNMI Public School System and HYSN started working together in 2009. At that time, HYSN was funded by the CDC to build the capacity of organizations to select, implement, and evaluate science based approaches to preventing teen pregnancy and HIV/STI. With success in Hawai'i, HYSN offered to assist the CNMI due to the concern about the high rate of CNMI teen births. HYSN conducted training on teen pregnancy prevention with the CNMI public school system in 2009 and 2010, and they worked together to design a CNMI-appropriate program.

In addition to training on sexual health, the public school staff and community partners, including the Maternal and Child Health Bureau within the Commonwealth Healthcare Corporation, identified other training needs. For example, in 2016, several students completing the "Making a Difference" curriculum then reported sexual abuse to school staff. As a result, HYSN recommended that school staff consider a prevention curriculum developed by the Sex Abuse Treatment Center (SATC) in Hawai'i. SATC allowed free access to curriculum materials and trained an HYSN staff member at no charge. The HYSN staff person then trained teachers and counselors in the CNMI. In addition, the CNMI public school staff organized meetings with all agencies involved in child sexual abuse to develop better-coordinated systems for handling children. The train-the-trainer model was utilized to sustain the program with successful and committed trainers.

CNMI school staff also were involved in gathering evaluation data and reviewing the findings to improve the program. For example, students completed pre- and posttests on each curriculum to gauge learning and identify areas for improvement. HYSN also worked with the Commonwealth Healthcare Corporation to review data from CNMI birth records and the Youth Behavioral Risk Survey to track the impact of the program on teen pregnancy and risk for pregnancy and STI. End-of-training surveys, as well as semiannual quality improvement meetings, also were conducted, and all stakeholders were invited to review and interpret the findings. Training and technical assistance also were provided on all aspects of federal grants. This included training on grant writing, program design, budgets, grants management, logic models, and evaluation. Engaging CNMI stakeholders in evaluation activities and data sharing also helped them build leadership and advocacy skills.

Outcomes

Positive outcomes were seen in several sexual health indicators. For example, the percentage of high school students who had sexual intercourse declined from 46% in 2011 to 33.6% in 2017. In the same time frame, the percentage of high school students who had first sexual intercourse before age 13 declined from 7% to 4%. Also, fewer students reported drinking or using drugs before sexual intercourse (30% to 24%). Most impressively, CNMI documented a steep decline in teen births and declines in youth risk behaviors. Specifically, in 2011, the teen birth rate in the CNMI was 97 per 1,000 girls aged 15–17; by 2017, it had dropped to 37 per 1,000 girls.

Important for sustainability, the program resulted in increased skills and capacities of CNMI stakeholders. Thus, the community and schools had new programs and resources for youth health. Teachers, counselors, and other service providers in the CNMI benefited from training, and many subsequently served as trainers, grant writers, evaluators, and advocates for youth health. Even parents gained knowledge and skills. When the program first started, many parents were concerned and refused to allow their children to participate in sexual health training at school. Increasingly, sexual health became a normal part of the school's curriculum, with some parents advocating for the program.

.hi project
demonstrated the importance of listening to community to identify issues of
local concern, as well as champions willing to lead the project. Community
engagement was critical to taking an evidence-based curriculum from elsewhere and adapting it to fit the local culture. Project sustainability was considered from the very beginning of the project by helping CNMI partners build
their own skills and secure and manage their own grants. Local stakeholders
identified training needs, which were met to build internal capacity in program
development, program delivery, evaluation, and organizational management.

Summary

prevalence of teen pregnancy and STI among Indigenous Peoples justify
attention to interventions in this area. Knowledge about the role of HPV in
cervical cancer and the effectiveness of the HPV vaccine is growing, but still
needs to be disseminated. Family and culture play a large role in sexual knowledge, attitudes, and practices, especially among youth. Thus, culture needs to
be reflected in appropriate sex education materials and curricula. This chapter
featured case studies of how researchers engaged with Indigenous communities as they designed, adapted, and tested sexual health education materials
and programs. Strategies included formulating a community advisory board,
seeking advice on materials as they develop, and training community members in curriculum delivery and testing.

References

1. Youth.gov. Risk and protective factors. Accessed February 8, 2021. https://youth.gov/youth-topics/pregnancy-prevention/risk-and-protective-factors.

2. Centers for Disease Control and Prevention. About teen pregnancy. Accessed September 1, 2020. https://www.cdc.gov/teenpregnancy/about/index.htm.

3. STDs and HIV—CDC Fact Sheet. Centers for Disease Control and Prevention. Accessed February 8, 2021. https://www.cdc.gov/std/hiv/stdfact-std-hiv.htm.

4. Dixon M, Roubideaux Y. *Promises to keep: Public health policy for American Indians and Alaska natives in the 21st century.* American Public Health Association, 2001.

5. Petereit DG, Rogers D, Govern F, et al. Increasing access to clinical cancer trials and emerging technologies for minority populations: The Native American project. *J Clin Oncol.* 2005;22:4452–4455.

6. Guadagnolo BA, Cina K. Helbig P, et al. Medical mistrust and less satisfaction with healthcare among Native Americans presenting for cancer treatment. *J Health Care Poor Underserved.* 2009;20(1):210–226.

7. Hoffman SD, Maynard RA, eds. *Kids having kids: Economic costs and social consequences of teen pregnancy, 2nd ed.* Urban Institute Press, 2008.

8. Centers for Disease Prevention and Control. Incidence, prevalence, and cost of sexually transmitted infections in the US. Accessed September 1, 2020. https://npin.cdc.gov/publication/incidence-prevalence-and-cost-sexually-transmitted-infections-united-states.

9. Centers for Disease Prevention and Control. Sexually transmitted diseases. Accessed September 1, 2020. https://www.cdc.gov/std/general/default.htm.

10. World Health Organization. Sexually transmitted diseases. Accessed September 1, 2020. https://www.who.int/news-room/fact-sheets/detail/sexually-transmitted-infections-(stis).

11. Centers for Disease Control. *Sexually transmitted diseases surveillance report, 2017.* Accessed September 1, 2020. https://www.cdc.gov/std/stats17/2017-STD-Surveillance-Report_CDC-clearance-9.10.18.pdf.

12. Walker FJ, Llata E, Doshani M, *et al.* HIV, Chlamydia, gonorrhea, and primary and secondary syphilis among American Indians and Alaska Natives within Indian Health Service areas in the United States, 2007–2010. *J Community Health.* 2015;40(3):484–492.

13. Centers for Disease Control and Prevention. Health disparities in HIV/AIDS, viral hepatitis, and TB: Native Hawaiian and other Pacific Islanders. Accessed September 1, 2020. https://www.cdc.gov/nchhstp/healthdisparities/hawaiians.html#STD.

14. Jarvis GA, Chang TL. Modulation of HIV transmission by Neisseria gonorrhoeae: Molecular and immunological aspects. *Curr HIV Res.* 2012;10(3):211–217.

15. Centers for Disease Control and Prevention. HIV basic statistics. Accessed May 19, 2021. https://www.cdc.gov/hiv/basics/statistics.html.

16. Centers for Disease Control and Prevention. Diagnoses of HIV infection in the United States and dependent areas, 2017. Accessed September 1, 2020. https://www.cdc.gov/hiv/pdf/library/reports/surveillance/cdc-hiv-surveillance-report-2017-vol-29.pdf.

17. Centers for Disease Control and Prevention. Syphilis. Accessed September 1, 2020. https://www.cdc.gov/std/stats17/syphilis.htm.

18. Steben M, Duarte-Franco E. Human papillomavirus infection: Epidemiology and pathophysiology. *Gynecol Oncol.* 2007;107(2 Suppl 1):S2–S5.

19. Leyden WA, Manos MM, Geiger AM, *et al.* Cervical cancer in women with comprehensive healthcare access: Attributable factors in the screening process. *J Natl Cancer Inst.* 2005;97(9):675–683.

20. Bell MC, Schmidt-Grimminger D, Jacobsen C, *et al.* Risk factors for HPV infection among American Indian and White women in the Northern Plains. *Gynecol Oncol.* 2011;121(3):532–536.

21. Bakir AH, Skarzynski M. Health disparities in the immunoprevention of Human Papillomavirus Infection and associated malignancies. *Front Public Health.* 2015;3:256.

22. Schmidt-Grimminger DC, Bell MC, Muller CJ, *et al.* HPV infection among rural American Indian women and urban white women in South Dakota: An HPV prevalence study. *BMC Infect Dis.* 2011;11:252.

23. Lee NR, Winer RL, Cherne S, *et al.* Human papillomavirus prevalence among American Indian women of the Great Plains. *J Infect Dis.* 2019;219(6):908–915.

24. Stanley M. HPV - immune response to infection and vaccination. *Infect Agent Cancer.* 2010;5:19.

25. National Cancer Institute. Cancer stat fact sheets: Cervical cancer. Accessed September 1, 2020. http://seer.cancer.gov/statfacts/html/cervix.html.

26. Watson M, Benard V, Thomas C, *et al.* Cervical cancer incidence and mortality among American Indian and Alaska Native women, 1999–2009. *Am J Public Health.* 2014;104(Suppl 3):S415–S422.

27. American Cancer Society. *Hawai'i cancer facts and figures, 2010*. Accessed September 1, 2020. https://health.hawaii.gov/about/files/2013/06/Hawaii_Cancer_Facts_and_Figures_2010.pdf.

28. Hawai'i State Department of Health. Hawai'i Health Data Warehouse. BRFSS data on Pap smear. Accessed September 1, 2020. http://ibis.hhdw.org/ibisph-view/query/result/brfss/Pap3Yr2165/Pap3Yr2165Crude11_.html.

29. Dela Cruz MRI, Tsark JAU, Chen JJ, *et al*. Human Papillomavirus (HPV) vaccination motivators, barriers, and brochure preferences among parents in multicultural Hawai'i: A qualitative study. *J Cancer Educ*. 2017;32(3):613–621.

30. Dela Cruz MRI, Tsark JA, Soon R, *et al*. Insights in public health: Community involvement in developing a human papillomavirus (HPV) vaccine brochure made for parents in Hawai'i. *Hawaii J Med Public Health*. 2016;75(7):203–207.

31. Elam-Evans LD, Yankey D, Singleton JA, *et al*. National, regional, state, and selected local area vaccination coverage among adolescents aged 13–17 years—United States, 2019. *MMWR Morb Mortal Wkly Rep*. 2020;69:1109–1116.

32. Lewis RM, Markowitz LE, Gargano JW, *et al*. Prevalence of genital human papillomavirus among sexually experienced males and females aged 14–59 years, United States, 2013–2014. *J Infect Dis*. 2018;217(6):869–877.

33. Schmidt-Grimminger D, Frerichs L, Bird AEB, *et al*. HPV knowledge, attitudes, and beliefs among Northern Plains American Indian adolescents, parents, young adults, and health professionals. *J Cancer Educ*. 2013;28(2):357–366.

34. Duran FT, Frerichs L. HPV Is Not a Tradition [Video file]. YouTube, June 2, 2009. Accessed February 12, 2021. https://www.youtube.com/watch?v=MvXT9UeaUaw&t=2s.

35. Shegog R, Craig Rushing S, Gorman G, *et al*. NATIVE-It's Your Game: Adapting a technology-based sexual health curriculum for American Indian and Alaska Native youth. *J Prim Prev*. 2017;38(1–2):27–48.

36. Shegog R, Craig Rushing S, Jessen C, *et al*. Native It's Your Game: Improving psychosocial protective factors for HIV/STI and teen pregnancy prevention among American Indian/Alaska Native Youth. *J Appl Res Child*. 2017;8(1):3.

37. Centers for Disease Control and Prevention, Youth Risk Behavior Surveillance System. Youth online: High school YRBS. 2013. Accessed February 12, 2021. http://nccd.cdc.gov/youthonline/App/Default.aspx?SID=HS.

38. Edwards S. Among Native American teenagers, sex without contraceptives is common. *Fam Plan Perspect*. 1992;24(4):189–191.

39. Desiderio G, Garrido M, Martínez, *et al*. *Lessons learned in providing health care services for Native Youth*. Healthy Teen Network, 2014. Accessed September 1, 2020. http://www.npaihb.org/images/epicenter_docs/aids/2014/Report_Interviews.pdf.

40. Rushing SC, Stephens D, Leston J, *et al*. Surfing and texting for health: Media use and health promotion targeting NW native youth. *NW Public Health J*. 2011 Spring/Summer;28(1):16–17.

41. Rushing SC, Stephens D. Use of media technologies by Native American teens and young adults in the Pacific Northwest: Exploring their utility for designing culturally appropriate technology-based health interventions. *J Prim Prev*. 2011;32(3–4):135–145.

42. Rushing SC, Stephens D. Tribal recommendations for designing culturally appropriate technology-based sexual health interventions targeting Native youth in the Pacific Northwest. *Am Indian Alsk Native Ment Health Res*. 2012;19(1):76–101.

43. Healthy Native Youth. Home - Healthy Native Youth. Accessed February 12, 2021. https://www.healthynativeyouth.org.

44. Tingey L, Chambers R, Rosenstock S, *et al*. The impact of a sexual and reproductive health intervention for American Indian adolescents on predictors of condom use intention. *J Adolesc Health*. 2017;60(3):284–291.

45. Rushing SNC, Hildebrandt NL, Grimes CJ, *et al*. Healthy & Empowered Youth: A positive youth development program for native youth. *Am J Prev Med*. 2017;52(3 Suppl 3):S263–S267.

46. Hafner SP, Rushing SC. Sexual health, STI and HIV risk, and risk perceptions among American Indian and Alaska Native emerging adults. *Prev Sci*. 2019;20(3):331–341.

47. Donovan DM, Thomas LR, Sigo RL, *et al*. Healing of the canoe: Preliminary results of a culturally tailored intervention to prevent substance abuse and promote tribal identity for native youth in two Pacific Northwest tribes. *Am Indian Alsk Native Ment Health Res*. 2015;22(1):42–76.

48. Alaska Native Tribal Health Consortium. Safe in the Village. Accessed September 1, 2020. https://www.iknowmine.org/for-providers-educators/Curriculum/safe-in-the-village.

49. We R Native. Accessed February 12, 2021. www.weRnative.org.

50. Rushing SNC, Stephens D, Dog Jr. TLG. We R Native: Harnessing technology to improve health outcomes for American Indian and Alaska Native youth. *J Adolesc Health*. 2018;62(2):S83–S84.

51. I Know Mine. Truthful, accurate information for you(th). Accessed February 12, 2021. https://www.iknowmine.org/.

52. Hawai'i Health Survey 2012. Gender, age, ethnicity, and poverty by county – population of Hawai'i, Hawai'i Health Survey. 2016 http://health.hawaii.gov/hhs/files/2015/07/1.1-Gender-Age-and-Ethnicity-By-County---Population-of-Hawaii-Table-and-Figure.pdf.

53. Braun KL, Tsark J, Santos L, *et al*. Building Native Hawaiian capacity in cancer research and programming: The legacy of 'Imi Hale. *Cancer*. 2006;107(8 Suppl):2082–2090.

54. Dela Cruz MRI, Braun KL, Tsark JU, *et al*. Prevalence of HPV vaccination and parental barriers and motivators to vaccinating children in multi-ethnic Hawai'i. *Ethn Health*. 2020;25(7):982–994.

55. Kulukulualani M, Braun KL, Tsark J. Using a four-step protocol to develop and test culturally targeted cancer education brochures. *Health Promot Pract*. 2008;9:344–355.

56. Aitaoto N, Tsark J, Tomayasu-Wong D, *et al*. Strategies to increase breast and cervical cancer screening among Filipina, Hawaiian, and Pacific Islander women in Hawai'i. *Hawai'i Med J*. 2009;68:215–222.

57. ETR Program Success Center for Sexual & Reproductive Health. Accessed September 1, 2020. https://www.etr.org/ebi/programs/.

7

Cancer and Survivorship in American Indians and Alaska Natives

Linda Burhansstipanov, Kathryn L. Braun, Jessica Blanchard,
Daniel Petereit, Avery Keller Olson, Priscilla R. Sanderson,
Lorencita Joshweseoma, Chiu-Hiseh (Paul) Hsu, Ken Batai,
Lloyd Joshweseoma, Dana Russell, Diana G. Redwood,
and Mark C. Bauer

Introduction

The American Cancer Society (ACS) estimated that there were more than 1.8 million new cancer cases in the United States (US) in 2020. Additionally, about 16.9 million Americans alive on January 1, 2019, had a history of cancer (i.e., were cancer survivors).[1,2] This chapter presents information on cancer in American Indian (AI) and Alaska Native (AN), Native Hawaiian (NH), and Pacific Islander (PI) populations. Information on AI/AN childhood, adolescent, and young adult (AYA) cancers is included to summarize the dearth of accurate data and interventions for AI/AN childhood and AYA cancer patients. Clinical trials are an important source of new treatments and information about cancer care, yet many do not include AI/AN participants in sufficient quantities to impact AI/AN care. Ways to increase AI/AN participation in clinical trials, as well as four examples of successful AI/AN community engagement cancer programs, are summarized. Examples from the NH and PI communities are included in Chapter 8.

Cancer in AI/ANs

Cancer Incidence

Cancer usually develops in older people, with 80% of all US cancers diagnosed in people 55 years of age or older.[1] However, in AI/AN populations, cancer is diagnosed at earlier ages and at more advanced stages than in other racial groups[3,4] In 2014, the National Institutes of Health (NIH), the Centers for Disease Control and Prevention (CDC), and the Indian Health Service (IHS) produced a report on AI/AN cancer incidence, noting, "The cancer burden continues to escalate among AI/AN, and importantly, AI/AN are not experiencing the decreases in cancer incidence that is occurring among other racial groups."[5] According to National Cancer Institute (NCI) 2020 SEER Cancer Statistics Review 1975–2016, the cancers with the highest incidence for AI men and women were colorectal, breast, and cervical cancers.[6] This may be in part due to lower screening prevalence among AI/AN. For example, in their 2018 report, the CDC identified that only 51.5% of AI women had a mammogram within the past 2 years, compared to 65.8% of White women; and only 60.9% of AI women had a Pap smear within the last 3 years, compared to 68.4% of non-Hispanic White women.[7]

There are distinctive and significant geographic patterns in AI/AN cancer incidence and mortality, while rates in Whites remain homogeneous across geographic regions.[8,9,10,11,12,13] For example, cancer incidence is higher among AN living in Alaska and AI in the Southern and Northern Plains.[9,12,14,15,16,17,18] Nationally, AI/AN have higher incidence rates of stomach, kidney, and liver cancer than the general population, with geographic variation.[19] Cancer incidence is significantly lower for AI living in the Southwest, but due to the higher numbers of AI in this region, the disease burden is elevated overall. Similarly, tribal differences within specific regions can vary. For example, the Navajo Nation in the Southwest has the highest incidence of prostate, breast, and colorectal cancer and more than three times the age-adjusted incidence rate for stomach cancer in comparison with non-Hispanic Whites in the same region.[20]

Cancer Mortality

Cancer is the second leading cause of death in all AI populations (both genders) over age 45.[21,22] The substantial progress in reducing cancer deaths seen in Whites has not been seen in AI/AN,[9] with cancer mortality rates the same or increased.[4,5,6,7,8,9,12,13,14,23,24,25] In many cases, increased mortality is due to diagnostic delays, resulting in an advanced stage of disease at diagnosis and an increased risk of dying from cancer.[26] AI/AN experience challenges in accessing cancer care that contribute to delays and later cancer stage at the time of diagnosis.[3,4,9,20]

Among AI/AN, those living in Alaska and in the Northern and the Southern Plains have the highest mortality rates, while rates are lowest among AI/AN in the Southwest and East.[9,24] Death rates are two times higher for AI/AN men living in the Northern Plains (338.1 per 100,000) compared to those in the Southwest (163.8 per 100,000) for all cancers combined. Northern and Southern Plains AI have higher mortality rates for breast, lung, colorectal, and cervix cancers than non-Hispanic Whites living in the same region. Cancer rather than heart disease is the leading cause of AN death and the leading sites were lung and colorectal.[27,28,29]

Cancer Survival

AI/AN have the poorest 5-year survival among all racial/ethnic groups for all cancers combined (e.g., 60% in AI/AN, compared to 68% in non-Hispanic Whites).[17,19,21,24,30,31] Disparities in survival from cancer is largely due to differences in access to treatment, stage at diagnosis, and comorbidities.[19] For example, about half of AI/AN must travel more than 100 miles one-way to access cancer care, and about 15% travel more than 400 miles one-way to access treatment.[26] For AN, such travel distances (400+ miles) are more the norm than the exception because almost all cancer care must be accessed in Anchorage, Fairbanks, or Seattle.

For individuals, the cancer burden includes managing illness, adjusting to lifestyle changes, changing self-care practices, and living with disruptions from treatments, side effects, and altered lifestyles. Cancer takes the lives of older adults and elders, who are the community's leaders, wisdom keepers, and irreplaceable resources for cultural continuity. A well-known comment is, "Every time an elder dies, a library burns."[26] Common survivorship themes include the importance of family support and the value of spirituality and cultural beliefs in coping with the cancer experience.[32]

Cancer in Native Hawaiians and Other Pacific Islanders

Native Hawaiians and other Pacific Islanders (NH/PI) in the US have higher cancer incidence and mortality than Whites and Asian subgroups.[33] Specifically, Native Hawaiian men have especially high mortality from prostate, lung, and colorectal cancers. Samoan men have especially high mortality from prostate, lung, liver, and stomach cancers. Native Hawaiian and Samoan women have especially high mortality from breast and lung cancers.[34] Cancer registry data from the other Pacific jurisdictions indicate that cancer is the second leading cause of death, and the most detected malignancies are breast, lung and bronchus, prostate, colorectal, liver, and cervical.

Like AI/AN, the NH/PI face barriers to timely cancer diagnosis and treatment, including lack of knowledge about cancer, lack of insurance, low income, and distance to services.[35] Thus, NH/PI people are more likely than other ethnic groups to be diagnosed with cancer in the late stages when treatment options are reduced. The geography of Hawai'i and the Pacific present challenges to accessing care as the bulk of cancer care resources are located in Honolulu. Although healthcare systems on the neighboring islands of Hawai'i, Kaua'i, Lana'i, Maui, and Moloka'i have been expanding cancer services in the past few years, many neighbor island cancer patients still travel or relocate to Honolulu for diagnosis and treatment, which can impose financial, physical, and mental stresses.[36]

A large proportion of cancer among residents of the US-affiliated Pacific is associated with US thermonuclear weapons testing in the region.[37] Although these jurisdictions use US dollars as currency and have access to US public health funding from the CDC, NIH, and other funders, socioeconomic conditions are poorer than in most areas of the US, and services are limited. Hospitals are located in capitals, and individuals living on outer atolls and islands may be unable to get to the capital more than once a year. Jurisdictional health departments support small clinics or lay health workers in population centers outside the capital, but they have limited services and supplies. A portion of the jurisdictions' limited health budgets is set aside to transport some of the complex cases to the Philippines for care. Limited awareness about cancer screening and limited equipment, supplies, trained personnel, and laboratory capabilities are major barriers to timely screening. Thus, many cancers are diagnosed at advanced stages, and the region has almost no capacity to treat cancer, especially late-stage cancer.[37]

Cancer in Childhood, Adolescents, and Young Adults

Cancer care professionals discuss cancer for three age groups—children (ages 0–14 years), adolescents and young adults (aged 15–39 years), and adults. In this section, data are presented first for children and then for young adults. In the general US population, cancer is the second leading cause of death for children aged 0 to 14 years. The ACS estimated that 11,050 new cancer cases will be diagnosed among children aged 0 to 14 years in the US in 2020, and about 1,190 children will die from cancer.[1] Following is a summary of the International Classification of Childhood Cancer (ICCC) and includes the percentages and symptoms of the more common cancers among children aged 0–14 years.[38]

The International Classification of Childhood Cancer (ICCC)

- Leukemia (28% of all childhood cancers) may cause bone and joint pain, fatigue, weakness, pale skin, bleeding or bruising easily, fever, or infection.
- Brain and other central nervous system tumors (26%) may cause headaches, nausea, vomiting, blurred or double vision, seizures, dizziness, and difficulty walking or handling objects.
- Neuroblastoma (6%), a cancer of the peripheral nervous system that is most common in children younger than 5 years of age, usually appears as a swelling in the abdomen.
- Wilms tumor (5%), also called nephroblastoma, is a kidney cancer that may appear as swelling or a lump in the abdomen.

- Non-Hodgkin lymphoma (5%; includes Burkitt lymphoma) and Hodgkin lymphoma (3%), often cause lymph nodes to swell and appear as a lump in the neck, armpit, or groin; other symptoms can include fatigue, weight loss, and fever.
- Rhabdomyosarcoma (3%), a soft tissue sarcoma that can occur in the head and neck, genitourinary area, trunk, and extremities, may cause pain and/or a mass or swelling.
- Retinoblastoma (2%), an eye cancer that usually occurs in children younger than 5 years of age, is often recognized because the pupil appears white or pink instead of the normal red color in flash photographs or during an eye examination.
- Osteosarcoma (2%), a bone cancer that most often occurs in adolescents, commonly appears as sporadic pain in the affected bone that may worsen at night or with activity and eventually progresses to local swelling.
- Ewing sarcoma (1%), another cancer usually arising in the bone in adolescents, typically appears as pain at the tumor site.

For children, the highest standard of care is provided by hospitals that specialize in treating children and through childhood clinical trials. However, anecdotal information reported to Native American Cancer Research Corporation's "Native American Cancer Education for Survivors" and four national AI/AN survivorship conferences from 1997 to 2017 suggest that few AI/AN children or young adults receive care from children's hospitals or are included in clinical trials. The reasons varied, but among the highest were that the children were misdiagnosed (typically as diabetic) in their local clinics. When these cases are finally referred via Purchased Referred Care (PRC), the children are in advanced stages of cancer and referred to cancer centers rather than children's hospitals. Because children's hospitals are the source of most data on childhood cancers, data on AI/AN children are underreported. Insufficient data greatly contributes to the dearth of research or programs that address Indigenous AI/AN childhood cancer interventions and outcomes. This is "a critical gap because the knowledge gained from survivorship research may not be generalizable to minority populations that are underrepresented in published studies."[39]

Based on the limited research that has included Indigenous children, it appears that cancer incidence in AI/AN children is similar to or less than what is reported for the general population (see ICCC list).[40] For example, AI/AN children in the US have a lower incidence of central nervous system (CNS) tumors and glioblastoma.[41] Leukemia is the most common type of cancer among children, with acute lymphoid leukemia (ALL) comprising 75% of all childhood leukemia cases.[42] While some studies suggest the incidence of ALL for AI/AN children is similar to or less than Whites and Asians,[43] others report AI/AN children have a greater risk of ALL compared with Whites.[44] The discrepancies are likely due to racial misclassification. Studies conducted since 2011 also suggest that AI genetic ancestry is predictive of relapse.[45,46,47,48]

There may be significant, geographic differences in incidence rates for AI/AN childhood cancers. For example, AI/AN children living in New Mexico have a lower incidence of neuroblastoma than Whites.[36,49] In contrast, a study among AI in Oklahoma reported a higher incidence of cancer among AI children compared to Whites in all pediatric age groups except for those aged 5–9, with significantly higher age-adjusted rates for AI youth aged 15–19.[50] Another study found that the significantly higher rate of hepatic tumors among AN children prior to 2000 was associated with elevated rates of hepatitis B.[4] Subsequently, a comprehensive hepatitis B immunization program eliminated transmission, and no AN born between 1991 and 2011 has received a diagnosis of hepatocellular carcinoma.[51] These may be significant differences than those summarized in the ICCC.

These findings document the variation that exists in diverse AI/AN populations and further highlighted the need for more robust and local investigations of AI/AN childhood cancers.[52] These studies also highlight the value of longitudinal data sets for AI/AN populations and the impacts of developing preventive practices and interventions that are responsive to local and population-specific needs.

Although incidence of childhood cancers among AI/AN may not be higher than for non-Hispanic Whites, Indigenous children appear to have the lowest survival from all cancers combined,[53] all leukemia types[54,55] (ALL in particular),[56,57] and neuroblastoma.[58] New Mexico documented that AI children with neuroblastoma had lower survival and worse event-free survival when compared with Whites. Although ALL survival for children of all racial/ethnic groups has markedly improved over the past two decades to nearly 88.5%,[59] AI/AN children may have the worst ALL survival probability of all race/ethnic groups.[60] Relapse is the primary cause of death in children with ALL.

The key to improving data on incidence and mortality rates associated with childhood cancers in AI/AN populations is to account for known regional variations, such as lower survival rates of AI/AN children with cancer in Minnesota and higher incidence of some cancers among AI/AN children in Oklahoma.[52] Data related to the burden and experience of cancer among Indigenous children worldwide are limited and inconclusive to identify the most pressing priorities for cancer research. Racial/ethnic differences in long-

Table 7.1. Incidence and Mortality Rates for Top Cancers among US Adolescents and Young Adults

Incidence		Mortality	
Breast	115.7	Breast	12.2%
Melanoma	103.1	Leukemia	12.1%
Thyroid	81.1	CNS	9.1%
Testicular	51.7	Colorectal	8.0%
Non-Hodgkin lymphoma (NHL)	39.7	Lung	6.3%
Hodgkin lymphoma	36.8	NHL	5.7%
Central nervous system (CNS)	34.1	Cervical	4.8%
Colorectal	32.0	Sarcoma	4.2%
Cervical	32.0	Stomach	4.1%
Leukemia	29.9	Melanoma	3.5%

term and disease-free survival for Indigenous and other minority children are linked to differences in disease biology, socioeconomic factors, and access to quality care associated with living in rural areas, pharmacogenetic differences, and sociocultural and environmental factors.[61]

There are about 70,000 adolescents and young adults aged 15–39 diagnosed with invasive cancer each year in the US.[62,63] There have been no national studies about Indigenous AYA, and this is a greatly understudied area in oncology. The prevalence of cancer among AYA of all races in the US are expected to increase from approximately 104 million in 2000 to 115 million in 2030.[64] The leading cancer incidence and age-adjusted mortality rates are listed in Table 7.1.

For AYA patients of all races, the mortality decreased from 8.3% for those diagnosed in 1975–1984 to 5.4% for those diagnosed in 2005–2011, primarily due to decreases in mortality from primary cancer.[65,66] Although there have been improvements in the inclusion of AYA in clinical trials, there continue to be access-to-care and psychosocial issues for this vulnerable population.

Cancer Clinical Trials

Cancer clinical trials are studies designed to answer a specific scientific question that will lead to better ways to diagnose, prevent, and treat cancer.[67] Cancer clinical trials offer patients the opportunity to receive the newest treatments to improve cancer-related health options. They help to progress cancer control outcomes and may shorten treatment times, therefore improving quality of life by reducing the burden of treatment. In 1993, the NIH Revitalization Act stated that steps must be taken for women and minority patients to be included in NIH-sponsored research.[68] However, studies continue to indicate low rates of enrollment in clinical trials among minority, rural, and low socioeconomic subgroups.[69,70,71,72,73] Across the US, AI patients are among the most underrepresented in clinical trials based on race/ethnicity[62] and are enrolled at rates disproportionately lower than their percentage of the US population.

Most of the time, clinical trials test a new intervention by randomly assigning eligible participants to either a treatment or control group. A common misconception among AI/AN is that one is a guinea pig when taking part in clinical trials and that Indigenous Peoples only receive sugar (placebo) treatments. Of note, potential participants in clinical trials must make an informed choice to be included. Similarly, there rarely are placebo groups in any NIH-sponsored cancer clinical trial, unlike in pharmaceutical-supported trials. Rather, NIH trials provide options for Indigenous patients to receive standard care even if they are randomized into a control group. Researchers need to be prepared to discuss randomization, what it is, and why it is necessary to truly benefit the community. Educational materials have been developed for AI.[74]

Often Indigenous Peoples are blamed for low participation in clinical trials. However, research suggests that once Indigenous Peoples learn about clinical trials, they want to participate. Most Native patients with whom the authors have discussed clinical trials say they want to help subsequent cancer patients have a better experience than they had. Although the research staff can never promise that an individual patient will personally benefit from taking part in a clinical trial, most people hope that they will have some improvement in their cancer. Tips for recruiting and retaining Indigenous Peoples in clinical trials include:

- Explain the trial in a relaxed manner and encourage patients to ask questions.
- Provide accurate information to eliminate misconceptions about clinical trials and to allow patients to make an informed choice regarding participation.
- Provide *culturally appropriate* education on clinical trials.
- Encourage discussion of clinical trial options with significant others.
- Provide access to community patient navigators that have sufficient in-service training to explain the purpose and processes involved in a clinical trial.
- Allow patients to talk with others from a similar cultural background who can translate the clinical trial information into easy-to-understand language.
- Provide resources that effectively address barriers that interfere with participation.
- Allow flexibility in eligibility criteria.[66]

Children and Clinical Trials

Because of clinical trials, the 5-year survival among all US children with cancer have dramatically increased from 62% in the mid-1970s to 83% in the 2000s. Children's hospitals provide the highest number of pediatric clinical trials and facilitate the highest quality of life among children diagnosed with cancers. Addressing the gap in access to clinical trials for Indigenous children with cancer is a priority for improving survivability rates and for improving the process whereby Indigenous pediatric cancer data are more accurately reported. Patient navigation has proven to be effective in improving rates of Indigenous participation in clinical trials.[75,76]

In addition to participation in clinical trials, it is important to engage tribal members in health interventions, so that benefits are spread more widely in Indigenous communities. Below are four examples of AI/AN cancer health interventions conducted in the US.

Successful Indigenous Community-Engaged Interventions
Walking Forward[i]

Description

The Walking Forward program was founded in 2002 by Dr. Daniel Petereit to combat the high cancer mortality rates observed in the AI population in Western South Dakota. The program aimed to assess barriers to cancer detection, increase community education, and increase access to clinical trials.[77] With funding from the National Cancer Institute and support from Monument Health Rapid City Hospital (MHRCH) and, since 2016 from Avera Cancer Care Institute, Walking Forward enrolled more than 4,000 AI in various research studies. Between 2009 and 2012, Walking Forward supplemented the care of more than 1,900 AI patients and survivors through patient navigation.[78] This success story focuses on one of the first funded programs of Walking Forward in 2006–2008, which aimed to increase AI participation in clinical trials.

Intervention

Monument Health Rapid City Hospital (MHRCH), formally known as Rapid City Regional Hospital, is the secondary and tertiary oncology care provider to 60,000 adult AI in Western South Dakota. It serves as the major secondary and tertiary cancer services provider for the Oglala Sioux Tribe (Pine Ridge),

---

i Funding from NIH NCI 1U54CA142157 and 5U56CA099010.

Cheyenne River Sioux Tribe, Rosebud Sioux Tribe, and the Rapid City AI population. According to the Index of Medical Underservice,[79] the entire population of Western South Dakota is considered underserved.

Before the initiation of Walking Forward, limited infrastructure for clinical trials existed in this region, and less than 4% of patients and virtually no AI were enrolled. Components of the intervention to increase AI participation in clinical trials included (a) a culturally tailored patient navigation program that facilitated access to innovative clinical trials in conjunction with a comprehensive educational program encouraging screening and early detection, (b) surveys to evaluate barriers to access, and (c) clinical trials focusing on reducing treatment length to facilitate enhanced participation. A nurse navigator working at MHRCH was trained to identify cancer patients that might be eligible for clinical trial enrollment. Each patient met with the principal investigator (PI), who was a radiation oncologist, to discuss the recommended cancer care and learn about clinical trial options appropriate for their cancer. This first appointment took 30–45 minutes, and included questions like "How would you or your family members travel to Rapid City for treatments if you were scheduled for several days for six weeks?" Concerns about coercion by the provider were addressed by excluding the opportunity to enroll in the clinical trial until the second visit. This ensured that the patient took the time to consider the treatment choices outside of the clinical setting with their support system, helping to secure commitment.[72]

Community Engagement

To recruit and retain AI cancer patients in clinical trials, it was necessary to engage community leaders and IHS physicians. Throughout the grant application process, the PI continued dialogue with the tribes, including frequent in-person visits to the community and tribal council presentations. In-person visits demonstrated commitment and respect toward community leaders and physicians while the commute of 2-plus hours allowed for a shared understanding of how driving time/conditions are significant barriers for patients. It was only after years of laying the foundation that patient recruitment began.[80]

Outcomes

Critical Walking Forward outcomes included establishing trust within tribal communities, identifying barriers to cancer screening, increasing patient satisfaction, and enrolling patients in phase II clinical trials. Walking Forward tracked clinical trial enrollment for new patients presenting at MHRCH from Pine Ridge, Cheyenne River Sioux, and Rosebud Reservations and Rapid City, South Dakota, between September 2006 and January 2008.[81] The study also aimed to identify reasons for nonparticipation in clinical trials in rural community hospital settings. All patients presenting for an initial evaluation were eligible for inclusion in this analysis. Of the 94 AI patients evaluated, 6 were placed on a clinical treatment trial. This effort resulted in an increase in the percentage of clinical treatment trial patients who were AI, from almost 0% at the start of the intervention to 8% afterward.

For the 88 AI patients who were not enrolled in cancer treatment trials, the primary reasons for nonenrollment were (1) advanced stage/poor performance status/comorbidities (27%), (2) no protocol for tumor site (24%), (3) other reasons for ineligibility after evaluation (23%), (4) physician judgment/trial treatment not appropriate (20%), (5) patient refused/preferred standard treatment/preferred no treatment (4%), and (6) contract health coverage (through IHS) denied trial treatment coverage (1%).[76]

Lessons Learned

Walking Forward has an extensive history in Western South Dakota, through which program leaders have learned major lessons. First, sociocultural factors and mistrust may play a role in hindering efforts to engage minority populations in research-related treatment regimens, and South Dakota AI patients exhibit higher levels of medical mistrust and higher levels of dissatisfaction with previous healthcare compared to their White counterparts.[82,83,84,85,86,87]

Second, little published data exist on successful trial recruitment programs, perhaps reflecting the heterogeneity of underserved populations, and what works in one vulnerable or underserved population may not serve another as well.[88] Recruitment for all clinical research is dependent upon trust, which must be built before grant submission to align community and academic priorities with a shared interest in potential outcomes. While waiting for grant decisions, communication must be maintained with frequent community visits. Throughout the process, remaining aware of changing tribal leadership is advantageous to avoid aligning with groups that may hinder recruitment. Sharing preliminary data with the community throughout the study reinforces the trusting relationship, allowing for future recruitment.

Third, patient navigator programs may provide a culturally competent avenue to actively engage vulnerable populations in the cancer care continuum, including clinical trial participation.[89,90,91,92,93] Walking Forward has two patient navigation programs, one at the community level, and one within the cancer center. These efforts have increased visibility and trust, which may be responsible for the improved rates of AI enrollment on clinical trials.

Fourth, when serving a rural population with low socioeconomic status, it is difficult to recruit patients to phase III trials involving emerging technologies due to the possibility of extended treatment times. When presented with an option for treatment regimens with a lower time burden (short-course radiation therapy) versus the possibility of weeks of protracted standard therapy, many patients simply opt for the shortest course of treatment rather than risk randomization to a longer regimen. In comparison, phase II clinical trials offer access to emerging treatments without the risk of being randomized into a longer treatment regimen. In the future, an increase in the number of short treatment time phase II trials may be better suited for limited access populations.

Namitunatya: *A Pilot Study to Increase Cancer Screenings of Hopi Men*[ii]

Description

The study aimed to assess the feasibility of a future intervention study using mobile health (mHealth) technology to increase preventive care utilization and cancer screening among Hopi men living on the reservation. Namitunatya, a Hopi word translated as "taking care of yourself," was used as a cultural vehicle to influence the health behaviors of Hopi men. This study was a collaborative project involving the Hopi Office of Prevention and Intervention (HOPI) Cancer Support Services, Northern Arizona University (NAU), and the University of Arizona (UA). The study was funded through an NIH grant to NAU and UA as part of the Partnership for Native American Cancer Prevention.

Studies showed that AI/AN men have higher death rates for many diseases, including cancer, than non-Hispanic White (NHW) men or AI/AN women.[94,95] Despite the heavy disease burden among AI/AN men, they have low healthcare utilization and poor access to care.[96,97,98] The Hopi Tribe is one of the 22 tribes in Arizona. There are approximately 14,000 persons enrolled in the Hopi Tribe, half of whom live on the Hopi reservation. There were approximately 2,081 households; 62% of the population spoke a language other than English at home, 20% of whom spoke English less than very well. Based on Hopi tribal enrollment record, there were approximately 910 men eligible for cancer screening in 2021.

The *Hopi Survey of Cancer and Chronic Disease* was conducted in 2012 with randomly selected 248 Hopi men and 252 Hopi women. Results revealed high blood pressure, diabetes, asthma, high cholesterol, and cancer as the five most preventable chronic diseases. Results revealed that Hopi men received

ii Funding from NIH NCI U54CA143924 and U54CA143925.

inadequate direction from healthcare providers and insufficient information about preventive care and cancer screenings.

Based on these data, the pilot study's intended population was Hopi adult men that resided on the Hopi Reservation in Arizona. A Hopi male Native patient navigator (NPN) conducted educational group sessions with Hopi men and used an audience response system (ARS) to collect needs assessment data specific to the use of cell phones. These assessments revealed Hopi male participants had minimal knowledge about cancer, colorectal cancer, and prostate cancer screening.

Intervention

The study used community-based participatory research principles to guide communication and collaboration among the three partners utilizing mHealth (text messaging). A review of the literature revealed limited information available for reservation residents who are AI men using mHealth technology and text messaging for preventive care and cancer screening reminders.

During the pilot study, the team developed a NPN-led mHealth program to test the effectiveness after consulting with expert NPN and the study's Community Advisory Committee (CAC). Focus group and survey results assisted to define the responsibilities of the male NPN in the HOPI Cancer Program. These were tested for cultural appropriateness with a small group of Hopi men. An example of a text message: "Do you know that colorectal cancer (CRC) is the leading cause of new cases of cancer among American Indians? According to our records, you are over 50 and/or have a family history of CRC. Contact HOPI Cancer Support Services navigator at 928-734-xxxx". The Native patient navigation program for men and the effectiveness of the text messaging and educational materials were pilot tested in coordination with an IHS facility on Hopi Reservation and a tribal-operated healthcare facility outside the Hopi Reservation border to track Hopi patient screening and follow-up during spring and summer 2019.

Community Engagement

This study was a community-initiated pilot study. The Hopi team gained Hopi tribal resolution approval and facility support, submitted a grant proposal to the NACP, recruited Hopi males to the CAC, and hosted quarterly CAC meetings. The CAC members reviewed the study protocol, consent forms, and focus group and survey questions to assess cultural appropriateness and provided suggestions for improvement as well as recruitment strategies. The Hopi team hired male NPN who lived on the Hopi Reservation, recruited and interviewed Hopi male participants, and retained signed informed consent documents. The university team did not get copies of the signed informed consent documents to maintain confidentiality. The university team assisted with meeting expenses, designed the surveys based upon literature reviews, received Institutional Review Board approvals, provided participants with a gift card, hired a Hopi focus group facilitator, ensured that approved research protocols were followed and implemented, and organized weekly phone meetings.

Men from racial/ethnic minority groups generally have low enrollment in biomedical studies.[99,100] To overcome this challenge, the team used several recruitment strategies. First, the Hopi team sent mass email messages and newsletters to Hopi tribal employees. Second, the team made announcements during community health events to advertise focus groups and ARS community surveys for men. The team also recruited focus group participants in front of village stores during the lunch hour. Finally, the NPN implemented door-to-door home recruitment and telephone calls to explain the benefits of cancer screening and the need to develop a Hopi men's cancer program. The Hopi men that the research team talked to in the community generally showed their concerns about increasing cancer diagnosis and an unhealthy lifestyle in the community and interest in participating in the study.

The NPN contacted an urban cancer center's Native American oncology nurse to post flyers and encourage the Hopi patients to contact the NPN. Additionally, the NPN conducted home visits to recruit Hopi men that were cancer survivors. Ten cancer survivors were recruited. The team conducted nine focus group sessions held in locations such as the Hopi Cultural Center, HOPI Cancer Support Services, and Village Community Development Office. Participants were offered transportation support, meals, and incentives (gift cards). Participants included 29 Hopi men without prior cancer diagnoses plus 10 Hopi men who were cancer survivors.

The pilot project team received two types of tribal resolution approvals. The Hopi Tribal Council resolution language included approval for Hopi eligible men to participate in the study and to disseminate results in the Hopi community. It also specified that all data were the property of the Hopi Tribe. The second resolution allowed the NPN to have access to the electronic patient records to assess cancer screening outcomes and results at the two participating health facilities.

Outcomes

The study enrolled 29 eligible men who were assigned to two groups; 14 men (48.3%) were assigned to a mHealth group to receive text messages from the NPN, and 15 men (51.7%) were assigned to a NPN-only group. The mHealth group was younger (average age of 58.7), while the average age of the NPN-only group was 67.9. In the NPN-only group, 53.3% of men were retired, while only 7.1% of men in the mHealth reported were retired.

During the pilot intervention period, six (20.7%) participants completed CRC screening (colonoscopy or fecal occult blood test (FOBT)), and seven participants (24.1%) either completed or scheduled prostate-specific antigen (PSA) screening. Among six who completed CRC screening, colonoscopy (5 men) was more common than FOBT (1 man). Three out of 14 (21.4%) in the mHealth group had CRC screening, while 3 out of 15 (20.0%) in the NPN-only group had CRC screening. Three out of 14 (21.4%) in the mHealth group completed PSA screening, and 4 out of 15 (26.7%) in the NPN-only group completed or scheduled PSA screening. The three-month pilot program evaluation indicated that mHealth and NPN-only approaches both may increase cancer screening among Hopi men living on Hopi Reservation.

Lessons Learned

The project team determined it was necessary to hire a Hopi male NPN from the start date of the project. The Hopi male NPN proved to be an invaluable asset to the overall pilot study. He assisted with project logistics, recruited eligible men for surveys and focus groups, and became the "face" of the project in the community. The team had difficulty recruiting Hopi male cancer survivors, especially with the eligibility criterion 50 years and older, and confusion as to what "cancer survivor" referred to. A focus group for cancer survivors had one participant who showed up and said he was a cancer survivor because close family members (mom, uncle) had cancer and passed away, which indicated there was a need for community-based cancer education.

Native American Cancer Education for Survivors (NACES)[iii]

Description

Native American Cancer Education for Survivors (NACES) was a web-based public health education program designed to increase the quality of life of AI/AN cancer survivors.[101,102,103,104,105,106,107] NACES began in 1996 with a focus on breast cancer survivorship, and later evolved into a culturally appropriate, interactive web-based education site for all AI/AN cancer survivors.[108] Between 1998 and 2019, an average of 800 users visited the website each month.

iii Funded by NIH NCI R25CA101938 and U01CA114609 and Susan G. Komen Foundation #POP0503920 and #POP0202135.

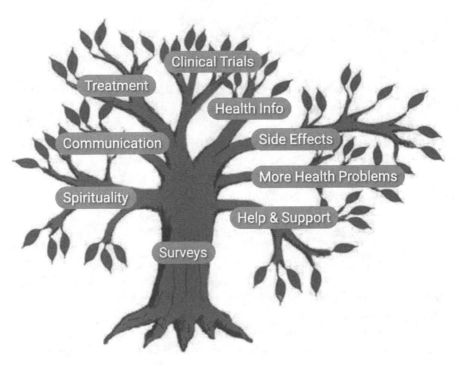

Fig 7.1. NACES QOL tree. Created by Linda Burhansstipanov.

Intervention

The NACES interactive website included several components. First, visitors could complete a quality of life (QOL) survey. The survey's 178 items solicited information on cancer history, cancer treatment, barriers to care, and QOL measures for mental/emotional, physical, social, and spiritual domains. These four domains represent the domains of the Medicine Wheel. In 2013, additional items from the NIH Patient-Reported Outcomes Measurement Information System (PROMIS®) measures were added. The content of NACES was organized as a QOL tree (Figure 7.1). The roots of the tree represented ancestry, family, and cultural strengths. Surveys were on the "trunk" of the NACES QOL tree. The "branches" included culturally modified and scientifically accurate content about cancer, presented at reading grade levels 5–7 for most pages.

Community Engagement

The development and testing of NACES was guided by a community advisory board (CAB). Members of the CAB included 12 AI/AN men and women living in diverse geographic regions of the US who were survivors of lymphoma, breast cancer, head and neck cancers, and other cancers. The advisory board and cancer survivors recommended people to create the content for the NACES branches. For example, Drs. Jennie Joe and DeeAnn DeRoin created the breast cancer and diabetes pages, Caren Trujillo created the content for spirituality, and Maxine Brings Him Back Janis developed the content for oral side effects. The NACES research team reviewed all content for cultural appropriateness and scientific accuracy before posting online.

Outcomes

There were 1,237 deidentified surveys collected between 1998 and 2017, with about 175 of them completed by family members on behalf of the cancer survivor. The research team quickly learned that information collected by family members was less accurate according to the survivors during subsequent conversations. For example, one survivor said, "Those answers about pain weren't correct. I didn't want my granddaughter to know that I was having trouble." For this reason, the NACES research team only included surveys completed by the survivors in data summaries.

Of the cancer survivors who visited the website and completed the surveys, 79.2% were female, 46.0% had a high school education or less, and 53.4% identified themselves as full-blooded AI or AN. Most were from the Southwest and the Northern and Southern Plains. In terms of residence, 37.1% lived in urban areas, 33.6% on reservations, 18.5% in rural communities (nonreservation), and 10.9% moved back and forth from city/rural/reservation. Most patients had significant comorbidity conditions that impacted their QOL.

Transportation (distances, duration, and expense) was the most consistent barrier to accessing quality cancer care.[109] Almost half (48.7%) traveled more than 100 miles *one-way* to access cancer care, and 15% traveled more than 400 miles *one-way* to access treatment. Another major barrier was the time it took, 6–9 months, to process referrals to care through the IHS/PRC service, previously called "Contract Health Services." On average, only 12% of the responding survivors received cancer care through IHS/PRC. Referrals to cancer care were greatly delayed via local clinics. There were more successful referrals to the Veterans Administration or Medicaid than through IHS. Medicaid was used frequently because many patients were younger than age 65 and, thus, not eligible for Medicare. Privately insured participants reported more barriers to access treatment than Medicaid participants, in part because many AI/AN with private health insurance were unfamiliar with how to use it.

Another common barrier identified was cultural differences between Western medicine and Native American culture. The more barriers the patient experienced, the more likely the patient was to report a poorer QOL. Social

QOL scores were significantly impacted when individuals encountered five or more barriers when accessing initial cancer care. Those who had less than a high school education reported more barriers than those who had higher educational attainment.

Patients who had the support of a NPN noted that they were helpful in overcoming barriers, especially logistic barriers and cultural mismatches between Western medicine and Native American culture. AI/AN cancer patients who received patient navigation had fewer interruptions during cancer treatment and reported higher satisfaction with healthcare, though medical mistrust was not significantly improved.

Areas associated with a positive QOL following a cancer diagnosis were strong feelings of spirituality and strong relationships with family and community. Finding strength in one's spirituality, Native identity, and traditions was critical in framing survivors' orientation to illness and healing and to improving survivors' cancer journeys. Also, nearly all survivors expressed feelings of deep responsibility to share their cancer stories with others to help Native communities.[110] They also almost universally put their family and other loved one's needs before their own. Many survivors emphasized the importance of "living both ways" by embracing both traditional modes of healing and Western medicine. These survivors felt that Western medicine alone was insufficient for healing the whole self, including the physical, mental/emotional, social, and spiritual domains of wellness.

Lessons Learned

As of 2018, about half of the NACES survivors still did not have private health insurance and still were limited in their access to cancer care services. AI/AN cancer survivors accessing NACES were younger at the time of diagnosis (~48% younger than age 50) than other racial groups and had significant comorbidity conditions that impacted their QOL. In the late 1990s and early 2000s, about two-thirds of the survivors reported being diagnosed at an advanced stage of disease—for example, stage 3 or 4, when cancer is more difficult to treat. However, between 2010 and 2019, 75% of NACES survivors were being diagnosed in stages 1 and 2. This represented significant improvement throughout Indian Country.

Survivors continued to need assertive strategies to gain timely access to quality cancer care. Most survivors welcomed assistance from the NPN, but others learned to advocate for themselves. More than half of all NACES survivors continued to have long and late effects from cancer or cancer treatment (e.g., pain, cognitive dysfunction) and needed continued support 5 years beyond their initial diagnoses.

Improving Colorectal Cancer Screening Among Alaska Native People[iv]

Description

AN people are a diverse population, with multiple cultures and languages throughout Alaska. However, AN people face one of the world's highest rates of colorectal cancer (CRC). CRC is the second leading cause of new cases of cancer among AN people, with rates of new cases and deaths two times higher than US Whites.[111] Incidence is higher in every age group, and as high in 40–49-year-old AN people as in the US White 50–59-year-old age group.[112] AN people also have higher CRC rates than AI living in the rest of the US.[18] CRC screening can prevent this cancer or identify it early when it is highly treatable,[2] but the vast geography of Alaska combined with small community sizes makes access to CRC screening difficult.

An effort by tribal health leadership led to a focus on cancer prevention within the Alaska Native Tribal Health System. Initiatives around CRC screening and prevention included training midlevel rural providers in flexible sigmoidoscopy,[113] providing itinerant colonoscopy services at rural tribal health facilities, and integrating a CRC screening patient navigator project within a CDC-funded tribal breast and cervical cancer early detection program. In addition, the creation and use of an AN CRC first-degree relative database facilitated CRC screening for those at increased risk.[114]

Intervention

These efforts were assisted from 2009 to 2015 when the CDC funded three Alaska tribal health organizations to establish CRC programs, including one at the Alaska Native Tribal Health Consortium (ANTHC).[115,116] The ANTHC CRC Control Program aimed to increase screening among AI/AN people living in Alaska through the provision of direct screening services, provider education, community outreach and education, and policy and systems-level improvements. Direct screening included setting up screening programs at rural/remote tribal health organizations. An important strategy for the program was to hire and train culturally knowledgeable AI/AN patient navigators who were able to connect with clients and help get them screened. The program held annual trainings for healthcare providers and others on patient navigation, social marketing, motivational interviewing, and health literacy; periodic teleconference in-services; and presentations at the statewide Community Health Aide Program annual training.

---

iv Funding from CDC 5U58DP002032.

Community Engagement

To improve community outreach, the ANTHC CRC Control Program collaborated with other tribal organizations and the State of Alaska to develop AN culturally relevant media. These included patient reminder cards, brochures, posters, newsletters, videos, and digital stories as part of "The Cancer I Can Prevent" campaign, which featured AN and non-Native people sharing their screening stories. As a result, ANTHC, along with the Alaska CRC Partnership, won the Prevent Cancer Foundation's 2014 National "Screening Saves Lives" Challenge.

The ANTHC CRC Control Program received feedback from elders and other AN community members that they wanted more humor in cancer prevention messaging. Subsequently, they purchased Nolan the Colon, a giant inflatable colon that traveled around the state with staff to promote CRC screening to community members. A study on the use of the giant colon at community events found that Nolan the Colon significantly increased knowledge of CRC screening, intention to screen, and comfort talking about screening with friends and family.[117]

Systems and policy changes included greater use of patient navigators at regional tribal health organizations to encourage screening, improvements in access to CRC screening including client and provider reminders in the electronic medical record, direct access to endoscopy, and improved clinical workflows to reduce system barriers to screening. There have been several collaborative research studies investigating the effectiveness of different CRC screening methods such as the fecal immunochemical test and the stool DNA test (Cologuard®) to improve screening test availability in the tribal health system.[118,119]

Outcomes

As a result of these combined efforts, CRC screening increased substantially among AN people. Before the CRC Control Programs, the AN CRC screening rate was about 10–15% lower than that of Alaska non-Natives. During the years of the program, the AN screening rate climbed to about 4% higher than Alaska non-Natives (66.4% vs. 62.0%).[120] While this progress is encouraging, the AN screening rate still did not meet the national Healthy People 2020 CRC screening goal of 70.5% or the National CRC Roundtable's 80% in every community goal. AN screening rates also vary substantially by Alaska tribal health region from 29% to 73%.[121]

Lessons Learned

Patient navigators and the need to address capacity and systems barriers to screening are vital to success. Given Alaska's many small and geographically isolated AN communities, the focus remains on developing programs to give all AN people access to some form of CRC screening. The Alaska Tribal Health System continues to work to find novel and innovative ways to increase CRC screening among AN people to ensure that fewer AN people suffer from this preventable disease.

Summary

This chapter provided an overview of cancer in AI/AN communities and provided four examples of successful and emerging programs designed to address cancer. Long-established programs, such as Walking Forward, document the commitment of healthcare providers and communities to collaborate to create the most successful clinical trial program for AI in the US. In the Hopi Men's Study, the community perceived men's health as a priority and developed cultural messages to increase cancer screening among men through a dynamic community-driven process. The development of the NACES website was guided by AI/AN community representatives and cancer survivors to provide education and collect data on QOL. The Alaska CRC screening program targeted hard-to-reach and high-risk AN and used humor (Nolan the Colon and people in polyp costumes) to get the community's attention and engagement. All four programs used or tracked the use of navigators (i.e., people from the community trained to educate about cancer and guide AI/AN to cancer screening and treatment programs), and more examples of successful use of cancer patient navigation are provided in the next chapter.

References

1. American Cancer Society. *Cancer facts and figures 2020*. Accessed February 28, 2021. https://www.cancer.org/content/dam/cancer-org/research/cancer-facts-and-statistics/annual-cancer-facts-and-figures/2020/cancer-facts-and-figures-2020.pdf.

2. American Cancer Society. *Colorectal cancer facts & figures 2020–2022*. Accessed May 14, 2021. https://www.cancer.org/content/dam/cancer-org/research/cancer-facts-and-statistics/colorectal-cancer-facts-and-figures/colorectal-cancer-facts-and-figures-2020-2022.pdf.

3. Burhansstipanov L, Dignan M, Jones KL, *et al.* Comparison of quality of life between Native and non-Native cancer survivors: Native and non-Native cancer survivors' QOL. *J Cancer Educ.* 2012;27(1 Suppl):S106–S113.

4. Cobb N, Espey D, King J. Health behaviors and risk factors among American Indians and Alaska Natives, 2000–2010. *Am J Public Health.* 2014;104 Suppl 3(Suppl 3):S481–S489.

5. Indian Health and Family Services. GPRA and other national reporting. Accessed May 23, 2021. https://www.ihs.gov/crs/gprareporting/.

6. Howlader N, Noone AM, Krapcho M, *et al. SEER cancer statistics review, 1975–2016*. National Cancer Institute. Accessed February 28, 2021. https://seer.cancer.gov/archive/csr/1975_2016/.

7. Kunitz SJ, Veazie M, Henderson JA. Historical trends and regional differences in all-cause and amenable mortality among American Indians and Alaska Natives since 1950. *Am J Public Health.* 2014;104:S268–S277.

8. Espey DK, Wu XC, Swan J, *et al.* Annual report to the nation on the status of cancer, 1975–2004, featuring cancer in American Indians and Alaska Natives. *Cancer.* 2007;110(10):2119–2152.

9. Espey D, Paisano R, Cobb N. Regional patterns and trends in cancer mortality among American Indians and Alaska Natives, 1990–2001. *Cancer.* 2005;103 (5):1045–1053.

10. Haverkamp D, Espey D, Paisano R, *et al. Cancer mortality among American Indians and Alaska Natives: Regional differences, 1999–2003.* Indian Health Service, 2008.

11. Wiggins CL, Espey DK, Wingo PA, *et al.* Cancer among American Indians and Alaska Natives in the United States, 1999–2004. *Cancer.* 2008;113(5 Suppl):1142–1152.

12. Cobb N, Paisano RE. Patterns of cancer mortality among Native Americans. *Cancer.* 1998;83(11):2377–2383.

13. White MC, Espey DK, Swan J, *et al.* Disparities in cancer mortality and incidence among American Indians and Alaska Natives in the United States. *Am J Public Health.* 2014;104:S377–S387.

14. Bauer UE, Plescia M. Addressing disparities in the health of American Indian and Alaska Native people: the importance of improved public health data. *Am J Public Health.* 2014;104(Suppl 3):S255–S257.

15. Colorado Department of Public Health and Environment. Inequity fact sheets. Accessed September 8, 2020. www.colorado.gov/pacific/cdphe/inequity-factsheets.

16. White A, Richardson LC, Li C, *et al.* Breast cancer mortality among American Indian and Alaska Native women, 1990–2009. *Am J Public Health.* 2014;104 Suppl 3(Suppl 3):S432–S438.

17. Watson M, Benard V, Thomas C, *et al.* Cervical cancer incidence and mortality among American Indian and Alaska Native women, 1999–2009. *Am J Public Health.* 2014;104(Suppl 3):S415–S422.

18. Perdue DG, Haverkamp D, Perkins C, *et al.* Geographic variation in colorectal cancer incidence and mortality, age of onset, and stage at diagnosis among American Indian and Alaska Native people, 1990–2009. *Am J Public Health.* 2014;104 Suppl 3(Suppl 3):S404–S414.

19. Siegel RL, Miller KD, Jemal A. Cancer statistics, 2017. *CA Cancer J Clin.* 2017;67(1):7–30.

20. Navajo Cancer Workgroup. *Cancer among the Navajo, 2005–2013.* Navajo Epidemiology Center, 2017.

21. Lanier AP, Redwood DG, Kelly JJ. The Alaska education and research towards health (EARTH) study: Cancer risk factors. *J Cancer Educ.* 2012;27(1 Suppl):S80–S85.

22. Health status of American Indians compared with other racial/ethnic minority populations—selected states, 2001–2002. *MMWR Morb Mortal Wkly Rep.* 2003;52(47):1148–1152.

23. Plescia M, Henley SJ, Pate A, *et al.* Lung cancer deaths among American Indians and Alaska Natives, 1990–2009. *Am J Public Health.* 2014;104 Suppl 3(Suppl 3):S388–S395.

24. Espey DK, Jim MA, Cobb N, *et al.* Leading causes of death and all-cause mortality in American Indians and Alaska Natives. *Am J Public Health.* 2014;104 Suppl 3(Suppl 3):S303–S311.

25. Hoffman RM, Li J, Henderson JA, *et al.* Prostate cancer deaths and incident cases among American Indian/Alaska Native men, 1999–2009. *Am J Public Health.* 2014;104 Suppl 3(Suppl 3):S439–S445.

26. Kaur JS, Burhansstipanov L, Krebs LU. Understanding the true burden of cancer in American Indian and Alaska Native communities. In: Jackson OT, Evans KA, eds. *Health disparities*. Nova Science Publishers, Inc., 2013:39–75. https://mayoclinic.pure.elsevier.com /en/publications/understanding-the-true-burden-of-cancer-in-american-indian-and-al.

27. Day GE, Provost E, Lanier AP. Alaska native mortality rates and trends. *Public Health Rep.* 2009;124(1):54–64.

28. Centers for Disease Control. Cancer statistics at a glance. Accessed January 29, 2022. https://gis.cdc.gov/Cancer/USCS/#/AtAGlance/.

29. Alaska Native Epidemiology Center. *Alaska Native mortality: 1980–2018*. Anchorage (US): Alaska Native Epidemiology Center; 2021.

30. Jemal A, Ward EM, Johnson CJ, et al. Annual report to the nation on the status of cancer, 1975–2014, featuring survival. *J Natl Cancer Inst.* 2017;109(9).

31. Cancer Trends Progress Report. National Cancer Institute, NIH, DHHS, Bethesda, MD, March 2020. Accessed September 8, 2020. https://progressreport.cancer.gov.

32. Bastian TD, Burhansstipanov L. Sharing wisdom, sharing hope: Strategies used by Native American cancer survivors to restore quality of life. *JCO Global Oncol.* 2020:6:161–166.

33. Braun KL, Kim BJ, Ka'opua LS, et al. Native Hawaiian and Pacific Islander elders: What gerontologists should know. *Gerontologist.* 2015;55:912–919.

34. Miller BA, Chu KC, Hankey BF, et al. Cancer incidence and mortality patterns among specific Asian and Pacific Islander populations in the US. *Cancer Causes Control.* 2008;19(3):257–258.

35. Tsark J. Cancer in Native Hawaiians. *Pac Health Dialog.* 1998;5:315–327.

36. Tsark JU, Braun KL. Eyes on the Pacific: Cancer issues of Native Hawaiians and Pacific Islanders in Hawai'i and the US-Associated Pacific. *J Cancer Educ.* 2009;24(Suppl 2):S68–S69.

37. Tsark JU, Cancer Council of the Pacific Islands. Braun KL. Reducing cancer health disparities in the US-associated Pacific. *J Public Health Manage Pract.* 2007;13:49–58.

38. National Cancer Institute Surveillance, Epidemiology, and End Results Program. International classification of childhood cancers. Accessed March 28, 2021. https://seer .cancer.gov/iccc/

39. Bhatia S, Gibson TM, Ness KK, et al. Childhood cancer survivorship research in minority populations: A position paper from the Childhood Cancer Survivor Study. *Cancer.* 2016;122(15):2426–2439.

40. Valery PC, Moore SP, Meiklejohn J, et al. International variations in childhood cancer in Indigenous populations: A systematic review. *Lancet Oncol.* 2014;15(2):e90–e103.

41. Johnson KJ, Cullen J, Barnholtz-Sloan JS, et al. Childhood brain tumor epidemiology: A brain tumor epidemiology consortium review. *Cancer Epidemiol Biomarkers Prev.* 2014;23(12):2716–2736.

42. U.S. Department of Health and Human Services National Institutes of Health. Analysis of the National Cancer Institute's Investment in Pediatric Cancer Research. National Cancer Institute, 2013. Accessed March 29, 2021. https://www.cancer.gov/types /childhood-cancers/research/pediatric-analysis.pdf.

43. Wang L, Gomez SL Yasui Y. Racial and ethnic differences in socioeconomic position and risk of childhood acute lymphoblastic leukemia. *Am J Epidemiol.* 2017;185(12):1263–1271.

44. Chow EJ, Puumala SE, Mueller BA, et al. Childhood cancer in relation to parental race and ethnicity: A 5-state pooled analysis. *Cancer.* 2010;116(12):3045–3053.

45. Lim JYS, Bhatia S, Robison LL, et al. Genomics of racial and ethnic disparities in childhood acute lymphoblastic leukemia. *Cancer.* 2014;120(7):955–962.

46. Yang JJ, Cheng C, Devidas M, *et al.* Ancestry and pharmacogenomics of relapse in acute lymphoblastic leukemia. *Nat Genet.* 2011;43(3):237–241.

47. Xu H, Cheng C, Devidas M, *et al.* ARID5B genetic polymorphisms contribute to racial disparities in the incidence and treatment outcome of childhood acute lymphoblastic leukemia. *J Clin Oncol.* 2012;30(7):751–757.

48. Willman CL, Cancer health disparities in AI and Alaska Native populations. *Cancer Res.* 2017;77(13 Suppl):SY14-04.

49. Lanier AP, Holck P, Day GE, *et al.* Childhood cancer among Alaska Natives. *Pediatrics.* 2003;112:e396.

50. Campbell JE, Martinez SA, Janitz AE, *et al.* Cancer incidence and staging among American Indians in Oklahoma. *J Okla State Med Assoc.* 2014;107(3):99–107.

51. Harpaz R, McMahon BJ, Margolis, HS, *et al.* Elimination of new chronic hepatitis B virus infections: Results of the Alaska immunization program. *J Infect Dis.* 2000;181(2):413–418.

52. Perez-Andreu V, Roberts KG, Xu H, *et al.* A genome-wide association study of susceptibility to acute lymphoblastic leukemia in adolescents and young adults. *Blood.* 2015;125(4):680–686.

53. Rotte L, Hansford J, Kirby M, *et al.* Cancer in Australian Aboriginal children: Room for improvement. *J Paediatr Child Health.* 2013;49:27–32.

54. Foucar K, Duncan MH, Stidley CA, *et al.* Survival of children and adolescents with acute lymphoid leukemia. A study of American Indians and Hispanic and non-Hispanic whites treated in New Mexico (1969 to 1986). *Cancer.* 1991;67:2125–2130.

55. Ridgway D, Skeen JE, Mauger DC, *et al.* Childhood cancer among the Polynesian population. *Cancer.* 1991;68:451–454.

56. Kadan-Lottick NS, Ness KK, *et al.* Survival variability by race and ethnicity in childhood acute lymphoblastic leukemia. *JAMA.* 2003;290:2008–2014.

57. Goggins WB, Lo FF. Racial and ethnic disparities in survival of US children with acute lymphoblastic leukemia: Evidence from the SEER database 1988–2008. *Cancer Causes Control.* 2012;23:737–743.

58. Henderson TO, Bhatia S, Pinto N, *et al.* Racial and ethnic disparities in risk and survival in children with neuroblastoma: A Children's Oncology Group Study. *J Clin Oncol.* 2011;29(1):76–82.

59. Smith MA, Seibel NL, Altekruse SF, *et al.* Outcomes for children and adolescents with cancer: challenges for the twenty-first century. *J Clin Oncol.* 2010;28:2625–2634.

60. Janitz AE, Campbell JE, Pate A, *et al.* Racial, ethnic, and age differences in the incidence and survival of childhood cancer in Oklahoma, 1997–2012. *J Okla State Med Assoc.* 2016;109(7–8):355–365.

61. Bhatia S. Disparities in cancer outcomes: Lessons learned from children with cancer. *Pediatr Blood Cancer.* 2011;56(6):994–1002.

62. Surveillance, Epidemiology, and End Results (SEER) Program. SEER incidence data, 1975 - 2017. Accessed May 2020. https://seer.cancer.gov/data/.

63. Close AG, Dreyzin A, Miller KD, *et al.* Adolescent and young adult oncology-past, present, and future. *CA Cancer J Clin.* 2019;69(6):485–496.

64. Go RS, Gundrum JD. Cancer in the adolescent and young adult (AYA) population in the United States: Current statistics and projections. *J Clinical Oncol.* 2011;29(15_suppl): 6072–6072.

65. Anderson C, Nichols HB. Trends in late mortality among adolescent and young adult (AYA) cancer survivors. *J Natl Cancer Inst.* 2020;112(10):994–1002.

66. Pollock BH. Where adolescents and young adults with cancer receive their care: Does it matter? *J Clin Oncol.* 2007;25(29):4522–4523.

67. National Cancer Institute. NCI dictionary of cancer terms: "Clinical trial." Accessed March 8, 2021. https://www.cancer.gov/publications/dictionaries/cancer-terms?expand=C.

68. National Institute of Health. S.1 - National institutes of health revitalization act of 1993. Accessed March 8, 2021. https://orwh.od.nih.gov/sites/orwh/files/docs/NIH-Revitalization-Act-1993.pdf.

69. Sateren WB, Trimble EL, Abrams J, et al. How sociodemographics, presence of oncology specialists, and hospital cancer programs affect accrual to cancer treatment trials. *J Clin Oncol.* 2002;20:2109–2117.

70. Murthy VH, Krumholz HM, Gross CP. Participation in cancer clinical trials: Race-, sex-, and age-based disparities. *JAMA.* 2004;291:2720–2726.

71. Baquet CR, Commiskey P, Daniel Mullins C, et al. Recruitment and participation in CTs: Socio-demographic, rural/urban, and health care access predictors. *Cancer Detect Prev.* 2006;30:24–33.

72. Stewart JH, Bertoni AG, Staten JL, et al. Participation in surgical oncology clinical trials: Gender-, race/ethnicity-, and age-based disparities. *Ann Surg Oncol.* 2007;4:3328–3334.

73. Gross CP, Filardo G, Mayne ST, et al. The impact of socioeconomic status and race on trial participation for older women with breast cancer. *Cancer.* 2005;103(3):483–491.

74. Native American Cancer Initiatives. Training: Clinical trials education for Native Americans. Accessed February 28, 2021. https://natamcancer.org/Training#trainings.

75. Guadagnolo BA, Boylan A, Sargent M, et al. Patient navigation for American Indians undergoing cancer treatment: Utilization and impact on care delivery in a regional healthcare center. *Cancer.* 2011;117(12):2754–2761.

76. Burhansstipanov L, Bad Wound D, Capelouto N, et al. Culturally relevant "navigator" patient support: The Native sisters. *Cancer Pract.* 1998;6(3):191–194.

77. Petereit DG, Rogers D, Govern F, et al. Increasing access to clinical cancer trials and emerging technologies for minority populations: The Native American project. *J Clin Oncol.* 2005;22:4452–4455.

78. Petereit DG, Guadagnolo BA, Wong R, et al. Addressing cancer disparities among American Indians through innovative technologies and patient navigation: The Walking Forward experience. *Front Oncol.* 2011;1:11.

79. The Index of Medical Underservice Indicators. Reviewing shortage designation applications. Accessed October 4, 2018. https://bhw.hrsa.gov/shortage-designation/muap-process.

80. Petereit DG, Burhansstipanov L. Establishing Trusting partnerships for successful recruitment of American Indians to clinical trials. *Cancer Control.* 2008;15:260–268.

81. Guadagnolo BA, Petereit DG, Helbig P, et al. Involving American Indians and medically underserved rural populations in cancer clinical trials. *Clin Trials.* 2009;6(6):610–617.

82. Corbie-Smith G, Thomas SB, St. George DM. Distrust, race, and research. *Arch Intern Med.* 2002;162:2458–2463.

83. Roberson NL. Clinical trial participation. Viewpoints from racial/ethnic groups. *Cancer.* 1994;74(9 Suppl):2687–2691.

84. Advani AS, Atkeson B, Brown CL, et al. Barriers to the participation of African-American patients with cancer in clinical trials: A pilot study. *Cancer.* 2003;97(6):1499–1506.

85. Wood CG, Wei SJ, Hampshire MK, et al. The influence of race on the attitudes of radiation oncology patients towards clinical trial enrollment. *Am J Clin Oncol.* 2006;29:593–599.

86. Clegg LX, Li FP, Hankey BF, *et al.* Cancer survival among us whites and minorities: A SEER (Surveillance, Epidemiology, and End Results) program population-based study. *Arch Intern Med.* 2002;162:1985–1993.

87. McClelland S 3rd, Leberknight J, Guadagnolo BA, *et al.* The pervasive crisis of diminishing radiotherapy access for vulnerable populations in the United States—Part 2: American Indian patients. *Adv Radiat Oncol.* 2018;3:3–7.

88. Lai GY, Gary TL, Tilburt J, *et al.* Effectiveness of strategies to recruit underrepresented populations into cancer clinical trials. *Clin Trials.* 2006;3:133–141.

89. Molloy K, Reiner M, Ratteree K, *et al.* Patient navigation and cultural competency in cancer care. *Oncol Issues.* 2007;22:38–41.

90. Rogers D, Petereit DG. Cancer disparities research partnership in Lakota Country: Clinical trials, patient services and community education for the Oglala, Rosebud and Cheyenne River Sioux Tribes. *Am J Public Health.* 2005;95:1–4.

91. Dohan D, Schrag D. Using navigators to improve care of underserved patients: Current practices and approaches. *Cancer.* 2005;104:848–855.

92. Freeman HP. Patient navigation: A community-based strategy to reduce cancer disparities. *J Urban Health.* 2006;83:139–141.

93. Regnante JM, Richie NA, Fashoyin-Aje LA, *et al.* Strategies associated with enhanced inclusion of racial and ethnic minorities in clinical cancer. *J Clin Oncol.* 2018;36(15_suppl):e18643–e18643.

94. Weir HK, Jim MA, Marrett LD, et al. Cancer in American Indian and Alaska Native young adults (ages 20–44 years): US, 1999–2004. *Cancer.* 2008;113(5 supple):1153–1167.

95. Howard BV, Lee ET, Cowan RB, *et al.* Rising tide of cardiovascular disease in American Indians. The Strong Heart study. *Circulation.* 1999;99(18):2389–2395.

96. Arizona Cancer Registry. *Cancer in Arizona: Cancer incidence and mortality 2008–2009.* Arizona Department of Health Services, Statistics BoPH, 2013. Accessed March 8, 2021. https://azdhs.gov/documents/preparedness/public-health-statistics/cancer-registry/reports/az-cancer-report-05-07.pdf.

97. Burhansstipanov L, Krebs LU, Dignan MB, *et al.* Findings from the Native Navigators and the Cancer Continuum (NNACC) study. *J Cancer Educ.* 2014;29(3):420–427.

98. Arizona Rural Policy Institute. Demographics of the Hopi Tribe. Accessed March 8, 2021. https://www.google.com/url?sa=t&rct=j&q=&esrc=s&source=web&cd=&ved=2ahUKEwiX-OzvrtzrAhXPuZ4KHa7gC4AQFjAAegQIAxAB&url=https%3A%2F%2Fgotr.azgovernor.gov%2Ffile%2F7276%2Fdownload%3Ftoken%3D1hYvsLMx&usg=AOvVaw20DtkF8h-vWbgsXwvTrpkT.

99. George S, Duran N, Norris K. A systematic review of barriers and facilitators to minority research participation among African Americans, Latinos, Asian Americans, and Pacific Islanders. *Am J Public Health.* 2014;104(2):e16–e31.

100. Oh SS, Galanter J, Thakur N, *et al.* Diversity in clinical and biomedical research: A promise yet to be fulfilled. *PLoS Med.* 2015;12(12):e1001918.

101. Burhansstipanov L, Hollow W. Native American cultural aspects of oncology nursing care. *Semin Oncol Nurs.* 2001;17(3):206–219.

102. Burhansstipanov L, Lovato MP, Krebs LV. Native American cancer survivors. *Health Care Women Int.* 1999;20(5):505–515.

103. Burhansstipanov L, Gilbert A, LaMarca K, *et al.* An innovative path to improving cancer care in Indian country. *Public Health Rep.* 2001;116(5):424–433.

104. Weiner D, Burhansstipanov L, Krebs LU, *et al*. From survivorship to thrivership: Native peoples weaving a healthy life from cancer. *J Cancer Educ*. 2005;20(1 Suppl):28–32.

105. Burhansstipanov L, Krebs LU, Seals BF, *et al*. Native American breast cancer survivors' physical conditions and quality of life. *Cancer*. 2010;116(6):1560–1571.

106. Burhansstipanov L, Dignan M, Jones KL, *et al*. Comparison of quality of life between Native and non-Native cancer survivors: Native and non-Native cancer survivors' QOL. *J Cancer Educ*. 2012;27(1 Suppl):S106–S113.

107. Goodwin EA, Burhansstipanov L, Dignan M, *et al*. The experience of treatment barriers and their influence on quality of life in American Indian/Alaska Native breast cancer survivors. *Cancer*. 2017;123(5):861–868.

108. Native American Cancer Initiatives. Native American Cancer Education and Survivors (NACES) quality of life (QOL) tree. Accessed April 18, 2021. https://natamcancer .org/Quality-of-Life-Tree.

109. Burhansstipanov L, Harjo L, Krebs LU, Marshall A, *et al*. Cultural roles of native patient navigators for American Indian cancer patients. *Front Oncol*. 2015;5:79.

110. Pelusi J, Krebs LU. Understanding cancer-understanding the stories of life and living. *J Cancer Educ*. 2005;20(1 Suppl):12–16.

111. Zimpelman GL, Miller KN, Carlo DD *et al*. *Cancer in Alaska Native people: 1969–2018, The 50-year report*. Alaska Native Tumor Registry, Alaska Native Epidemiology Center, Alaska Native Tribal Health Consortium, 2021.

112. Kelly JJ, Alberts SR, Sacco F, *et al*. Colorectal cancer in Alaska Native people, 2005–2009. *Gastrointest Cancer Res*. 2012;5(5):149–154.

113. Redwood D, Joseph DA, Christensen C, *et al*. Development of a flexible sigmoidoscopy training program for rural nurse practitioners and physician assistants to increase colorectal cancer screening among Alaska Native people. *J Health Care Poor Underserved*. 2009;20(4):1041–1048.

114. Redwood D, Provost E, Perdue D, *et al*. The last frontier: Innovative efforts to reduce colorectal cancer disparities among the remote Alaska Native population. *Gastrointest Endosc*. 2012;75(3):474–480.

115. Joseph DA, Redwood D, DeGroff A, *et al*. Use of evidence-based interventions to address disparities in colorectal cancer screening. *MMWR Suppl*. 2016;65:21–28.

116. Seeff LC, Major A, Townsend JS, *et al*. Comprehensive cancer control programs and coalitions: Partnering to launch successful colorectal cancer screening initiatives. *Cancer Causes Control*. 2010;21(12):2023–2031.

117. Redwood D, Provost E, Asay E, *et al*. Giant inflatable colon and community knowledge, intention, and social support for colorectal cancer screening. *Prev Chronic Dis*. 2013;10:E40.

118. Redwood DG, Asay ED, Blake ID, *et al*. Stool DNA testing for screening detection of colorectal neoplasia in Alaska Native people. *Mayo Clin Proc*. 2016;91(1):61–70.

119. Redwood D, Provost E, Asay E, *et al*. Comparison of fecal occult blood tests for colorectal cancer screening in an Alaska Native population with high prevalence of Helicobacter pylori infection, 2008–2012. *Prev Chronic Dis*. 2014;11:E56.

120. Alaska Department of Health and Social Services. *Alaska behavioral risk factor surveillance system*. Alaska Department of Health and Social Services, 2017.

121. Federal Reserve. Government performance and results act data, 2017. Accessed September 9, 2020. https://www.federalreserve.gov/publications/gpra.htm.

Cancer Patient Navigation Community Engagement Programs

Kathryn L. Braun and Linda Burhansstipanov

Introduction

Cancer patient navigators (CPN) are individuals trained to help people through the full continuum of cancer care—from providing cancer information, helping people access cancer screening, helping individuals with positive screens get a definitive diagnosis, and helping those with cancer through cancer treatment, quality of life, survivorship, and end of life (Figure 8.1).[1] This definition is much broader than the definition of "navigation" specified in the Affordable Care Act, which reduces the patient navigator role to that of an insurance enrollment specialist.[2] CPN may be professionals (e.g., licensed nurses and social workers), paraprofessionals (e.g., community health workers and lay navigators), or recognized community leaders and peers (including cancer survivors).[3] They may be based in a clinical or community setting. This chapter provides information about cancer patient navigation and shares examples of three community-engaged cancer navigation programs within and for Indigenous communities.

Brief History of Cancer Patient Navigation

Dr. Harold Freeman, a surgical oncologist and the former chair of the President's Cancer Panel, started the CPN movement in response to the American Cancer Society *National Hearings on Cancer in the Poor* conducted in seven American cities in 1989.[4] His goal was to improve outcomes in underserved populations by eliminating barriers to timely cancer diagnosis and treatment in a culturally sensitive manner.[5] CPN services soon were extended throughout the oncology care continuum, from outreach/prevention to survivorship and end of life.[6,7] Since Dr. Freeman's initial cancer-focused programs, navigation programs have documented improvements in resource sharing, continuity and quality of care, health outcomes, and patient satisfaction.[6] Also, the concept of patient navigation has significantly evolved beyond cancer into other chronic diseases, and the patient navigation movement has embraced

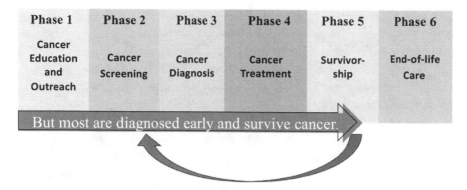

Fig 8.1. Cancer care across a continuum. Created by Kathryn Braun and Linda Burhansstipanov.

the idea that nonclinical staff members can play a key role in reducing health disparities.[8,9]

Research has documented that cancer patient navigation is appreciated by patients and that navigated patients are more likely than nonnavigated patients to receive timely screening and follow through with diagnostic tests.[3,10,11,12,13] CPN provide prevention education,[14] help increase screening,[7,9,15,16] save health-care costs,[17,18] facilitate access to care,[19] and improve patient satisfaction.[20,21] They assist with financial and insurance issues,[22] transportation, childcare, and community resources.[9] CPN hired from within the community built trust by speaking the same language as the client[23] and addressing cultural beliefs.[24] Research has suggested that cancer patient navigation programs decrease healthcare resource use, including emergency department visits and hospitalization.[25,26] Other studies demonstrate that these programs are cost-effective in addressing breast and cervical cancer screening[13,27] and lung cancer.[28] Other cost analyses performed on government-funded navigation programs also have shown promising results.[29,30]

Roles of Cancer Patient Navigators

The CPN can play an important role in every phase of the cancer care continuum (Figure 8.1). In phase 1, cancer education and outreach, CPN use their knowledge of the community to increase awareness of the value of early detection. The CPN can help community members learn about cancer and the importance of early detection and treatment. In phase 2, cancer screening, CPN use different approaches to increase screening among underserved individuals—for example, helping them make appointments and arranging transportation and childcare if needed. The majority of people who are screened have a negative finding, meaning that cancer is not suspected. CPN can help remind their clients to repeat cancer screening at appropriate time intervals depending on screening type. In phase 3, diagnosis and staging, CPN help clients understand the different tests that may be done to make a definitive diagnosis of cancer and to determine how advanced the cancer is. These findings are needed to create a treatment plan. In phase 4, cancer treatment, CPN perform tasks to reduce the elapsed time between diagnosis and treatment, help cancer patients understand treatment options, make informed decisions about treatment, and complete treatment. CPN help patients access treatment facilities and medications and they understand behaviors that may reduce potential side effects. In phase 5, survivorship, CPN help individuals adjust to living with cancer, address long-term/chronic or late effects from cancer or cancer treatments, and learn ways to improve both their quality and quantity of life. They also help patients return to a regular cancer screening routine posttreatment. In phase 6, end-of-life care, CPN help patients designate a healthcare decision-maker (usually from within the family) and talk about wishes for comfort care, cultural and religious ceremony, and burial.[1]

Table 8.1. summarizes some of the distinctive roles of navigators who are licensed CPN (e.g., nurse navigators and social workers), community health workers, and lay CPN. In addition to training and licensure, CPN roles may vary by state, funding source, and clinic/hospital rules. For example, in large, tertiary hospitals, typically only CPN who also are licensed nurses and social workers are allowed to access the electronic health records (EHR). Some clinics and community programs have their own CPN tracking system that may or may not interface with the EHR.

Community Health Workers as Cancer Patient Navigators

As noted, several different positions share some of the roles of CPN, including professional nurses, social workers, and case managers. However, most CPN, especially those working in Indigenous communities, are paraprofessional workers, including community health workers, peer educators, lay navigators, and *Promotores de Salud*.

According to the World Health Organization, community health workers are community-based workers that educate community members about various health issues and help them access health and social services. The US Department of Labor has defined community health workers as paraprofessionals that work in the community to assist individuals and communities in adopting healthy behaviors.[32] The American Public Health Association's

Table 8.1. Roles of CPN Who Are Licensed, Community Health Workers, or "Lay" Navigators[31]

	Clinically Licensed CPN (Nurse or Social Worker)	Community Health Worker CPN	"Lay" or Nonlicensed CPN
Knowledge	Knowledge of cancer clinical resources, interpretation of clinical findings and recommendations for follow-up care, ability to intervene to manage symptoms and assess functional status or psychosocial health	General knowledge and culturally appropriate outreach, prevention, linking to resources for health	Knowledge of cancer outreach, prevention, screening guidelines, diagnostic processes, treatment options, survivorship issues, palliative, and end-of-life care and related physical, psychological, cultural, and social issues; conduct needs assessments and other surveys (e.g., distress); do not provide individual medical information
Documentation	Provide active documentation in the medical records	Document outreach and education activities within an unofficial or official client record as allowed	Document patient encounters, barriers to care, and resources or referrals within a client or medical record or tracking system(s) as allowed

definition is similar, defining a community health worker as a "frontline public health worker who is a trusted member of and/or has an unusually close understanding of the community served. This trusting relationship enables the community health worker to serve as a liaison/link/intermediary between health/social services and the community to facilitate access to services and improve the quality and cultural competence of service delivery."[33] Thus, community health workers should be members of the communities where they work, selected by the communities, answerable to the communities for their activities, and appreciated by the local health system. Community health workers conduct outreach for medical personnel or health organizations and implement community programs that promote, maintain, and improve individual and community health. Community health workers provide patients with information on available resources, social support, informal counseling, and services such as first aid and blood pressure screening, as well as advocate for individual and community health needs.

CPN function similarly to community health workers. However, depending on their organizational scope of work, they may cross the threshold of the healthcare facility and continue providing cultural support within clinical departments (e.g., radiation, surgery, adjuvant care).[34] Community health workers and CPN frequently team up for the benefit of the patient, with a community health worker or community-based CPN in a rural area providing a friendly hand-off to a CPN based at the hospital.

The Need for Indigenous Navigators

As noted in Chapter 2, Indigenous populations are more likely to live in geographically isolated and environmentally challenging communities than White Americans and do not have equal access to healthcare and cancer screening. As a result, these populations tend to be diagnosed with cancer at younger ages and more advanced stages and are more likely to die from cancer than White Americans.[35]

Because many people have questioned the need to train and support navigators from within Indigenous communities, five of the most common reasons are listed here. First, Indigenous Peoples often lack trust in the healthcare system and providers from the dominant US culture. This is because of their historical experiences with loss of land, language, power, and human rights under US rule.[36,37] A second reason is that communication patterns are unique to each Indigenous group. Communication includes verbal (words), vocal (tone, volume), and non-verbal (body language) ways of interacting. For example, non-Indigenous Peoples sometimes stereotype American Indians (AI) as being stoic and lacking expressions, but such nonverbal patterns are unique to each tribal culture. Local subtleties may include avoiding direct eye contact or constructing sentences with words, word order, and phrasing that are different from English.

A third reason is a variation in the perceptions of the word "cancer." Most Indigenous cultures do not have a native word for "cancer," and some have a cultural norm to avoid speaking the word "cancer."[38] Fourth, Indigenous cultures have unique traditional frameworks for understanding disease, as well as unique practices for treating disease. The latter could include local complementary medicine and spiritual ceremonies or practices. Finally, many Indigenous Peoples use health services that may be targeted to them, including the Indian Health Service (IHS), the Native Hawaiian Health Care Systems (NHHCS), and the Alaska Tribal Health Corporations. Local navigators would best know how to navigate their local healthcare system.

To address these issues, cancer patient navigation programs attempting to serve Indigenous communities should hire, train, and nurture CPN from or familiar with and trusted by the local community. These individuals will be more likely to respect local cultures and spiritual practices, respect and use local communication styles, understand traditional conceptualizations of disease and treatment, and link patients with the best combination of traditional and Western providers to meet their cancer care needs.[39]

Standardized Competencies for Cancer Patient Navigators

CPN training, regardless of its trainees (e.g., nonlicensed paraprofessional workers or licensed social workers and nurses) should address competencies that require attainment of basic CPN skills.[1,40,41] In 2016, the Academy of Oncology Nurse and Patient Navigators (AONN+) identified core competencies for nurse navigators and patient navigators (paraprofessionals). These core competencies have been supported by national organizations, including but not limited to the following:

- American Cancer Society's National Navigation Roundtable
- American College of Surgeons Commission on Cancer
- The American Society of Clinical Oncology's Quality Oncology Practice Initiative
- Center for Medicare and Medicaid's Oncology Care Model
- Merit-based Incentive Payment System / Alternative Payment Models
- National Accreditation Program for Breast Centers
- Oncology Nursing Society

These groups expanded the definition of cancer patient navigation to *individualized assistance offered to patients, families, and caregivers to help overcome healthcare system barriers and facilitate timely access to quality health and psychosocial care from pre-diagnosis through all phases of the cancer experience.*[42] Also, the Institute of Medicine recommended that quality care be measured using a core set of metrics.[43] These metrics were used to evaluate whether patient navigation can improve care—from outreach throughout end of life—and overall value in healthcare. They also are being used as criteria for patient navigation accreditation certification and programs.

As part of the American Cancer Society's National Navigation Roundtable (NNRT), the "Workforce Development" Task Force came to a consensus on standardized competencies around which CPN training should be framed (Table 8.2.). The Task Group members also identified potential roles and

Table 8.2. National Navigation Roundtable Task Force Domains for Training and Certification Competencies

I. Ethical, cultural, legal, and professional issues	Demonstrate sensitivity and responsiveness to a diverse patient population, including but not limited to respecting confidentiality, organizational rules and regulations, ethical principles, and diversity in gender, age, culture, race, ethnicity, religion, abilities, sexual orientation, and geography.
II. Client and care team interaction and communication skills	Apply insight and understanding concerning human emotional responses to create and maintain positive interpersonal interactions leading to trust and collaboration between patient/client/family and the healthcare team. Patient safety and satisfaction is a priority.
III. Health knowledge	Demonstrate breadth of health, the cancer continuum, psychosocial and spiritual knowledge, attitudes and behaviors specific to their patient navigator (PN) role.
IV. Patient care coordination	Participate in the development of an evidence-based or promising/best practice patient-centered plan of care, which is inclusive of the client's personal assessment and health provider/system and community resources. The PN acts as a liaison among all team members to advocate for patients to optimize health and wellness with the overall focus to improve access to services for all patients. PN conducts patient assessments (needs, goals, self-management, behaviors, strategies for improvement) integrating clients' personal and cultural values.
V. Practice-based learning	Optimize navigator practice through continual professional development and the assimilation of scientific evidence to continuously improve patient care, based on individual PN gaps in knowledge, skills, attitudes, and abilities.
VI. Systems-based practice	Advocate for quality patient care by acknowledging and monitoring needed (desirable) improvements in systems of care for patients from enhancing community relationships and outreach through end of life. This includes enhancing community relationships, developing skills and knowledge to monitor and evaluate patient care and the effectiveness of the program.
VII. Communication/ interpersonal skills	Promote effective communication and interactions with patients in shared decision-making based on their needs, goals, strengths, barriers, solutions, and resources. Resolution of conflict among patients, family members, community partners, and members of the oncology care team is demonstrated in professional and culturally acceptable behaviors.

responsibilities relevant to each competency for possible inclusion in a CPN job description (Table 8.3.). A cancer navigation program can use this job description to identify the specific competencies, roles, and responsibilities for employees that are most relevant to its particular setting, patient population, type of cancer, focus along the cancer continuum (e.g., screening or treatment or both), and type of employee that will serve as the navigator (e.g., professional or paraprofessional). These collaborative efforts will further the standardization of CPN practice and thereby enhance patient care.[44]

The American College of Surgeons, Commission on Cancer (CoC) is "a consortium of professional organizations that ensures the delivery of quality cancer care by setting standards to address cancer prevention, research, education, treatment, and survivorship. It also accredits more than 1,200 US cancer programs that demonstrate a commitment to delivering high-quality, safe, patient-centered care through a multidisciplinary team."[45,46,47] In 2016, CoC Standard 3.1 required cancer programs to put a cancer navigation system in place to address barriers to care. This standard was significantly relaxed in 2020, no longer specifying the need for a cancer navigation system, but the 2020 Standard 8.1 focuses on barriers to care. Since the primary role of patient navigators is to help the patient overcome barriers, a role for the CPN is implied within the new standard. These standards are relevant to community, nurse, and social work patient navigators and are relevant to diverse settings that provide CPN services, including hospitals, community clinics, rural and reservation clinics, and community organizations.

Examples of Successful Indigenous Community-Engaged Interventions

Native Navigators and the Cancer Continuum[i]

Description

Native Navigators and the Cancer Continuum (NNACC) was implemented to help address the growing cancer health disparity among AI, funded from 2008 to 2014 by the National Institutes of Minority Health and Health Disparities. It was a community-based participatory research (CBPR) study among five partners: Native American Cancer Research Corporation in Colorado, Inter-Tribal Council of Michigan, Rapid City Regional Hospital's Walking Forward in South Dakota, Great Plains Tribal Chairman's' Health Board in South Dakota, and Muscogee Creek Nation in Oklahoma. Native CPN were trained in these

---

i Funding from NIH R24MD002811.

Table 8.3. American Cancer Society National Navigator Roundtable Workforce Development Sample Cancer Patient Navigator Job Description

Ethical, cultural, legal, and professional issues
- Maintain patient confidentiality and privacy when working with clinical and professional staff both within and outside of systems of care and community-based programs.
- Use assessment information to develop a plan to address health and related patient needs in cooperation with the patient and based on patient priorities.
- Demonstrate culturally respectful knowledge and behaviors when assisting patients with ceremonies or special services (that are pertinent to the patients' cultural healthcare values, beliefs, and practices).
- Demonstrate respect for Limited English Proficiency and English Language Learner by providing access to medical interpretation at the health systems level.

Client and Care Team Interaction
- Participate in healthcare team discussions about ways to proactively address patient barriers and improve overall patient care.
- Provide support for patients' healthcare decisions when interacting with healthcare professionals.
- Communicate with health systems staff and social service organizations to help them understand and accept the community and individual conditions, culture, and behavior to develop policies and plans that support individual and community health efforts.
- Identify how the social determinants of health impact a client's ability to access healthcare.

Health Knowledge
- Conduct assessment of patient's understanding of their treatment options.
- Identify gaps in patient's knowledge of self-management of their health conditions.
- Enhance patient knowledge on treatment for informed decision-making.
- Assist patients to identify their personal strengths and problem-solving abilities.
- Provide emotional support or identify sources of support in the community.
- Provide culturally and linguistically appropriate information relevant to the patient and their family's culture, health literacy level.
- Effectively use coaching techniques to enhance patient knowledge.
- Enhance knowledge of patients on treatment summary and follow-up posttreatment.
- Conduct health education.
- Identify sources of spiritual support in the community that are respectful of the patient's religious and cultural practices.
- Document health education activities and in a Health Insurance Portability and Accountability Act–compliant manner.
- Apply knowledge of cancer pathophysiology, disease process, and treatments.

Patient Care Coordination
- Provide care coordination, including basic care planning (prepare questions to ask provider, treatment options clarifications) with individuals and families based on engagement and needs/barriers assessments, and facilitate care transitions.

- Use a formal tool to assess risk/acuity, clinical, emotional, spiritual, psychosocial, financial, and other patient needs and quality improvement initiatives such as the National Comprehensive Cancer Network or equivalent distress thermometer. Re-evaluate and update assessment regularly.
- Implement strategies that assist patients in identifying and prioritizing their personal, family, and community needs for new resources.
- Develop relationships with relevant agencies and professionals to address health needs and inequities.
- Schedule and/or accompany patients to medical appointments when appropriate.
- Provide support for patients to follow professional caregiver instructions or advice.
- Provide support, information, and referrals to family and healthcare providers/ professional caregivers.
- Coordinate one's roles with other local programs to prevent duplication of services.
- Inform patients about clinical trials and share information regarding appropriate clinical trials. Provide referrals for clinical trials.

Practice-Based Learning
- Maintain appropriate boundaries that balance professional and personal relationships while recognizing dual roles as both navigator and community members.
- Use appropriate technology, such as computers and database systems, for work-based communication in accordance with employer requirements.
- Document client tracking information, program evaluation, and sustainability data to help patients achieve their goals. Engage in quality improvement initiatives.
- Pursue personal ongoing continuing education on navigation, community resources, and specific oncology education needs.
- Use outreach methods to engage individuals and groups in diverse settings including underserved and rural populations.

Systems-Based Practice
- Conduct baseline and ongoing needs assessments of communities and their members with clearly defined goals and objectives.
- Utilize a database or electronic medical record system to collect service information and inform program statistics.

Communication/Interpersonal Skills
- Assist patients in identifying what changes in services they believe are needed to diminish said barriers.
- Demonstrate the ability to effectively communicate with clients, families, and members of the healthcare team. Effectively adjust communication style to the needs of the audience.
- Demonstrate the ability to communicate using nonjudgmental language that conveys respect and empathy.
- Identify cultural and language needs of patients and effectively use resources.
- Encourage communication interchange between patients/families and healthcare providers to optimize patient outcomes.

communities, but were not widely accessed. The goal of the study was to work in partnership with the five AI communities to raise awareness of healthy behaviors, including those related to cancer screening and treatment, and how the Native CPN could help.

Intervention

The study intervention implemented and evaluated community education workshops at each of the five participating sites. Each 24-hour workshop included topics within the cancer care continuum (Figure 8.1) to increase knowledge of cancer screening and treatment. The workshops also highlighted the role of the Native CPN who were available to schedule screening appointments, carry out follow-up recommendations, and provide support and education for those diagnosed with cancer.

Community Engagement

Each of the five communities established a Community Advisory Committee. Individuals on these committees were involved with planning, recruiting, implementing the education intervention, and disseminating the findings. During the grant planning stage, committee members, in consultation with their broader communities, gave ideas for the intervention and the research design for testing it. When funding was received, the Community Advisory Committees helped adapt the curricula to their communities and identified potential community partners. Each community created a memorandum of agreement with two other AI organizations in their local areas who took the lead for coordinating each 24-hour workshop series for each year during the implementation phase. Partners provided the staff to facilitate and evaluate each workshop.

Native CPN implemented and evaluated the workshops using an audience response system to collect demographics, pre- and postworkshop knowledge, attitudes and behaviors, and workshop evaluation and satisfaction. Each partner had an independent online evaluation program for uploading workshop data and summaries, as well as to document Native CPN interactions with workshop participants related to obtaining cancer screening or receiving supportive navigation care.

In addition to the workshop series, each partner coordinated and implemented two Family Fun Events—one at the start of the workshop series (baseline) and another 3–6 months following the final workshop. All workshop participants, their families, and the local organization's community-at-large were invited. These events lasted 2–3 hours and included food and family activities such as bingo, dance competitions, and health fairs. Easy-to-understand summaries of the findings were described orally, and hard copies were provided to all participants at the follow-up Family Fun Event.[48]

Outcomes

Community participants primarily were AI (83%) ranging in age from 18 to 95. The majority (70%) were females. Their interest and willingness to take part in the education intervention was much greater than anticipated. Rather than the intended 738 participants, the final participant count was 1,964 individuals. The workshop intervention was effective regardless of the community members' gender, age, race, and education level. Evaluation data suggested that the workshops increased participants' knowledge by 23%, surpassing the 20% estimated in the grant proposal. The workshops also increased the visibility and availability of the Native CPN to help local community members find healthcare assistance and resources and obtain cancer screening services. Finally, the project resulted in improved access to quality cancer care, with 77 cancer patients assisted by the Native CPN to obtain cancer care services promptly.

Lessons Learned

The NNACC education intervention successfully increased community members' knowledge in all five sites. The intervention also resulted in increased visibility and use of Native CPN. Because these navigators were from the local community and familiar with local culture, customs, and healthcare systems, they were able to help clients overcome barriers often confronted in the mainstream health services available to AI. These barriers included lack of trust of conventional services due to a history of AI mistreatment, unique cultural perspectives and communication styles of specific tribal populations, desire to use complementary medicines unique to specific tribal nations or geographic regions, and logistic issues associated with the IHS.[49,50]

Kukui Ahi on the Island of Moloka'i[ii]

Description

In 2005, 'Imi Hale Native Hawaiian Cancer Network ('Imi Hale) assisted Moloka'i General Hospital (MGH) to secure grant funds to navigate island residents to cancer screening and cancer treatment. 'Imi Hale was 1 of 23 Community Network Program Centers funded by the National Cancer Institute's Center to Reduce Cancer Health Disparities and operated from 2000 to 2017. 'Imi Hale's

---

ii Funding from CMS 500–00–0024; NIH NCI U01CA86105, U01CA114630, U54CA153459.

work was guided by principles of CBPR, emphasizing community involvement, capacity building, respect for cultural values, and information sharing.[51] This project with MGH was initiated and evaluated with funding from the Centers for Medicare and Medicaid Services (CMS).[52]

MGH serves the island of Moloka'i, which is one of seven inhabited islands in the state of Hawai'i. It has a very small population (less than 8,000), and more than 92% of the island's population is Native Hawaiian (NH) or Filipino.[53] Approximately 18% of the Moloka'i population live below the federal poverty level, compared with approximately 10% of the state population. Moloka'i is a medically underserved area and a primary healthcare professional shortage group area, as designated by HRSA. Screening prevalence for breast, cervical, and colorectal cancers on Moloka'i are below the state average, and cancer mortality is high.

Intervention

The program was named Kukui Ahi, a Hawaiian phrase meaning "to show the way." MGH employed lay CPN from the community, one NH and one Filipino, along with a supervisor. The navigators were not certified healthcare providers, but they completed a 48-hour navigator training program sponsored by 'Imi Hale and participated in quarterly continuing education sessions to extend their navigation skills.[54] Early in the project, a nurse supervised them, but starting from the second year, a young woman with a college degree in business and two physicians affiliated with the hospital supervised them. The Kukui Ahi CPN provided services across the cancer care continuum (Figure 8.1), from providing outreach and education about cancer, to helping individuals get screened, to assisting patients diagnosed with cancer to complete their treatment, to assisting with survivorship and end-of-life care.

Community Engagement

Relationships between MGH and 'Imi Hale were established in 2000. Between 2000 and 2003, Moloka'i providers and patients helped in the development and pretesting of a set of cancer screening brochures tailored to NH.[55] In 2003, 'Imi Hale helped the community sponsor an 'Ohana Day event, at which community members could meet with a cadre of NH physicians flown in from Honolulu for a day of education, music, food, and cancer screening.[56] In 2006, Moloka'i health providers were engaged in the development of 'Imi Hale's 48-hour CPN training. However, the leaders of 'Imi Hale had been engaged with Moloka'i health providers for decades. These trusting relationships allowed the team to move quickly to write the proposal for CMS funding.

Once funding was received, 'Imi Hale trained the MGH navigators and provided educational materials. MGH staff were partners in dissemination and publication about the program and presented their program at conferences in Hawai'i, in the Pacific, and in the Continental US.

Outcomes

The CMS Cancer Prevention and Treatment Demonstration operated from 2006 to 2010. With funding from CMS and other sources, MGH CPN assisted all island residents diagnosed with cancer. In addition, MGH conducted a randomized clinical trial of Kukui Ahi's screening navigation services. Over the course of four years, 488 Medicare beneficiaries were randomized to navigation for cancer screening (n = 242) or cancer education (n = 246).[55] For those in the navigation group, CPN provided outreach and education, made screening appointments, sent reminders, provided transportation to appointments, facilitated communication between patients and providers, and completed paperwork. At the beginning of the study, the intervention and control groups were similar in demographic characteristics and baseline screening prevalence of breast, cervical, prostate, and colorectal cancers.[55]

At study exit, however, cancer screening prevalence was much higher in the navigated group compared to the control group. Specifically, 57.0% of women in the experimental arm compared to only 36.4% of controls had a Pap test in the past 24 months (p = .001), 61.7% of women in the experimental arm compared to 42.4% of controls had a mammogram in the past 12 months (p = .003), 54.4% of men in the experimental arm compared to only 36.0% of controls had a prostate-specific antigen test in the past 12 months (p = .008), and 43.0% of both sexes in the experimental arm compared to only 27.2% of controls had a flexible sigmoidoscopy or colonoscopy in the past 5 years (p < .001).[55] Additionally, participants were overwhelmingly satisfied with navigation services. Specifically, 94% reported that they valued working with the navigator, 95% would recommend this service to others, and 93% rated their overall experience with the navigator as excellent.

Kukui Ahi navigators also reported major changes in receptivity to screening. In Hawaiian culture, there was a belief that saying the word cancer may bring it on and that cancer screening procedures were painful.[47] Hence, elders initially were reluctant to discuss cancer or participate in screening. This was overcome by continuous outreach and education and finding those elders willing to "take a leap of faith to get screened." Of course, the majority of those screened did not have or get cancer. Elders then communicated to others that the procedures were "not so bad." Men were especially surprised at the ease of the PSA test.

Lessons Learned

Long-term engagement between 'Imi Hale and employees at MGH supported a quick response to the CMS call for proposals and subsequent good working relationships between the two organizations. The hospital chose to hire CPN from the community who were not professionals, but were trusted community members. The CPN were receptive to training and able to ask for help from their supervisors when needed. Because they were community members, they had access to hard-to-reach groups and were able to be "heard" by them. Their demonstrated helpfulness and their ability to maintain confidentiality about the people they helped earned them respect and trust from the community, which increased their ability to reach more people. Because the hospital saw good results in terms of increased community screening and earlier-stage cancer diagnoses, they decided to fund the program internally. The navigators extended their services to help noncancer patients as well, especially those that needed to travel off-island for care.

Women to Women, with Micronesians United[iii]

Description

In 2005, a nonprofit organization in Honolulu called Micronesians United approached 'Imi Hale to develop a cancer patient navigation program with and for Micronesian migrants in Hawai'i. Hawai'i attracts many migrants from the US-Affiliated Pacific, including about 20,000 from the Federated States of Micronesia, Palau, and the Republic of the Marshall Islands. As explained in Chapter 2, these nations have signed Compacts of Free Association (COFA) with the US. COFA gives the US access to and military control of these island nations in exchange for support for governmental, educational, and healthcare services. This relationship with the US dates back to World War II, and it was in these jurisdictions that the US tested its nuclear weapons, polluting environments, displacing islanders, and increasing cancer risk. COFA migrants are often referred to as Micronesians.[57] As stipulated in the COFA, they may freely migrate to the US, and many do so in pursuit of education, work, and healthcare opportunities, which are limited in their home countries.[58,59,60] Discussions between Micronesians United and 'Imi Hale resulted in the Woman to Woman program, through which Micronesian women were trained to navigate their compatriots to cancer screening.[61]

---

iii Funding from NIH NCI U01CA86105, U01CA114630, U54CA153459.

Intervention

The intervention included a culturally tailored training curriculum and toolkit for Micronesian lay CPN. The 6-hour training included information about breast cancer, Micronesian women's high risk of cancer due to nuclear weapons testing in their home islands, and local cancer screening services. Trainees heard from physicians and cancer survivors, visited mammography clinics, and met with staff who conducted breast cancer screening. They also practiced making referrals by phone and documenting peer contacts.

The trainees helped to choose and adapt culturally appropriate breast cancer education materials and tools to help them educate their communities. For example, they chose to adopt a portable education flip chart that they could use to help with educational presentations. They also chose to distribute breast education brochures and shower hangers and two tactile breast cancer education pieces—a beaded key chain distributed by the American Cancer Society Hawai'i Chapter and a multiple-sized beaded necklace produced by 'Imi Hale. The beads in the necklace kit and keychain demonstrated the sizes of cancerous lumps found through mammography (the smallest bead), by clinical breast examination, and by breast self-examination (the largest bead). Also developed were a resource card with phone numbers of breast cancer screening providers, referral slips, and a journal for lay educators to record information, questions, and concerns to discuss at weekly meetings. All materials were tailored for Micronesian women and translated into four different Micronesian languages.

Once trained, each CPN received a name badge, business cards, and a toolkit in a distinctive colorful bag. They began providing cancer educational presentations to Micronesian women, and each woman was given the bead necklace kit and bead keychain. Women aged 40 or older who needed a mammogram were assisted in screening. Women who were not accompanied to screening showed their mammography results to the lay CPN as proof of screening. Grant funding was available to pay each lay CPN a stipend of $100 per month to offset costs associated with outreach. Many women used the stipend toward transportation for themselves and the women they educated and navigated.

Community Engagement

The relationship between the two organizations began in 2001, when 'Imi Hale began to participate with Micronesians United in grant writing, educational workshops, and health fairs. Thus, a trusting relationship had been established between the two organizations by 2005, when Micronesians United asked for help to increase breast cancer awareness and screening in their community.

Each group identified champions for the project, and they worked together to conduct focus groups in October 2005 with 16 women representing four Micronesian cultural groups— Marshallese, Pohnpeian, Chuukese, and Kosraean. Sessions were started with a prayer, food was served, and the group was allowed to determine the amount of time spent on each question. Questions included (1) What are your leading health concerns? (2) What are the barriers to good health? and (3) What cultural strengths can help improve the health of Micronesian women in Hawai'i?

Fifteen of the 16 participants identified breast cancer as a leading concern, relating their knowledge of friends and family who had been diagnosed with breast cancer. Most participants knew that the US tested nuclear weapons on their islands but did not understand the relationship between cancer and radiation from nuclear testing. They also noted that there were no cancer education materials in their languages and very limited cancer care services on their home islands. Thus, many cancers in Micronesia were diagnosed late and caused death, leading Micronesians to have fatalistic attitudes toward cancer. Only half knew about the breast and cervical cancer screening programs funded by the Centers for Disease Control and Prevention in their home countries or Hawai'i.

Participants also said that local providers were unfamiliar with Micronesian culture. For example, it is not usual for Micronesians to talk to others about their "private parts," and participants wished healthcare providers would apologize before asking questions about women's issues. Also, women who wanted to have a mammogram felt hesitant to make appointments by telephone and anticipated difficulties arranging transportation, taking time for appointments, and paying for services.

The participants also identified cultural strengths. The collectivistic orientation and strong affiliation with family, church, and community would make it easy to find and educate Micronesians about cancer. Women in these cultures have responsibility for the health of the family, and they felt they could give health advice to friends as they gathered together for church, childcare, and other activities. Therefore, the group decided to provide peer education on breast cancer and to navigate Micronesian women to screening.

Outcomes

Of the 16 women who started the training, 11 completed it and served as CPN. They started by educating and navigating their relatives, friends, and neighbors. Once they were comfortable with their presentations, they extended their outreach to churches, Micronesian neighborhoods, homeless shelters, and other places where Micronesian women gather.

In the first 3 months, 567 Micronesian women aged 18 to 75 were educated about breast cancer. Of these, 324 were under age 40, and they were taught about the importance of the clinical breast exam and of encouraging older women to get mammograms. Among the 202 women aged 40 or older and eligible for mammography screening, 166 (82%) had never had a mammogram and were assisted in screening appointments. After 6 months, 146 (88%) of the women who had never had a mammogram had received one. Therefore, the percentage compliant with mammography screening recommendations increased from 18% (36/202) to 90% (182/202). CPN found that the most successful practice was to arrange back-to-back mammogram appointments for 5 to 10 women at a time, with women going together to the clinic and staying until the last woman was screened.

The CPN reported an increase in self-esteem and confidence. During weekly meetings, they expressed their pride in serving in traditional roles of health promoters and, in this way, being useful to their communities in Hawai'i.

Lessons Learned

CBPR processes were critical in engaging the community and developing a culturally appropriate intervention. Materials were tailored to the community and improved through extensive pretesting. The lay educator training was respectful of Pacific customs, processes, and practices. Involving women with a range of ages in education sessions and scheduling back-to-back mammogram appointments for a group of women fit well with Micronesian values of collectivity and mutual support. The Pacific manner of reciprocity and gifting also was respected. Lay educators expressed pride in their new but traditionally expected roles of caretaker and healer.

Summary

Cancer patient navigation programs helped increase cancer awareness, screening, and treatment among Indigenous Peoples. Identifying, training, and supporting Indigenous Peoples as CPN also built community capacity to understand and navigate the cancer care continuum. Findings from the community-engaged CPN projects highlighted in this chapter attested to the good outcomes achievable by and in Indigenous communities. The primary challenge to establishing and maintaining CPN programs was the lack of permanent funding. The Moloka'i program was initially supported by grants funds, and the hospital decided to support the program after funding ended. However, most programs, like the 'Imi Hale-Micronesians United program and the Native Navigator program, had to continue to secure grant funding to maintain their services. Now that CPN competencies have been developed, it is hoped that CPN training can be standardized and CPN services can become a reimbursed service under major health insurers.

References

1. Braun KL, Kagawa-Singer M, Holden AE, et al. Cancer patient navigator tasks across the cancer care continuum. *J Healthcare Poor Underserved.* 2012;23(1):398–413.

2. Centers for Medicare & Medicaid Services, Department of Health and Human Services. Patient Protection and Affordable Care Act: Exchange and insurance market standards for 2015 and beyond. Final rule. *Fed Regist.* 2014;79(101):30239–30353.

3. Wells KJ, Battaglia TA, Dudley DJ, et al. Patient navigation: State of the art or is it science? *Cancer.* 2008;113(8):1999–2010.

4. Freeman HP. Cancer in the socioeconomically disadvantaged. *CA Cancer J Clin.* 1989;39(5):266–288.

5. Freeman HP. The Harold P. Freeman Patient Navigation Institute. Accessed June 14, 2020. www.hpfreemanpni.org.

6. Freeman HP, Rodriguez RL. History and principles of patient navigation. *Cancer.* 2011;117(15 Suppl):3539–3542.

7. Burhansstipanov L, Shockney LD, Gentry S. History of oncology patient and nurse navigation. In: Shockney L, ed. *Team-based oncology care: The pivotal role of oncology navigation.* Springer Publishing, 2018:13–42.

8. Winch PJ, Gilroy KE, Wolfheim C, et al. Intervention models for the management of children with signs of pneumonia or malaria by community health workers. *Health Policy Plan.* 2005;20(4):199–212.

9. Chowdhury AM. Rethinking interventions for women's health. *Lancet.* 2007;370(9595):1292–1293.

10. Battaglia TA, Roloff K, Posner MA, et al. Improving follow-up to abnormal breast cancer screening in an urban population: A patient navigation intervention. *Cancer.* 2007;109(2 Suppl):359–367.

11. Ell K, Vourlekis B, Lee PJ, et al. Patient navigation and case management following an abnormal mammogram: A randomized clinical trial. *Prev Med.* 2007;44(1):26–33.

12. Ferrante JM, Chen PH, Kim S. The effect of patient navigation on time to diagnosis, anxiety, and satisfaction in urban minority women with abnormal mammograms: A randomized controlled trial. *J Urban Health.* 2008;85(1):114–124.

13. Robinson-White S, Conroy B, Slavish KH, et al. Patient navigation in breast cancer: A systematic review. *Cancer Nurs.* 2010;33(2):127–140.

14. Wang ML, Gallivan L, Lemon SC, et al. Navigating to health: Evaluation of a community health center patient navigation program. *Prev Med Rep.* 2015;2:664–668. Published 2015 August 13.

15. Ladabaum U, Mannalithara A, Jandorf L, et al. Cost-effectiveness of patient navigation to increase adherence with screening colonoscopy among minority individuals. *Cancer.* 2015;121(7):1088–1097.

16. Taylor VM, Hislop TG, Jackson JC, et al. A randomized controlled trial of interventions to promote cervical cancer screening among Chinese women in North America. *J Natl Cancer Inst.* 2002;94(9):670–677.

17. Markossian TW, Calhoun EA. Are breast cancer navigation programs cost-effective? Evidence from the Chicago Cancer Navigation Project. *Health Policy*. 2011;99(1):52–59.

18. Enard KR, Ganelin DM. Reducing preventable emergency department utilization and costs by using community health workers as patient navigators. *J Healthc Manag*. 2013;58(6):412–428.

19. Roland KB, Milliken EL, Rohan EA, *et al*. Use of Community health workers and patient navigators to improve cancer outcomes among patients served by Federally Qualified Health Centers: A systematic literature review. *Health Equity*. 2017;1(1):61–76.

20. Jean-Pierre P, Cheng Y, Wells KJ, *et al*. Satisfaction with cancer care among underserved racial-ethnic minorities and lower-income patients receiving patient navigation. *Cancer*. 2016;122(7):1060–1067.

21. Wells KJ, Winters PC, Jean-Pierre P, *et al*. Effect of patient navigation on satisfaction with cancer-related care. *Support Care Cancer*. 2016;24(4):1729–1753.

22. Darnell JS. Navigators and assisters: Two case management roles for social workers in the Affordable Care Act. *Health Soc Work*. 2013;38(2):123–126.

23. Ramirez A, Perez-Stable E, Penedo F, *et al*. Reducing time-to-treatment in underserved Latinas with breast cancer: The Six Cities Study. *Cancer*. 2014;120(5):752760.

24. Harjo LD, Burhansstipanov L, Lindstrom D. Rationale for "cultural" native patient navigators in Indian country. *J Cancer Educ*. 2014;29(3):414–419.

25. Colligan EM, Ewald E, Ruiz S, *et al*. Innovative oncology care models improve end-of-life quality, reduce utilization and spending. *Health Aff*. 2017;36(3):433–440.

26. Seaberg D, Elseroad S, Dumas M, *et al*. Patient navigation for patients frequently visiting the emergency department: A randomized, controlled trial. *Acad Emerg Med*. 2017;24(11):1327–1333.

27. Li Y, Carlson E, Villarreal R, *et al*. Cost-effectiveness of a patient navigation program to improve cervical cancer screening. *Am J Manag Care*. 2017;23(7):429–434.

28. Shih YC, Chien CR, Moguel R, *et al*. Cost-effectiveness analysis of a capitated patient navigation program for Medicare beneficiaries with lung cancer. *Health Serv Res*. 2016;51(2):746–767.

29. Bir A, Smith K, Kahwati L, *et al*. *Healthcare Innovation Awards (HCIA) meta-analysis and evaluators collaborative annual report: Year 3*. RTI International, 2018. Accessed June 14, 2020. https://downloads.cms.gov/files/cmmi/hcia-metaanalysisthirdannualrpt.pdf.

30. Bensink ME, Ramsey SD, Battaglia T, *et al*. Costs and outcomes evaluation of patient navigation after abnormal cancer screening: Evidence from the patient navigation research program. *Cancer*. 2014;120(4):570–578.

31. Willis A, Reed E, Pratt-Chapman M, *et al*., Development of a framework for patient navigation: Delineating roles across navigator types. *J Onc Navigation Survivors*. 2013;4(6):20–26.

32. US Bureau of Labor Statistics. Occupational employment and wages, community health workers. Accessed May 23, 2021. https://www.bls.gov/oes/current/oes211094.htm.

33. Community Health Workers Section, American Public Health Association. Accessed June 14, 2020. https://www.apha.org/apha-communities/member-sections/community-health-workers.

34. Burhansstipanov L, Harjo L, Krebs LU, *et al*. Cultural roles of native patient navigators for American Indian cancer patients. *Front Oncol*. 2015;5:79.

35. Cobb N, Espey D, King J. Health behaviors and risk factors among American Indians and Alaska Natives, 2000–2010. *Am J Public Health.* 2014;104(Suppl 3):S481–S489.

36. Brave Heart MY, Chase J, Elkins J, *et al.* Historical trauma among Indigenous peoples of the Americas: Concepts, research, and clinical considerations. *J Psychoactive Drugs.* 2011;43(4):282–290.

37. Sotero M. A conceptual model of historical trauma: Implications for public health practice and research. *J Health Disparities Res Pract.* 2006;1(1):93–108.

38. Braun KL, Mokuau N, Hunt GH, *et al.* Supports and obstacles to cancer survival for Hawai'i's native people. *Cancer Pract.* 2002;10(4):192–200.

39. Burhansstipanov L, Harjo L, Krebs LU, *et al.* Cultural roles of native patient navigators for American Indian cancer patients. *Front Oncol.* 2015;5:79.

40. Valverde PA, Burhansstipanov L, Patierno S, *et al.* Findings from the National Navigation Roundtable: A call for competency-based patient navigation training. *Cancer.* 2019;125(24):4350–4359.

41. National Navigation Roundtable. Patient navigator training competency domains. Accessed June 14, 2020. https://navigationroundtable.org/about/how-we-work/workforce-development/patient-navigator-training-competency-domains/.

42. Oncology Nursing Society, Association of Oncology Social Work, National Association of Social Workers. Oncology Nursing Society, the Association of Oncology Social Work, and the National Association of Social Workers joint position on the role of oncology nursing and oncology social work in patient navigation. *Oncol Nurs Forum.* 2010;37(3):251–252.

43. Institute of Medicine and National Research Council. *Ensuring quality cancer care.* The National Academies Press, 1999.

44. National Navigation Roundtable. How we work. Accessed June 15, 2020. https://navigationroundtable.org/about/how-we-work/.

45. Oncology Nursing Society Voice. Commission on cancer revises its standards: Here are the takeaways for oncology nurses. Accessed June 15, 2020. http://voice.ons.org/news-and-views/commission-on-cancer-revises-its-standards-here-are-the-takeaways-for-oncology.

46. Burhansstipanov L. Team-based oncology care. In: Shockney L, ed. *Team-based oncology care: The pivotal role of oncology navigation.* Springer Publishing, 2018:1–11.

47. Johnston D. Navigation across the continuum of care. In: Shockney L, ed. *Team-based oncology care: The pivotal role of oncology navigation.* Springer Publishing, 2018:111–124.

48. Burhansstipanov L, Krebs LU, Dignan MB, *et al.* Findings from the Native Navigators and the Cancer Continuum (NNACC) study. *J Cancer Educ.* 2014;29(3):420–427.

49. Harjo LD, Burhansstipanov L, Lindstrom D. Rationale for "cultural" native patient navigators in Indian country. *J Cancer Educ.* 2014;29(3):414–419.

50. Watanabe-Galloway S, Burhansstipanov L, Krebs LU, *et al.* Partnering for success through community-based participatory research in Indian country. *J Cancer Educ.* 2014;29(3):588–595.

51. Braun KL, Tsark JU, Santos L, *et al.* Building Native Hawaiian capacity in cancer research and programming. A legacy of 'Imi Hale. *Cancer.* 2006;107(8 Suppl):2082–2090.

52. Braun KL, Thomas WL Jr, Domingo JL, *et al.* Reducing cancer screening disparities in Medicare beneficiaries through cancer patient navigation. *J Am Geriatr Soc.* 2015;63(2):365–370.

53. Cluett C, Hibner L. Tracking Molokai's population 2010 [online]. Accessed June 15, 2020. http://d3c8esugncvql9.cloudfront.net/wp-content/uploads/Molokai_Stats1.jpg.

54. Braun KL, Allison A, Tsark JU. Using community-based research methods to design cancer patient navigation training. *Prog Community Health Partnerships*. 2008;2(4):329–340.

55. Kulukulualani M, Braun KL, Tsark JU. Using a participatory four-step protocol to develop culturally targeted cancer education brochures. *Health Promot Pract*. 2008;9(4):344–355.

56. Gellert K, Braun KL, Morris R, et al. The 'Ohana Day Project: A community approach to increasing cancer screening. *Prev Chronic Dis*. 2006;3(3):A99.

57. Yamada S. Cancer, reproductive abnormalities, and diabetes in Micronesia: The effect of nuclear testing. *Pac Health Dialog*. 2004;11(2):216–221.

58. Tsark JU, Braun KL, Pacific Islands Cancer Council. Reducing cancer health disparities in the US-associated Pacific. *J Public Health Manag Pract*. 2007;13(1):49–58.

59. Aitaoto N, Tsark JU, Tomiyasu DW, et al. Strategies to increase breast and cervical cancer screening among Hawaiian, Pacific Islander, and Filipina women in Hawai'i. *Hawaii Med J*. 2009;68(9):215–222.

60. Pobutsky AM, Buenconsejo-Lum L, Chow C, et al. Micronesian migrants in Hawai'i: 2005 health issues and culturally appropriate, community-based solutions. *Calif J Health Promot*. 2005;3(4):59–72.

61. Aitaoto N, Braun KL, Estrella J, et al. Design and results of a culturally tailored cancer outreach project by and for Micronesian women. *Prev Chronic Dis*. 2012;9:E82.

9

Reducing Prediabetes and Diabetes

Francine C. Gachupin, Jennie R. Joe, Christina L. Interpreter,
Noshene Ranjbar, Christina (Kiki) Stinnett, JoAnn 'Umilani Tsark,
Marjoree Neer, and Kathryn L. Braun

Introduction

Type 2 diabetes mellitus (T2DM) is a complex, chronic illness that requires
continuous medical and self-management. Historically, it was an adult-onset
disease, but it has increased substantially among children and adolescents, primarily due to increased poverty, food availability, and obesity in the United
States (US). It also has been linked to heredity genes, classifying it as an intergenerational health problem. Prevalence tends to be higher among Indigenous
Peoples than Whites. Several Indigenous communities have engaged with universities and infrastructure-supporting organizations to address T2DM in their
regions. After more detail about diabetes, three examples are shared of Indigenous community–engaged interventions that demonstrate the importance of
education and empowerment in the control of T2DM.

Description of Diabetes Mellitus

Diabetes mellitus (or diabetes) is a chronic, lifelong condition that affects the
body's ability to use the energy found in food. Normally, the pancreas secretes
insulin, a hormone that assists with the breakdown of food to glucose. Glucose
fuels the cells in the body, and the cells need insulin in the bloodstream to
absorb glucose and use it for energy. With diabetes mellitus, either the pancreas does not make enough insulin, the body cannot use the insulin produced
by the pancreas, or a combination of both.[1] This leads to increased levels of
glucose in the bloodstream, causing symptoms of hyperglycemia, including
increased thirst, frequent urination, increased hunger, fatigue, blurred vision,
and weight loss. If left untreated, irreversible damages occur to body systems,
including the heart, small and large blood vessels, the nervous system, the
eyes, and most importantly, the kidneys. Failure to manage diabetes can
lead to frequent hospitalizations, lower-extremity amputations, major heart
disease, blindness, neuropathy, and end-stage renal disease, which requires
dialysis.

In their 2020 report, the Centers for Disease Control and Prevention (CDC) estimated that 34.2 million people (10.5% of the US population) have diabetes.[2] There are three major types of diabetes. *Gestational diabetes* is diabetes that occurs during pregnancy and usually resolves after childbirth. It occurs in 2–10% of pregnancies and is a risk factor for developing T2DM later in life for both the child and the mother.[3] *Type 1 diabetes* occurs when the body does not produce insulin at all. This type of diabetes is usually diagnosed in childhood, and 5–10% of all people with diabetes have type 1 diabetes.[4] *Type 2 diabetes* is the most common type, and it occurs if the body loses the ability to use insulin efficiently.[5] People who smoke, are overweight, do not exercise, and/or have an unhealthy diet are at increased risk of developing T2DM, and scientists estimate about 90% of T2DM cases could be prevented by avoiding these risk factors. All types of diabetes are complex conditions and require continuous medical management.

The medical cost of living with diabetes is high. An American Diabetes Association report estimated that the total cost of diagnosed diabetes in the US was $327 billion in 2017, including $237 billion in direct medical costs and $90 billion in reduced productivity. On the individual level, people with diabetes have medical expenditures that are about 2.3 times higher than for people without diabetes.[6]

Prevalence of Diabetes in Indigenous Peoples

According to the 2017–2018 data, the CDC estimated the prevalence of diabetes among American Indians (AI) and Alaska Natives (AN) to be 14.7%, compared to 7.5% in non-Hispanic Whites.[2] Data collected in Hawai'i from 2011 to 2017 estimated that 10% of NH adults and 10% of other PI adults had diabetes, compared to 5% of Whites in the state.[7,8] Across the US-Affiliated Pacific Island (USAPI) jurisdictions, data published in 2013 estimated that diabetes affected 47% of adults in American Samoa, 32% in Pohnpei State in the Federated States of Micronesia (FSM), 23% in Yap State (FSM), 22% in Palau, 20% in the Marshall Islands, 13% in Kosrae State (FSM), 10% in the Commonwealth of the Northern Mariana Islands (CNMI), and 9% in Guam.[9]

Globally, the prevalence of T2DM among Indigenous adults began to increase after the introduction of processed foods and wage-based economies by colonizers, and by the 1980s, about 50% of Pima Indians above age 35 were recorded as having T2DM. Starting in the mid-1980s, physicians began reporting increases in T2DM among AI/AN and NH/PI children and adolescents. Today, high proportions of Indigenous grandparents, parents, and children have T2DM, making this an intergenerational health problem.[10] For young people, being diagnosed with T2DM is especially costly, as it lowers their quality of life, precipitates early development of diabetic-related complications, and shortens life expectancy.[11]

Adverse Childhood Experiences as a Risk Factor for T2DM

The high prevalence of T2DM in Indigenous Peoples has been linked to several risk factors, including adverse childhood experiences (ACE), as well as genetics, environment, poverty, obesity, and lifestyle choices. ACE are upsetting and stressful events that occur before the age of 18, including abuse (physical, sexual, emotional), neglect (physical, emotional), domestic violence, parental substance misuse, household mental illness, parental separation or divorce, and incarcerated household member.[12] The 1998 Adverse Childhood Experiences Study included more than 17,000 individuals who were asked about their experience of these events in childhood, and a dose-response pattern was found. Specifically, the more ACE in childhood, the greater the likelihood of experiencing complex health and behavioral issues across one's lifespan, including stroke, cancer, heart disease, pain, obesity, diabetes, autoimmune diseases, metabolic syndrome, addiction, depression, anxiety, and other mental health conditions. Results also demonstrated strong associations between ACE and risky health behaviors, such as inactivity, substance misuse, violence, overeating, and smoking.[13,14,15] Follow-up studies have broadened adverse experiences to include the death of a parent, sibling and peer victimization, property crimes, community violence, and spanking.[16,17,18] ACE also have been associated with increased risk in adulthood of internalizing psychopathologies, such as social withdrawal and self-blame, and externalizing psychopathology, including physical aggression.[19,20] A meta-analysis of seven articles reporting risk estimates for diabetes by ACE found significant odds ratios of 1.92 for victims of childhood neglect, 1.39 for victims of childhood sexual abuse, and 1.30 for victims of childhood physical abuse.[21]

ACE disproportionately affect Indigenous communities. Data from the National Child Health Survey in 2011–2012 suggested that AI/AN children were much more likely to have a parent who served time in jail (18% versus 6% of non-Hispanic White children), to have observed domestic violence (15.5% versus 6.3%), and to have lived with a substance abuser (23.6% versus 11.6%). Additionally, they were 1.5 times more likely to live in families with difficulty paying for basic needs, including food or housing (35.7% versus 22.8%), to have lived with a divorced or separated parent (33% versus 21.4%), and to have experienced the death of a parent (4.2% versus 2.5%). About 40% of AI/AN children were reported to have experienced two to five ACE, compared to only 9.9% of non-

Hispanic White children, and 10% of AI/AN children were treated or judged unfairly based on race, compared to only 1.4% of non-Hispanic White children.[22]

Using a different methodology, researchers in Hawai'i added questions probing for eight different ACE to the Behavioral Risk Factor Surveillance Survey in 2010. This survey was administered to adults, who were asked to recall ACE from their youth. The findings suggested 74.9% of Native Hawaiian adults (age 18 or older) reported experiencing at least one ACE compared to 63.8% of Whites, and 40–50% of Asians. Even more startling, 38.4% of NH reported experiencing four or more ACE, compared to 29.0% of Whites, and 10–15% of Asians.[23]

Importance of Resiliency Skills

Many factors affecting Indigenous Peoples cause stress, including racism, poverty, living in under-resourced areas, high prevalence of ACE in childhood, and a high prevalence of chronic conditions in childhood and adulthood. Chronic stress leads to maladaptive, stress-related behaviors, such as overeating, use of drugs and alcohol, social isolation, and a sedentary lifestyle, which also can contribute to chronic disease. For example, when one's biological system reacts to high or sustained stress, there is a negative impact on the function of the central and autonomic nervous systems. This increases the allostatic load, negatively affects inflammatory and immune processes, upregulates the hypothalamic–pituitary–adrenal axis, influences gene expression (epigenetics), and diminishes the capacity to self-regulate.[24,25]

Historically, Indigenous cultures promoted a lifestyle that was in nature "anti-inflammatory" and built resiliency to stress. For example, traditional lifestyles involved hunting, gathering, farming, and fishing, and these activities kept people physically active. People traveled on foot or by canoe or horseback. They slept and woke following the natural rhythms of the earth, ate nature-based foods, and practiced ceremonies and rituals that provided nurturance and a sense of meaning, purpose, and belonging as part of the tribe or community. These activities inherently promoted resiliency in children and youth into adulthood and beyond. Many of these protective factors are now lacking in the world in which Indigenous Peoples are living today. Furthermore, a sense of connectedness to Indigenous cultural traditions is lacking for many youths and adults, who find themselves torn between their ancestral culture and the modern ways of life that surround them.

A foundational approach to addressing chronic disease prevention and management from both an individual and a public health perspective is building stress management and resiliency skills for the mind, body, emotion, and spirit. Due to the numerous stress-inducing experiences confronting

Indigenous Peoples, wellness models for these communities must extend their focus and reach to address historical, cultural, and social determinants that lead to adverse childhood and community experiences. Relational support combined with strength-based, culturally sensitive, and trauma-informed care, education, and resiliency skills building may buffer against these negative effects. The following interventions were developed by Indigenous researchers to increase diabetes awareness and education in their communities.

Examples of Successful Indigenous Community–Engaged Interventions

American Indian Youth Wellness Camp[i]

Description

The American Indian Youth Wellness Camp is a 6-day residential program for AI youth with T2DM.[26] Funds for the camp come from private charitable donations, tribal contributions, and tribal diabetes prevention programs. The camp started in 1991 to address concerns of healthcare providers serving tribal communities in the Southwestern US who felt unprepared to deal with this emerging, noncontagious, chronic disease among young people.[27,28] They cited the lack of resources to develop diabetes control interventions to slow the incidence of potential diabetic-related complications.[29,30] Due to the rather rapid emergence of this problem, a consensus on the treatment of children and adolescents with T2DM was neither clear nor well addressed.[31] Like most T2DM treatments, most of the existing diabetes educational programs and prevention resources were targeted to adults. The major federal healthcare delivery system for AI/AN, Indian Health Service (IHS), did not have diabetic-related health resources for its young patients with diabetes. The most common medical treatment, in addition to advising newly diagnosed patients to be physically active and eat healthy meals, was oral medication, like Metformin.

Intervention

The American Indian Youth Wellness Camp includes multiple components. Youth stay overnight at the camp, so food and sleeping accommodations are provided. Activities are structured and include anthropometric and risk

i Funding from the Arizona Area Health Education Centers Program Career Development Award, University of Arizona Cancer Center Partnership for Native American Cancer Prevention [U54CA143924], Association of American Indian Affairs, Diabetes Action Research and Education Foundation, Marin Community Foundation, Mayo Clinic Spirit of EAGLES, and the National Institute of Minority Health and Health Disparities [R01MD014127].

behavior assessments, education sessions, physical engagement, and health messaging to increase healthy lifestyles among AI youth at risk for overweight, obesity, diabetes, and cardiovascular disease.[32] Volunteer medical providers lead the health education sessions to increase understanding of T2DM.[33] During instruction, the medical providers use approaches that contribute to the "ah-ha moments" like the acronym PIG-E, which stands for pancreas, insulin, glucose, and energy. All instruction and care are delivered using culturally appropriate examples to encourage youth to remember health promotion messages and to enable the youth to teach family members or friends. Including medical providers at camp provides an unparalleled opportunity for youth to get to know their local providers better and a chance for providers to meet tribal community members.

In 2016, Mind-Body Skills Groups (MBSG) were added as one of the camp activities. MBSG is an experiential skills-based model that incorporates the use of drawing, concentrative and active meditations, guided imagery, biofeedback, movement, body awareness, and expressive writing. Active skills building and sharing occur within the context of small groups (8–12 participants) and are based on principles of relational attunement and facilitation of both expressive and receptive domains of communication. The model addresses the impact of stress and enables individuals to take charge of their physiological functioning and build resilience by mobilizing a wide range of mental, emotional, imaginative, and physical abilities. Beyond the evidence base of the individual mind–body medicine modalities, research on this specific model suggests that it increases the ability to manage stress experienced by culturally diverse populations.[34,35,36] The MBSG component also fits well within the culture, beliefs, and practices of AI communities.[34]

Initially, the MBSG component was a 3-hour workshop at camp and, in 2018, it was expanded to cover 1.5 days of the 6-day camp. In its expanded form, the MBSG components provide youth with both a self-regulation toolkit and an enhanced sense of connection to others, self-awareness and self-efficacy, thereby enhancing wellness efforts over time. Because peer pressure and the need for belonging are important for this age group, the sharing of health-promoting skills and tools are accompanied by facilitated discussion within small groups. Much of the structure and content of the model itself is linked to ancient and Indigenous practices and concurrently validated by research. When combined with local cultural beliefs and approaches, it reflects a state-of-the-art approach for addressing both historical and ongoing trauma and resiliency in AI communities.

After camp, classes and programming helps transition students back to daily life. Progress is monitored through personal check-ins, supporting both students and parents after the safety net of the camp is gone. Connections with parents are especially important since their habits and actions largely influence the health of children.

The cost of the camp remains affordable because of donations. At the heart of the program is the goal to make the camp a meaningful diabetes education encounter and for AI youth to experience the educational offerings in a safe and fun environment. The camp provides an environment that includes exposure to tribal cultures and involves volunteers who work with tribal communities.

Community Engagement

In 1991, faculty members at the Department of Family and Community Medicine within the University of Arizona's College of Medicine collaborated with several healthcare providers working with tribes in Arizona to plan a medical camp for youth either diagnosed with T2DM or deemed at high risk for developing diabetes. The initial planning committee included tribal health personnel, including a pediatrician, a physician assistant, a registered nurse, two registered dietitians, several certified physical activity instructors, tribal wellness coordinators, and a tribal diabetes program director. The committee also included several tribal community health representatives (CHR), who are community members trained and compensated to provide education and outreach in their communities within the IHS. The model of a diabetes camp for young people was considered, but at the time most diabetes camps served only young people with type 1 diabetes. Based on research and community discussions, the planning committee decided to establish a 6-day residential medical camp for AI children and adolescents aged 10 to 15 years, as this was the age range in which many the tribal youth were being diagnosed with T2DM.

While several aspects of the camp have changed over time, it remains embedded in a collaborative model, a partnership between the university and participating tribal communities. The participation of the tribes also has changed, with several of the larger tribes establishing their own camps. Tribes that have little or no infrastructure to support their camp continue to collaborate with the university. The local wellness and/or diabetes program staff members coordinate the partnership within the tribal communities. The team members not only assist by identifying potential campers but also assist the families with enrollment requirements, such as medical examination and gathering pertinent diet and social information.

The American Indian Youth Wellness Camp has been operating continually since 1991. As funding became more competitive, the need for rigorous evaluation became evident and, since summer 2013, the program became more outcomes oriented. With full approval by participating tribes, more emphasis was placed on showing improvement in health risk behaviors (including exercise and diet patterns) and anthropometric measures, and the program has been expanded to 6 months with inclusion of parents.[37]

Outcomes

In any given summer, 35–60 youth attend camp. About 40% of youth return from one summer to the next. Between 2013 and 2020, 289 AI youth attended the residential camp. Youth who attend camp are self-selected or referred by local tribal health programs because of the presence of risk factors for T2DM that include strong family history (T2DM in first- and second-degree relatives), obesity, impaired glucose tolerance, hyperinsulinemia, or metabolic syndrome. In any given summer, about 11% of the campers are diagnosed with T2DM. Based on data from youth attending this camp between 2011 and 2014, 66% of girls and 87% of boys aged 10–15 years had a Body Mass Index (BMI)-for-age greater than the 95th percentile.

Data from the 2016 Youth Risk Behavior Survey of middle and high school students in these communities estimated that only 50% of youth lived with both parents, 17.9% sometimes did not have enough to eat, 76.8% were physically active for less than 60 minutes per day, 35.7% played video or computer games for 3 or more hours a day, 26.8% watched DVDs or videos for 3 or more hours a day, 39.3% were bullied on school property over the preceding 12 months, and only 35.7% had a friend about their age that cared about them.

Table 9.1. presents clinical characteristics associated with risk for metabolic syndrome and T2DM for youth attending camp in 2016. The average age was 11.9 years, with a range of 10–14 years. Most (78%) of the participants were classified as overweight or obese. Fasting plasma glucose concentrations averaged 91 mg/dL, which is the higher end of the normal (70–100 mg/dL). The hemoglobin A1c test (HbA1c) presented the average level of blood sugar over the past 2 to 3 months. and the average HbA1c was 5.8%, whereas the normal range is below 5.7%. A blood sugar level between 5.7 and 6.4 indicates a prediabetic state. Over 40% of the youth had HbA1c values that met the criteria for prediabetes or T2DM (between 5.7 and 6.4).

Reported dietary intakes of total energy, fiber, and various macro- and micronutrients for girls and boys, reported before camp, are shown in Table 9.2. Overall, the youth reported diets that were high in calories, fats, and sodium, and low in fiber, calcium, and potassium.[38] In assessing the percent of youth meeting the recommendations outlined in the Dietary Guidelines for Americans 2015–2020,[39] very few youth met the recommendations, with observed intake differences between girls and boys. More girls met the recommended intake of fruits and vegetables than boys, while more boys meet the

Table 9.1. Clinical Characteristics of Participants, Summer 2016 ($n = 26$)

Mean + SD or (range)	Value
Height, cm	155.1 ± 8.9
Weight, kg	68.3 ± 22.1
BMI, kg/m^2	28.1 (18–40)
BMI percentile	89.1 ± 16.2
BMI z-score	1.7 ± 0.9
Waist circumference, cm	90.9 ± 17.1
Fasting total cholesterol, mg/dL	171 (143–258)
Fasting glucose, mg/dL	91.0 (70–163)
Hemoglobin A1c, %	5.8 (4.7–11.1)
Height percentile	68.8 ± 23.6
Z-score	0.1 ± 1.2
Percentile	50.1 ± 32.5
Height percentile	68.8 ± 23.6
Z-score	1.0 ± 0.73
Percentile	79.4 ± 18.3
Heart rate (beats per minute)	95.4 ± 16.8

Table 9.2. Average Reported Dietary Intake of Total Energy, Fiber, and Various Macro- and Micronutrients for Girls and Boys

Dietary Intake	Girls ($n = 17$) mean ± SD	Boys ($n = 9$) mean ± SD	Total ($n = 26$) mean ± SD
Total energy, kcal	1,911.8 ± 555.7	1,721.1 ± 479.2	1,845.8 ± 533.6
Energy from fat	686.9 ± 234.6	696.8 ± 384.8	690.3 ± 291.6
Energy from saturated fat	226.0 ± 86.8	199.6 ± 61.3	216.8 ± 79.3
Energy from protein	294.8 ± 103.9	259.6 ± 91.6	282.6 ± 101.7
Fiber, g	14.2 ± 4.5	13.0 ± 6.5	13.8 ± 5.2
Calcium, mg	712.5 ± 340.3	736.3 ± 340.6	720.7 ± 337.2
Iron, mg	11.7 ± 4.5	12.5 ± 7.9	11.9 ± 5.9
Sodium, mg	3,106.1 ± 1,118.4	3,028.8± 923.8	3,079.3 ± 1,046.5
Potassium, mg	2,066.6 ± 701.1	1,689.7 ± 1014.9	1,936.1 ± 833.2
Vitamin A, RE	490.9 ± 303.8	479.1 ± 355.7	486.8 ± 319.3
Vitamin B12, mcg	3.6 ± 1.8	3.6 ± 2.2	3.6 ± 1.2
Folate, mcg	278.5 ± 145.0	269.6± 215.9	275.4 ± 170.8
Vitamin C, mg	95.0 ± 86.6	59.0 ± 39.5	82.5 ± 75.3
Vitamin D, mcg	3.5 ± 2.8	3.8 ± 3.3	3.6 ± 3.0
Vitamin E, mg	1.8 ± 4.2	0.6 ± 0.9	1.4 ± 3.5

Table 9.3. Wrist Accelerometer Data for American Indian Youth, Summer 2014

	Day 1 N = 27	Day 2 N = 27	Day 3 N = 27	Day 4 N = 27
Active Time (H:M)	4:06 (1:42–6:32)	9:06 (4:51–12:26)	9:10 (3:53–12:00)	6:56 (4:36–11:27)
Steps taken	10,942 (3,927–17,456)	27,781 (13,880–41,037)	27,526 (12,759–39,084)	17,768 (12,398–35,329)
Kilocalories burned	2,455 (1,312–3,979)	3,563 (1,864–6,353)	3,636 (1,545–7,101)	2,744 (1,418–5,460)
Sleep last night (H:M)	–	7:37 (2:27–9:07)	8:42 (7:33–9:58)	7:50 (5:24–9:02)
Restful sleep (H:M)	–	6:12 (1:51–7:28)	6:58 (5:03–8:44)	6:22 (4:19–7:36)
Restless sleep (H:M)	–	1:24 (0:36–2:12)	1:43 (0:44–2:57)	1:27 (0:47–2:28)
% Restful sleep	–	81.3% (75–92%)	80% (65–90%)	81.4% (69–90%)

recommended intake of dairy than girls. The Dietary Guidelines for Americans recommend that less than 10% of calories per day come from added sugars and less than 10% of calories per day from saturated fats. Empty calories, defined as calories from solid fats and added sugars, accounted for about 40% of total energy intake in these youth.

Increasingly, mobile health (mHealth) technology is used to track individual daily fitness,[40,41,42,43,44] and social networking sites are being utilized to promote adolescent health.[45] In summer 2014, Polar Loop physical activity monitors, worn on the wrist, were provided to AI youth attending camp, and the intensity and duration of physical activities and sleep were recorded for each participant (Table 9.3.). On the first full day of wearing devices, the monitors showed the youth achieved an average active time of 9 hours (range 5–12.50 hours). Healthy activity guidelines recommend 10,000 steps a day. Camp participants' average daily number of steps was 27,781, and the average daily number of kilocalories burned was 3,563. The average number of hours of sleep was 7.5 hours, with 81.3% experiencing restful sleep. The youth responded positively to these devices and received support to synchronize and charge their devices while at camp.

Lessons Learned

The community engagement model in the wellness camp delivers diabetes education in a culturally oriented and child-friendly environment. The success of the program is enhanced by the ongoing collaboration with tribal medical providers and diabetes program staff members, providers, and staff members who work with the campers and their families in their respective communities. The inclusion of medical providers within community-based diabetes prevention program efforts underscore health promotion messages and lessen the potential fear of community members of taking part in preventive and routine healthcare upon returning home. The health data collected and utilized by the collaborative partners provide invaluable reference data for decision-making, program planning, and feedback on the respective communities' efforts in decreasing the problem of diabetes.

Within AI/AN populations, family and culture are core. Teaching future generations about their rich traditions and including these components in health education programs are crucial aims of the program. Education on how to understand and break the cycle of T2DM is critical to reducing the impact of diabetes on future generations. Based on the evidence and experience, the provision of self-awareness, self-regulation, self-expression, and prosocial behavior training help youth recognize and reduce maladaptive coping behaviors such as unhealthy overeating and/or inactivity resulting in poor moods.

Diabetes Primary Prevention Programs at Toiyabe Indian Health Project[ii]

Description

The Toiyabe Indian Health Project (TIHP) is an IHS-supported healthcare system with three clinics (Bishop, Lone Pine and Coleville, CA) serving seven AI tribes and two AI communities in the Sierra Nevada Mountains of rural eastern California. Since the late 1990s, the TIHP Special Diabetes Program for Indians has provided services for Toiyabe Native patients who are on the diabetes registry. With funding through the CDC's Tribal Public Health Capacity Building and Quality Improvement program, TIHP expanded its capacity to identify and assist AI community members in the prevention of diabetes.

Intervention

A process framework was established to work toward building capacity in diabetes prevention. This started with communicating the vision and strategy of

ii Funding from CDC Grant U38 OT000252.

this project throughout the organization and to the communities served by TIHP, as well as building relationships with community partners. The community health representatives (CHR) employed by TIHP were key players in the quality improvement project, as these staff members provided outreach, education, case management, home visits, transportation, and other services to TIHP patients. Next, CHR and other TIHP staff were trained to increase their competence around diabetes prevention, to assure consistency of messaging through case management, and to develop culturally competent educational tools. Then, community members were engaged in outreach and education, and the organization was assisted in the development of policies and procedures around collaboration for diabetes prevention.

The TIHP staff worked to nurture communication and collaboration between the medical providers and the public health staff, as well as to define the issue of prediabetes clearly. An early task was to implement the 26 modules of the CDC Diabetes Prevention Program (DPP) curriculum to be tribally and geographically appropriate for the Sierra Nevada region of California. The subsequent program provided at least 22 of the 26 biweekly modules and met the criteria to achieve CDC recognition. Both clinical staff and CHR were trained to provide a common approach for patients to support their efforts to prevent diabetes. The diabetes prevention program staff also developed a method to track individuals' blood sugar levels, weight, and diabetes prevention needs and activities.

Another program, Family Spirit, was introduced in 2014 to help pregnant women have a healthy and informed pregnancy and prevent gestational diabetes, as well as education on parenting. This program delivered a strong home visiting curriculum that focused on pregnancy through the first 36 months of life of the baby.[46] Eight of the Toiyabe public health staff completed the weeklong training. The full 63-lesson curriculum was too difficult to implement, and the project team made significant modifications and tailored the curriculum to the individual woman. The revised version was referred to as Family Spirit Lite and allowed for more flexible scheduling and selection of topics of greatest interest to participants. There were clinical goals as well, which included identifying and assisting community members who had prediabetes or were at risk for developing diabetes to meet clinical and behavioral goals through education and self-management support.

Community Engagement

The population involved in this project lived in an area that occupies over 13,000 square miles in the eastern Sierras Nevada mountains of California. The CHR traveled upward of 150 miles one-way to meet and engage individual families and small groups of families in diabetes prevention. This effort created relationships between the CHR and the community members and helped to build trust. For pregnant women, Family Spirit Lite provided culturally respectful information to help them personally and to improve the health and development of their babies. The process of communicating the vision and strategy of this project helped create a new culture around health.

Outcomes

Before the grant, the term "prediabetes" was not being used in a consistent or meaningful way at TIHP and was sometimes referred to as early diabetes or metabolic disorder. To change this, the public health staff collaborated with clinic staff to standardize definitions, adopt diagnostic criteria and to use the same phrasing orally and in printed materials. Reference cards were made with A1c criteria, ICD-10 codes, and other information for providers, support staff, and CHR so that all were using the same language when working with each other and with the community. An advisory board for the grant and monthly case review meetings with the medical department increased the collaboration and communication between the medical, nursing, public health, and CHR staff. CHR were trained to upload and document patient visits within the electronic health record (EHR).

Eight CHR and public health staff completed the training for the CDC Diabetes Prevention Program and became certified lifestyle coaches. All were involved in teaching one or more year-long classes. The CHR staff was able to document visits and class education directly into the EHR and receive referrals and notifications directly. CHR also received education and training in the Lifetime of Wellness project, which guided outreach to community members on prediabetes, blood pressure control, and self-management. Subsequently, CHR felt comfortable leading classes, and they interacted with more than 70 community members about taking care of their health. The CHR initiated and participated regularly in blood pressure and blood sugar screening events to identify community members at risk for prediabetes and hypertension and to provide one-on-one follow-up education and referrals.

CHR staff conducted many healthy lifestyle outreach activities, for example on healthy eating and active living, through one-on-one and small group activities. From 2013 to 2018, more than 300 rural community members participated in health screenings and education about health screenings and prediabetes. The adapted DPP curriculum was delivered successfully at the three clinics. The Lifetime of Wellness project was provided to individuals who were referred from medical providers or were patients known to have prediabetes or hypertension beginning in 2018. That project contributed to the infrastructure by providing blood pressure cuffs to community members. The CHR received additional training on hypertension and prediabetes.

About 20 families took part in the Family Spirit Lite program. Information and referral packets were developed for women with a positive pregnancy test. Infrastructure and quality improvement were supported by a strong working relationship with the OB/GYN practice in town and at the clinic with CHR and public health staff. These relationships increased the number of patients that were referred to TIHP.

The employees of TIHP also were patients. For several years, there was an active Employee Wellness Program, which encouraged fitness and healthy eating. Although inactive for several years, this program was revived in 2017 and contributes to increased wellness among the TIHP staff.

Lessons Learned

The CDC's Tribal Public Health Capacity Building and Quality Improvement Project allowed TIHP the opportunity to address the issue of prediabetes and diabetes prevention to provide a more comprehensive approach to the issue of diabetes in the Native American population in the eastern Sierra of California. CHR were certified as lifestyle coaches and felt comfortable leading classes and talking to community members about taking care of their health. Communication and collaboration between medical providers and the public health staff were improved. Both the prediabetes and lifestyle change education classes were more effective and efficient than were one-on-one education sessions. They also provided the most effective way to have consistent contact between the CHR and interested AI community members. More than 300 rural AI community members were reached through screenings and education sessions about prediabetes, diabetes, and lifestyle change classes. Overall, the TIHP created the infrastructure for future programs to prevent diabetes among AI living in the Sierras and rural areas.

The Pacific Diabetes Today Resource Center and its Spin-Offs[iii]

Description

T2DM is excessive among NH/PI. Even more startling is the prevalence of overweight and obesity among NH/PI adults. Data from 2016 in Hawai'i suggested that 78% of NH and 84% of other PI are overweight or obese.[47] Data from a 2013 assessment in the USAPI region estimated an overweight/obesity prevalence of 93% in American Samoa, 90% in Palau, 87% in the CNMI, 70%

---

iii Funding from CDC NU58DP006370 and 200-98-0425.

in the FSM, and 63% in the Marshall Islands.[9] Given the high prevalence of diabetes among adults and the high prevalence of overweight/obesity among NH/PI, the CDC and the governments of each jurisdiction were very interested in engaging with NH/PI communities to address T2DM.

As described in Chapter 2, Hawai'i and the USAPI region are composed of thousands of small islands and atolls within about 4 million square miles of ocean. These islands share a history of colonization. All of these jurisdictions use US dollars as currency, are served by the US Postal Service, and receive US federal funding for infrastructure, health, and education. They also may apply for additional federal funding—for example, from CDC. However, access to healthcare varies across the region. For example, excellent healthcare services are available in Honolulu, but less available on neighbor islands and the capitals of the USAPI jurisdictions, and are nonexistent on many atolls and islands. Many health programs depend on grants, so it is essential to develop local leadership and capacity to secure grants and operate programs.

Intervention

The Pacific Diabetes Today Resource Center (PDTRC) was an initiative funded by the CDC to train NH/PI communities in coalition building and program planning skills using CDC's Diabetes Today curriculum. The resource center, funded from 1998 through 2003, was hosted by Papa Ola Lōkahi, a community-based organization in Honolulu, Hawai'i, composed of a consortium of NH organizations and public agencies focused on improving the health and wellness of NH. The project worked with community groups in Hawai'i's four counties, American Samoa, the four culturally distinct states of the FSM (Chuuk, Kosrae, Pohnpei, and Yap), Guam, the CNMI, Palau, and the Marshall Islands.[48,49]

Guided by the principles of community building, and led by two NH/PI health professionals, the mission of PDTRC was to build capacity in Pacific communities to address the high and growing prevalence of T2DM. The resource center achieved this mission by providing training, technical assistance, and funding to community groups to learn about diabetes, to develop an idea for a program around diabetes prevention and control, and then to implement and evaluate that program. Technical assistance also was provided to help these communities secure grants to continue and expand their programming.

Community Engagement

Community engagement was evident in each of the steps taken to carry out the mission of the program. First, PDTRC hired an individual of NH/PI ancestry who spoke Hawaiian, Samoan, Carolinian, and several other NH/PI languages. Next, PDTRC staff identified agencies and champions within partner communities who already were committed to addressing diabetes or some other health or social issue. These champions joined PDTRC's Advisory Council, and their first task was to review the existing CDC curriculum for relevancy, cultural competency, health literacy, and acceptability for the Pacific communities they served. These individuals brought together additional community members, who participated in focus groups and other needs assessment activities related to diabetes. This resulted in the development of a new curriculum that incorporated Pacific stories, culture, and health-seeking behaviors. The curriculum also was designed to include healthcare providers and community members in the collection of assessment data and the implementation of the training, thereby increasing local awareness and capacity. Finally, PDTRC subcontracted with community-based agencies to host and cofacilitate a 6-day training on how to prioritize needs, plan programs, and secure resources to address diabetes in ways acceptable and relevant to their respective communities. PDTRC provided technical assistance to implement, evaluate, and secure funds to continue or expand them.

Outcomes

By 2003, at the end of PDTRC funding, 11 communities had mobilized stakeholders, conducted training, and developed diabetes initiatives. These initiatives included community outreach programs to increase screening, diabetes prevention education campaigns, diabetes training for local healthcare providers, and fundraising activities to purchase and provide medical supplies.[46] In 2008, PDTRC coalitions were revisited to see if they had been able to sustain their work. Of the 11 coalitions, 9 were still active. For example, in Kosrae State (FSM), PDTRC participants had formed the Kosrae Diabetes Today Coalition to increase diabetes awareness and prevent the onset of diabetes and its complications. A major focus was physical activity. The group had secured resources to equip each large village with volleyballs and nets and was sponsoring island-wide competitions. The group also influenced mayors and traditional leaders to improve streetlights and walkways to encourage physical activity and to allocate part of the workday to exercise. Regular volleyball games were being played in all four municipalities, and health providers began to use volleyball game sites to promote weight loss.[48]

The work of PDTRC also led to subsequent grants from CDC to continue work to address diabetes in the region, including the Pacific Diabetes Education Program (PDEP), which operated from 2005 to 2009. A spin-off of the PDEP was the Pacific Chronic Disease Coalition (PCDC), which included Indigenous representatives from across the Pacific region. This group continues to operate with support funding from the National Association of Chronic Disease Directors.

In 2017, another CDC grant was obtained by the same NH/PI health educators who worked to implement PDTRC and PDEP. This project was called Pacific Islands—Diabetes Prevention Program (PI-DPP), and it worked with several of the same communities. The rest of this "success story" focuses on one of the programs of the Chuuk Women's Council (CWC), a nonprofit organization that engaged with PDTRC (1998–2003), continued its work in diabetes in collaboration with PDEP (2005–2009), and later joined PI-DPP (2017–2022).

The CWC is an organization comprised of women's groups throughout Chuuk State, one of four states of the FSM (population 50,000). These women's groups are associated with churches, neighborhoods, and women's clubs, and each pays a small membership fee of $20 per year to CWC. In 2020, the Council had 63 organizational members representing more than 1,000 women in 39 municipalities across the 40 inhabited islands of Chuuk. Members are mostly housewives. The group meets monthly, and members communicate with each other through text, radio station announcements, word of mouth, and letters sent by cargo ships or water taxis.

Founded in 1993, the group's mission is to assist women in becoming more productive and self-sufficient members of society through comprehensive programs that enhance the social, economic, and physical well-being of women and their families in Chuuk. Initial activities focused primarily on economic opportunities for women. However, about the time the group learned about PDTRC in 1998, it had decided to expand activities into health-related areas. The CWC was subcontracted to translate the PDTRC curriculum into Chuukese and identify Chuukese healthcare providers to serve as training faculty and deliver portions of the curriculum, especially those related to diabetes pathology. This allowed trainees to develop a relationship with providers, who subsequently helped support diabetes outreach, education, and screening activities.

Representatives from over 20 women's organizations in Chuuk attended the initial PDTRC training, through which they wrote a proposal to develop local diabetes education materials (including measuring cups to teach portion control) and to train local women as educators. They also started a walking group, distributed pedometers, and challenged members to reach 10,000 steps a day.

After PDTRC funding ended in 2003, CWC agreed to partner in PDEP (2005–2009), and these resources helped the group expand its educational activities. As the first step with PDEP, the group conducted a needs assessment to learn about residents' concerns related to diabetes. One area of concern was the high number of amputations related to diabetes. In response, CWC decided to focus on foot care and worked with PDEP to develop foot-care kits. Each kit included a mirror to allow viewing of the bottom of the foot, toenail clippers, and a file that came in a waterproof, zippered bag with foot-care instructions printed on the outside. An education piece from Australia on "how to take care of your feet" was adapted, translated, and culturally tailored for the Chuukese audience. CWC members were trained to educate people with diabetes about foot care, and an assessment conducted 4 years later reported a significant reduction in amputations. CWC also sponsored annual health fairs and educational events on Diabetes International Day in collaboration with the Chuuk Health Department.

In 2017, the CWC partnered with PI-DPP to provide a 12-month lifestyle change program developed and promoted by CDC for prediabetic individuals. Trained lifestyle coaches, all Chuukese, conducted the program using a CDC curriculum that the CWC helped to translate and tailor to their community, incorporating local pictures and foods. This prevention program offered lifestyle coaching to help people at risk for diabetes to reduce their weight by 5–7% through healthy eating and increased physical exercise.

With grant writing and program management experiences initially gained through PDTRC, CWC applied for other health-related grants from the World Health Organization, the South Pacific Commission, and the Australian government. These funds allowed CWC to develop programs to address other community issues, including sex trafficking, human rights, youth employment, and home gardening for food security. The group recognized that programs support multiple agendas—for example, the gardening project addressed diabetes by offering opportunities for physical activity and access to healthy foods, as well as food security. Today, the CWC has a reputation as an association that can manage grants and actualize money into programs that work for Indigenous Peoples.

Lessons Learned

Diabetes prevalence is high among NH/PI in Hawai'i and the USAPI jurisdictions. While CDC's diabetes programs have been available to them, these programs needed to be tailored to fit NH/PI communities. To be successful, programs also must engage and build capacity of local stakeholders to plan, implement, and evaluate projects to address their diabetes needs. In building partnerships, outsiders, including NH/PI individuals from other jurisdictions, must demonstrate deep respect for the group being served. When the cultural and societal norms of the community are respected and include community voices and community wisdom in the development and execution of programs, then resources not previously considered are discovered, such as the power of an organized women's group willing to embrace health issues in their community.

Summary

The programs described in this chapter are unique in that they were developed by Indigenous researchers, involved high levels of community engagement, and worked to address feelings of disempowerment experienced by Indigenous Peoples through colonization. The American Indian Youth Wellness Camp focused on building resilience in youth by teaching about healthy eating, exercise, and the mind–body connection in an AI context and deeply rooted in AI culture. The Toiyabe Indian Health Project built individual, clinical, and community capacity to prevent and manage diabetes in AI tribes in eastern California. The Pacific Diabetes Today Resource Center focused on building community efficacy and competence by supporting community coalitions and transferring skills needed to plan programs, secure funding for programs, and to implement and evaluate them. In all three examples, Indigenous Peoples and organizations gained the capacity to better manage their health and improve the health of their communities. All three models demonstrate the continuing success of the initiatives, in large part due to the community-based partnerships and addition of other resources to build on and expand local health promotion efforts.

References

1. WebMD. Types of diabetes. Accessed July 12, 2020. https://www.webmd.com/diabetes/guide/types-of-diabetes-mellitus#1.

2. Centers for Disease Control and Prevention. *National diabetes statistics report, 2020.* Accessed September 14, 2020. https://www.cdc.gov/diabetes/library/features/diabetes-stat-report.html.

3. Centers for Disease Control and Prevention. Gestational diabetes. Accessed July 10, 2020. https://www.cdc.gov/diabetes/basics/gestational.html.

4. Centers for Disease Control and Prevention. Type 1 diabetes. Accessed July 10, 2020. https://www.cdc.gov/diabetes/basics/type1.html.

5. Mayer-Davis EJ, Lawrence JM, Dabelea D, *et al.* Incidence trends of type 1 and type 2 diabetes among youths, 2002–2012. *N Engl J Med.* 2017;376(15):1419–1429.

6. American Diabetes Association. Economic costs of diabetes in the US in 2017. *Diabetes Care.* 2018;41(5):917–928.

7. Hawai'i State Department of Health. Hawai'i Health Matters. Diabetes prevalence by race/ethnicity. Accessed September 14, 2020. http://ibis.hhdw.org/ibisph-view/query/result/brfss/DXDiabetes/DXDiabetesCrude11_.html.

8. Uchima O, Wu YY, Browne C, *et al.* Disparities in diabetes prevalence among Native Hawaiians/Other Pacific Islanders and Asians in Hawai'i. *Prev Chronic Dis.* 2019;16:E22.

9. Aitaoto N, Ichiho HM. Assessing the health care system of services for non-communicable diseases in the US-Affiliated Pacific Islands: A Pacific regional perspective. *Hawaii J Med Public Health.* 2013;72(5 Suppl 1):106–114.

10. Harris SB, Tompkins JW, TeHiwi B. Call to action: A new path for improving diabetes care for Indigenous peoples, a global review. *Diabetes Res Clin Pract.* 2017;123:120–133.

11. National Institutes of Health. Rates of new diagnosed cases of type 1 and type 2 diabetes on the rise among children, teens. Accessed July 12, 2020. https://www.nih.gov/news-events/news-releases/rates-new-diagnosed-cases-type-1-type-2-diabetes-rise-among-children-teens.

12. Felitti VJ, Anda RF, Nordenberg D, *et al.* Relationship of childhood abuse and household dysfunction to many of the leading causes of death in adults. The Adverse Childhood Experiences (ACE) Study. *Am J Prev Med.* 1998;14(4):245–258.

13. Anda RF, Felitti VJ, Bremner JD, *et al.* The enduring effects of abuse and related adverse experiences in childhood. A convergence of evidence from neurobiology and epidemiology. *Eur Arch Psychiatry Clin Neurosci.* 2006;256(3):174–186.

14. Scott KM, Korff MV, Angermeyer MC, *et al.* Association of childhood adversities and early-onset mental disorders with adult-onset chronic physical conditions. *Arch Gen Psychiatry.* 2011;68(8):838–844.

15. Merrick MT, Ports KA, Ford DC, *et al.* Unpacking the impact of adverse childhood experiences on adult mental health. *Child Abuse Negl.* 2017;69:10–19.

16. Finkelhor D, Shattuck A, Turner H, *et al.* Improving the adverse childhood experiences study scale. *JAMA Pediatr.* 2013;167(1):70–75.

17. Cronholm PF, Forke CM, Wade R, *et al.* Adverse childhood experiences: Expanding the concept of adversity. *Am J Prev Med.* 2015;49(3):354–361.

18. Afifi TO, Ford D, Gershoff ET, *et al.* Spanking and adult mental health impairment: The case for the designation of spanking as an adverse childhood experience. *Child Abuse Negl.* 2017;71:24–31.

19. Williamson DF, Thompson TJ, Anda RF, *et al.* Body weight and obesity in adults and self-reported abuse in childhood. *Int J Obes Relat Metab Disord.* 2002;26(8):1075–1082.

20. Barch DM, Belden AC, Tillman R, *et al.* Early childhood adverse experiences, inferior frontal gyrus connectivity, and the trajectory of externalizing psychopathology. *J Am Acad Child Adolesc Psychiatry.* 2018;57(3):183–190.

21. Huang H, Yan P, Shan Z, *et al.* Adverse childhood experiences and risk of type 2 diabetes: A systematic review and meta-analysis. *Metabolism.* 2015;64(11):1408–1418.

22. Kenney MK, Singh GK. Adverse childhood experiences among American Indian/Alaska Native children: The 2011–2012 National Survey of Children's Health. *Scientifica (Cairo).* 2016;2016:7424239.

23. Ye D, Reyes-Salvail F. Adverse childhood experiences among Hawai'i adults: Findings from the 2010 Behavioral Risk Factor Survey. *Hawaii J Med Public Health.* 2014;73(6):181–190.

24. Danese A, McEwen BS. Adverse childhood experiences, allostasis, allostatic load, and age-related disease. *Physiol Behav.* 2012;106(1):29–39.

25. Danese A, Lewis SJ. Psychoneuroimmunology of early-life stress: The hidden wounds of childhood trauma. *Neuropsychopharmacology.* 2017;42(1):99–114.

26. Gachupin FC, Joe JR. American Indian youth: A residential camp curriculum for wellness. *J Health Dispar Res Pract.* 2017:10(4):152–163.

27. Joe JR. Personal communication. May 24, 2018.

28. Burrows NR, Geiss LS, Engelgau MM, *et al.* Prevalence of diabetes among Native Americans and Alaska Natives, 1990–1997: An increasing burden. *Diabetes Care.* 2000;23(12):1786–1790.

29. Dixon M, Roubideaux Y. *Promises to keep: Public health policy for American Indians and Alaska Natives in the 21st century.* American Public Health Association, 2001.

30. Bohlen SA, Rapp D. Congress needs to finish the job and renew the Special Diabetes Program. *The Hill,* February 2, 2018. Accessed July 12, 2020. https://thehill.com/blogs/congress-blog/healthcare/372039-congress-needs-to-finish-the-job-and-renew-the-special.

31. Jones KL. *Type 2 diabetes in American Indian youth: An emerging epidemic.* Unpublished monograph. University of Arizona, Native American Research and Training Center, 2000.

32. Gachupin FC, Joe JR, Steger-May K, *et al.* Severe obesity among American Indian tribal youth in the Southwest. *Public Health.* 2017;145:4–6.

33. Interpreter C. Personal communication. August 28, 2018.

34. Gordon, JS, Staples JK, He DY, *et al.* Mind–body skills groups for posttraumatic stress disorder in Palestinian adults in Gaza. *Traumatol.* 2016;22(3):155–164.

35. Staples JK, Attai JAA, Gordon JS. Mind-body skills groups for posttraumatic stress disorder and depression symptoms in Palestinian children and adolescents in Gaza. *Int J Stress Manage.* 2011;18(3):246–262.

36. Gordon JS, Staples JK, Blyta A, *et al.* Treatment of posttraumatic stress disorder in postwar Kosovar adolescents using mind-body skills groups: A randomized controlled trial. *J Clin Psychiatry.* 2008;69(9):1469–1476.

37. Gachupin FC, Caston E, Chavez C, *et al.* Primary disease prevention for Southwest American Indian families during the COVID-19 pandemic: Camp in a box. Front. Sociol. 2021. https://doi.org/10.3389/fsoc.2021.611972.

38. Gachupin FC, Brown C, Torbzadeh E, *et al.* Usual dietary intake and adherence to dietary recommendations among Southwest American Indian youth at risk for type 2 diabetes. *Curr Dev Nutr.* 2019;3:nzz111.

39. U.S. Department of Health and Human Services and U.S. Department of Agriculture. *2015–2020 dietary guidelines for Americans, 8th ed.* 2015. Accessed July 12, 2020.http://health.gov/dietaryguidelines/2015/guidelines/.

40. Mercer K, Li M, Giangregorio L, *et al.* Behavior change techniques present in wearable activity trackers: A critical analysis. *JMIR Mhealth Uhealth.* 2016;4(2):e40.

41. Bravata DM, Smith-Spangler C, Sundaram V, et al. Using pedometers to increase physical activity and improve health: A systematic review. *JAMA.* 2007;298(19):2296–2304.

42. Naslund JA, Aschbrenner KA, Scherer EA, *et al.* Wearable devices and mobile technologies for supporting behavioral weight loss among people with serious mental illness. *Psychiatry Res.* 2016;244:139–144.

43. Patel MS, Asch DA, Volpp KG. Wearable devices as facilitators, not drivers, of health behavior change. *JAMA.* 2015;313(5):459–460.

44. Piwek L, Ellis DA, Andrews S, *et al.* The rise of consumer health wearables: Promises and barriers. *PLoS Med.* 2016;13(2):e1001953.

45. Francomano JA, Harpin SB. Utilizing social networking sites to promote adolescents' health: A pragmatic review of the literature. *Comput Inform Nurs.* 2015;33(1):10-E1.

46. Barlow A, Varipatis-Baker E, Speakman K, *et al.* Home-visiting intervention to improve child care among American Indian adolescent mothers: A randomized trial. *Arch Pediatr Adolesc Med.* 2006;160(11):1101–1107.

47. Hawai'i State Department of Health. Hawai'i Health Matters. Prevalence of obesity 2016. Accessed July 12, 2020. http://www.hawaiihealthmatters.org/?module=indicators&controller=index&action=view&comparisonId=&indicatorId=1219&localeTypeId=1&localeId=14.

48. Aitaoto NT, Braun KL, Ichiho HM, *et al.* Diabetes today in the Pacific: Reports from the field. *Pac Health Dialog.* 2005;12(1):124–131.

49. Braun KL, Ichiho HM, Kuhaulua RL, *et al.* Empowerment through community building: Diabetes Today in the Pacific. *J Public Health Manag Pract.* 2003;Suppl:S19–S25.

10

Addressing Heart Disease in Indigenous Communities

Kathryn L. Braun, JoAnn 'Umilani Tsark, Noa Emmett Aluli, Martha Pearson, and Marcia O'Leary

Introduction

Heart disease, also known as cardiovascular disease, is an umbrella term for a range of conditions that affect the heart. These include coronary artery disease, coronary heart disease, arrhythmias (abnormal heart rhythms), conditions that affect the valves of the heart, and heart defects. Heart disease is the leading cause of death for adults in most racial and ethnic groups in the United States (US), accounting for one in every four deaths.[1] In 2014 and 2015, the cost of heart disease in the US was estimated at $219 billion per year when accounting for healthcare services, medicines, and lost productivity due to premature death.[1] Indigenous Peoples have a high prevalence of heart disease and/or its risk factors. In this chapter, the causes and risk factors of heart disease are reviewed, and prevalence of heart disease and its risk factors among Indigenous groups are provided and compared with Whites in the US. Three examples are provided of community-engaged programs in Indigenous communities to address heart disease and reduce its prevalence and impact.

Causes and Risk Factors

The most common cause of heart disease is atherosclerosis, through which fatty plaques build up in the arteries. The artery walls can become thick and stiff, and the arteries themselves can become narrowed or blocked, restricting the flow of blood through the arteries to the other organs and tissues of the body. Narrowed or blocked blood vessels can lead to myocardial infarction (heart attack), angina (chest pain), and stroke.[2]

There are several risk factors for heart disease, some are modifiable and some are not. Risk factors that are not modifiable include age, sex, and family history. Specifically, aging increases the risk of damage to the heart, men are generally at higher risk of heart disease than women, and heart disease can run in families.[3]

Modifiable risk factors are those that, when managed or eliminated, can reduce the risk of heart disease. These include tobacco use, poor diet, physical inactivity, obesity, hypertension, high cholesterol, and diabetes.[3] For example, the nicotine found in tobacco can constrict blood vessels, and the carbon monoxide from smoking can damage the inner lining of the blood vessels. Exposure to nicotine and carbon monoxide both increase the risk of atherosclerosis.[4] Hyperlipidemia (high cholesterol levels) can hasten the formation of plaques that cause atherosclerosis. High blood glucose from prediabetes and diabetes can damage blood vessels and the nerves that control the heart and blood vessels. Hypertension (high blood pressure) also can contribute to the hardening, thickening, and narrowing of blood vessels. A diet high in fat, salt, and sugar can contribute to the development of hyperlipidemia, high blood glucose, and hypertension, which contribute to heart disease. Consuming the recommended amounts of fruits and vegetables tends to reduce the amount of fat, salt, and sugar in the diet, in addition to reducing the risk of obesity. Physical activity also helps reduce the risk of heart disease because it can lower blood pressure, blood cholesterol, and blood sugar, and reduce obesity.[4]

About half of all Americans (47%) have at least one of these three risk factors for heart disease: high blood pressure, high cholesterol, and smoking.[4] Using national data from the Behavioral Risk Factor Surveillance Survey (BRFSS) from 1995 to 1996 and from 2005 to 2006, Jernigan and colleagues found that 79% of American Indians (AI) and Alaska Natives (AN) had one or more of the six risk factors for heart disease (diabetes, obesity, hypertension, cigarette smoking, sedentary behavior, and low vegetable or fruit intake), and 46% had two or more.[5]

Another modifiable risk factor is poor hygiene. Viral and bacterial infections can irritate the heart, and regular hand washing can help reduce the chance that a viral or bacterial infection can affect the heart. Opportunities to wash hands may be limited for Indigenous Peoples who are houseless, lack indoor plumbing, or living in substandard housing. The National Congress on AI estimates that 40% of housing on reservations are substandard (vs. 6% elsewhere), less than 50% are connected to public sewer systems, and 16% lack indoor plumbing.[6]

Stress also has been implicated as a risk factor for heart disease.[7] In response to stress, the body releases a hormone called cortisol. Constant exposure to stress results in long-term exposure to high levels of cortisol, which can increase blood cholesterol, triglycerides, blood sugar, and blood pressure and can promote the buildup of plaque in the arteries.[8] Long-term stress also can make the blood stickier, which increases the risk of stroke. Also, people who have a lot of stress may choose to smoke, eat unhealthy foods, forego physical activity, or abuse substances, all of which can increase the risk for heart disease.[8] Stress can be caused by many of the social determinants of health, including unemployment, poverty, poor living and working conditions, and racism.

Prevalence of Heart Disease and Risk Factors in Indigenous Peoples

Heart Disease

National prevalence data from 2018 estimated the age-adjusted prevalence of heart disease among AI/AN adults at 14.6%, compared to 11.5% for White Americans.[9] Interestingly, individuals aged 18 and older who claimed both AI/AN and White ancestry had an even higher prevalence of heart disease, at 17.7%. In Hawai'i, data from the Hawai'i BRFSS in 2011–2014 suggested that 4.2% of NH adults were told by a physician they had heart diseases, compared to 3.4% of White adults in the state.[10] In an examination of Hawai'i insurance claims data from 1999 to 2009, Juarez and colleagues found that the prevalence of heart disease among NH deviated from that of Whites beginning at age 45 years. Based on these data, at age 60 years, about 15% of NH had heart disease, compared to 10% of Whites. By age 75, however, almost 35% of NH had heart disease, compared to only 20% of Whites in the state.[11] National estimates from 2018 suggested that death rates from heart disease for NH/PI were similar to those of Whites, about 168.0 per 100,000, but that death rates for PI living in Guam and the CNMI were higher, about 293.9 and 201.0 per 100,000 respectively.[12]

Tobacco Use

Based on data from the National Survey on Drug Use and Health, the prevalence of tobacco use among AI/ANs was significantly higher than for Whites in 2010–2015. Specifically, 43.3% of AI/AN adults reported using any tobacco product, compared to 30% of Whites. More than a third of AI/AN (37.3%) reported smoking already-rolled cigarettes, compared to 25% for Whites, and 7.1% of AI/AN rolled their tobacco, compared to 4% for Whites. More AI/AN adults (6.6%) reported using smokeless tobacco than White adults (4.5%).[13]

In Hawai'i, an estimated 27.0% of NH adults and 27.4% of other PI adults smoked cigarettes in 2014, compared to only 12.0% of White residents.[14] Although smoking prevalence has declined for NH in Hawai'i following the increases in the tobacco tax and restrictions to where one can smoke, 2018 data showed that NH continued to have a higher prevalence of smoking, at 22.8%, compared to about 13% for the general population.

Obesity

The prevalence of obesity among AI/AN adults has increased over time, with national BRFSS estimates increasing from about one in four (24.9%) in 1995–1996 to about one in three (31.2%) in 2005–2006.[5] More recent estimates from the 2018 National Health Interview Survey (NHIS) suggest that obesity among AI/AN has further increased and is now closer to half (48.1%) of all AI/AN adults, compared to about 31% of White Americans.[15] Hawai'i BRFSS data suggest that 43.5% of NH adults and 41.6% of other PI adults were obese in 2018, compared to only 18.9% of White adults.[16]

It should be noted that many Indigenous communities are challenged by a number of social and environmental barriers to maintaining a healthy weight. Social factors include low income and food insecurity, which are both linked to obesity.[17] Environmental factors include living in areas with poor access to affordable healthy foods, and limited time for, and safe places to engage in physical activity.[18]

Hypertension

Data from the NHIS estimated that 27.2% of AI/AN and 31.7% of mixed AI/AN-White individuals had hypertension in 2018, compared to about 23.9% of White Americans.[19] The same national report suggested that 24% of NH/PI adults had hypertension in 2018. Data from the Hawai'i BRFSS suggested that 29.7% of NH were hypertensive, compared to 23% of Whites in the state.[20]

Diabetes

According to the Centers for Disease Control and Prevention (CDC),[21] the prevalence of diabetes was 14.7% in AI/AN in 2017–2018. This compared to 11.7% in non-Hispanic Blacks, 12.5% in Hispanics, 9.2% in non-Hispanic Asians, and 7.5% in non-Hispanic Whites. Hawai'i BRFSS data from 2011 to 2015 demonstrated that NH/PI adults had a higher prevalence of diabetes in the state compared to Whites, even after controlling for demographic and diabetes risk factors. Additionally, the diabetes prevalence increases more rapidly with age among NH/PI, with significant disparities appearing in the 35–44 age group.[22]

Stress

Existing data suggest that AI/AN suffer from disproportionate mental health problems compared with other Americans, including a higher prevalence of substance abuse, posttraumatic stress disorder (PTSD), violence, and suicide. For example, from the National Comorbidity Survey, Gone and colleagues estimated a lifetime PTSD prevalence of between 16% and 22% for AI/AN groups, compared to a lifetime prevalence of 7–8% for Whites.[23] A subsequent review of the broader research literature confirmed a significantly higher prevalence of PTSD among AI/AN, with combat experience and interpersonal violence as leading contributors to PTSD and related symptoms in this population.[24] The experience of being taken from one's home and forced to attend boarding schools also contributed to PTSD among AI/AN. As was emphasized in Chapter 9, ACEs are significant contributors to unmanaged stress among AI, AN, NH, and PIs. Working with AI with type 2 diabetes, Walls and colleagues documented a dose-response relationship between stress accumulation and worse health outcomes (including heart conditions).[25] This team also developed a typology of stresses experienced by AI adults managing chronic illness, including stresses resulted from colonization, poverty, discrimination, social roles, and health management.[26]

Lifetime PTSD prevalence for NH veterans was found to be 38%, compared to 20% of US White veterans.[27] In Hawai'i, studies demonstrated higher levels of stress among NH/PI than among other groups.[28,29] Similar to AI adults, much of this stress is linked to historical trauma, systemic racism, and reduced opportunities for quality education, work, housing, and healthcare access. In cohort studies in NH communities, higher levels of perceived racism were associated with self-reported hypertension, higher systolic blood pressure, lower diurnal cortisol levels, and greater body mass index.[30,31] In addition, those who strongly identified with being NH perceived more racism than those who did not.

The three examples below demonstrate why community engagement and community control are critical to addressing disparities in cardiovascular disease, as well as inequities in the research enterprise. Community engagement helps overcome myopic approaches to addressing chronic diseases in the US as separate from social determinants of health, which perpetuates a power differential in research, programming, and resources to populations most in need.

Examples of Successful Indigenous Community-Engaged Interventions

The Strong Heart Study in the Dakotas[i]

Description

The Strong Heart Study was the largest study of heart disease in AI populations. The study started in 1988 and was continuously funded, in whole or in

---

i Funding from NIH NHLBI contract numbers 75N92019D00027, 75N92019D00028, 75N92019D00029, & 75N92019D00030, research grant numbers R01HL109315, R01HL109301, R01HL109284, R01HL109282, and R01HL109319, and cooperative agreement numbers U01HL41642, U01HL41652, U01HL41654, U01HL65520, and U01HL65521.

part, by the National Institutes of Health (NIH) National Heart, Lung, and Blood Institute (NHLBI). Phase VII of the Strong Heart Study began in 2019. About 4,500 AI from tribes in Arizona, Oklahoma, and the Dakotas enrolled in the study.

Missouri Breaks Industries Research, Inc. (MBIRI), a small, AI-owned and AI-operated research firm, conducted the Strong Heart Study in the Dakotas. The three participating Dakota tribes included the Oglala Lakota Nation, the Spirit Lake Nation, and the Cheyenne River Sioux Nation. The Oglala and Cheyenne River Nations are each the size of the state of Connecticut but sparsely populated (three people per square mile). These tribes once lived along the "breaks" (river-fed areas) in the Dakotas but, with colonialization, were pushed westward to lands on which it was hard to sustain the population. Thus, colonization changed the lifestyles and reduced the economic stability of the tribes. As a result, the life expectancy of these tribes is 10–15 years lower than for the majority US population.

Intervention

Strong Heart was essentially a longitudinal, observational study. Participants enrolled and agreed to provide demographic, behavioral, and clinical data about themselves that were tracked by researchers. Analyses of these data have led to important discoveries about the risk factors for cardiovascular disease among AI.

Equally important, Strong Heart data have been used to support intervention studies. For example, Strong Heart data showed that diabetes was a significant contributing risk factor for cardiovascular disease among AI. If not prevented or controlled, diabetes can lead to chronic kidney disease. Dr. Stacey Jolly, an AN physician, partnered with Strong Heart to test an educational intervention for its ability to increase behaviors to protect one's kidneys from disease.

Strong Heart data showed a smoking prevalence of 50% among AI. These data were used to stimulate the establishment of a group called the Canli (tobacco) Coalition that worked to pass tribal legislation to reduce exposure to tobacco smoke. Over 7 years of work, the Cheyenne River Sioux Tribe adopted a "no smoking in public places" law and became the third tribal nation in the US to go smoke-free. As of 2021, the Canli Coalition model was used to support tobacco coalition groups in other tribal nations.

Strong Heart data also showed a high prevalence of stroke among tribal members, with more extensive suffering among those who lived too far from healthcare services to receive treatment within the window for maximum treatment effectiveness. Small medical facilities in rural locations were unable to provide rehabilitation services for tribal members recovering from a stroke because reimbursement rates were not equitable to the costs. As a result, these services were located in facilities several hours away from their homes, making it extraordinarily difficult for individuals recovering from stroke to utilize them. An intervention called Rhythm and Timing Exercises for Cerebral Vascular Disease in AI was developed and involved 30–60 minutes of tapping and clapping to the beat of a metronome. It was tested by Dr. Steven Verney (Tsimshian) and Dr. Lonnie Nelson (Eastern Band of Cherokee) for delivery in the home by community health workers and public health nurses.

Strong Heart data showed that a high level of arsenic was a risk factor for diabetes.[32] Dr. Anna Navas-Acien from Columbia University and Dr. Christine George from Johns Hopkins University tested an intervention called Participatory Interventions to Reduce Arsenic in AI Communities. Also called the Strong Heart Water Study, all participants received a water filtration system, and the researchers tested the best amounts and types of health education to provide around water, arsenic, and filtration.

Community Engagement

Community control of research was integral to the Strong Heart Study. Tribal leadership guided and approved each phase of Strong Heart, as well as each supplemental observational study and intervention. Each tribal nation had its approval process requirements. Some had research review boards, while others worked with their legal teams for recommendations for edits and approval. Every tribal nation took the task of participation in research that could influence the health outcomes of its members very seriously.

Data sharing was an example of the importance of tribal oversight. The NIH data-sharing policy required research data to be shared. Although most tribal nations were not opposed to the practice of data sharing, historical examples of misuse of data were still very real. As a result, tribal nations were extremely cautious about ceding their responsibility for oversight of how data on their members were used. The Strong Heart researchers recognized that the relationships between the NIH and tribal nations were government-to-government relationships, requiring negotiations between the two entities to determine appropriate data use processes. As a result of uncertain negotiations between the tribal nations and NIH, funding was significantly cut for Phase VI. In 2019, NHLBI director Dr. Gary Gibbons traveled to the Dakotas to meet one on one with tribal leadership. He expressed his commitment to reducing health disparities experienced by tribal nations. In Phase VII, NIH came back to tribes with a fully funded contract for Strong Heart. The data-sharing requirements ensured tribal control of their data as an ongoing discussion, with tribal consultation continuing with tribal leadership.

An important aspect of Strong Heart was a commitment to building research capacity among tribal members and supporting students in research education, as its leaders felt there was no reason why local people could not be the drivers of the research. Shared ownership of data increased opportunities that research results were translated into best practices, informed legislation, and supported interventions. Trickle down research results through publications was not a practical data dissemination plan outside of academia.

Outcomes

Strong Heart had several successes. First, the prevalence of heart disease among tribes involved in Strong Heart began trending downward.[33] Although the exact mechanism of change is not known, it was believed that this was being accomplished in part through raising awareness and changing lifestyles.

Second, the study maintained an 85–95% retention rate, depending on the site. This spoke to the tribal-appropriate approach of Strong Heart and a continuous commitment to share information and data, and ensured everyone understood what they were participating in and why. By engaging in these partnerships, tribes and tribal members were willing to participate in research. When tribal members fully understood that research could be for and about them, they wanted to participate to generate findings that helped their children and grandchildren.

Third, findings from Strong Heart research were used to inform policy and programming. For example, data supported the development and passage of smoke-free legislation with specific tribes, and this helped to protect community members from exposure to tobacco and vaping products. Data also influenced the IHS to develop a Special Diabetes Program for Indians. This initiative provided annual funding to support programs to combat diabetes in AI communities.[34] The Spirit Lake Nation utilized their funding to renovate a fitness center that in 2020 had more than 800 members.

Fourth, Native researchers were developed, and they began proposing and conducting their own intervention studies. For example, Dr. Amanda Fretts, a researcher and member of the Eel Ground First Nation of New Brunswick, Canada, identified a relationship between eating processed meat and developing heart disease and diabetes.

Lessons Learned

Three major lessons emerged from the Strong Heart Study. First, Native people are willing to participate in research if treated as true partners, which means they are provided respect, given educational opportunities, and allowed autonomy over their data. Second, research data must be made available to inform policy change, program change, and intervention research. When research partnerships are true and findings lead to beneficial programs and policy change, Native people are enthusiastic about partnering with researchers. Third, Native people are very resilient. Although poverty levels are high in many tribal communities, poverty has not taken away hope.

Alaska WISEWOMAN[ii]

Description

WISEWOMAN, a program of the Southeast Alaska Regional Health Consortium (SEARHC), is dedicated to reducing risk for heart disease among women living in small, isolated communities in Southeast Alaska. SEARHC itself is a consortium of 15 tribes in Southeast Alaska, a region that includes islands and shorelines in the part of the state that stretches along the Western side of Canada. The region includes Juneau, the capital of the state, and Sitka, the hospital base for SEARHC.

Altogether, the region covers an area the size of Florida, but with a population of only 72,000. In the region's 15 tribal communities, village populations range in size from a few dozens to a few thousand, and, with virtually no roads, access to these communities is by plane or boat. Additionally, the people of Southeast Alaska cope with extreme climate. Weather conditions can ground boats and planes, delaying the departure of emergency cases and requiring travelers to stay until the weather clears.

The risk of heart disease is high among these communities, as assessments conducted in 2000 estimated that 70% of women were overweight or obese, 74% did not eat the daily recommended five or more servings of fruit and vegetables, and 40% did not get the recommended amount of physical activity. The WISEWOMAN program started in 2000 to improve women's heart health. From 2002, the program was supported by funding from the CDC to provide services in nine primary clinics in the region. Other sites were reached through a mobile mammography screening service. The target population for the program was low-income women of all races, aged 40–64, who were uninsured or underinsured. An estimated 45% of these women were of AI/AN ancestry, and the percentage living in poverty approached 40% in some of the region's isolated communities.

Intervention

The program recognized that many things can contribute to heart disease, and subsequently the program took a broad approach to health. The first step was

---

ii Funding from CDC NU58DP006647.

the annual health assessment, during which multiple aspects of a woman's health and life were reviewed to understand health risks.

The program aimed to "add value to women's lives." Thus, providers asked each woman about her priorities for health, and these priorities helped set the agenda for change. Once a woman decided to make lifestyle changes, WISE-WOMAN provided health coaching, access to medication that was needed to reduce high blood pressure and cholesterol, and linkages to sister programs providing breast and cervical cancer screening, diabetes screening and management, tobacco cessation, organized fitness activities, gardening, tips on food harvest and preservation, cooking lessons, stress management, and other wellness programs.

Health coaches emphasized making "small steps" toward a healthier life. These included making simple changes to diet, eating smaller portions, increasing participation in enjoyable physical activities, and building relationships with other women for mutual support of lifestyle changes.

The program also honored WISEWOMAN champions. These were women who made lifestyle changes and were willing to share their stories with others through personal testimonials, digital stories, posters, television ads, and social media. Champions inspired others to join the program and begin a journey toward a healthier lifestyle.

Community Engagement

Through SEARHC, the 15 tribes in Southeast Alaska agreed to pool funds received from the IHS, Medicare, Medicaid, CDC, and other sources to provide a network of health services in the area. Pooling funds was the only way to support a hospital in the region, which provides emergency and hospital care and is accredited by the Joint Commission. SEARHC is guided by an advisory board of representative members from each of the 15 communities. This group meets quarterly and makes decisions related to all organizational governance.

In addition to staffing services in Sitka and Juneau, SEARHC employs health educators through nine community clinics, and these employees serve the villages within their subregions. Some communities also have a case manager, usually a nurse. Health professionals from the SEARHC regional office in Sitka are sent to the villages as well, bringing mobile mammography and other screening expertise. It is a practice of SEARHC to hire people from the community or village if possible, and about 45% of SEARHC's employees are AN. Employees are encouraged to increase their professional skills through tuition reimbursement of $4,000 per year.

When SEARHC staff want to implement a change in a village, they first ask permission from the local community council or other tribal leaders. Once in the community or village, the staff of the SEARHC and the WISEWOMAN programs are trained to "go where people will trip over you." In other words, they are encouraged to participate in community activities at the senior centers, schools, and churches and to sponsor group activities that engage entire families. In this way, they can learn about the needs and assets of the community, build trust, and engage with community to improve health.

Outcomes

Since the program's inception in 2000, WISEWOMAN provided more than 14,000 screenings to about 5,000 women. Based on the results of the screening, women were linked to other services. For example, a woman with diabetes who came to the clinic for a Pap smear was connected to WISEWOMAN and engaged in the group session for weight loss provided by the program. She also brought her daughter with her to the weight-loss sessions.

The program viewed success as "one woman at a time." Thus, case studies and success stories were the primary currency of outcome evaluation. One such success, featured in a CDC publication, was J.I., a 57-year-old woman who lives on Prince of Wales Island in Southeast Alaska. "She was uninsured and hadn't had a physical exam in many years. After working with the program, J.I. was able to get an overall assessment of her health. Her cholesterol values were the highest the program had ever seen, and between that and a family history of heart disease and stroke, J.I. decided it was time to make a healthy change. Through health coaching, J.I. was immediately able to focus on nutrition to control her weight and that of her family. Her first steps were to include more fruits and vegetables in her meals each day and to reduce saturated fats and sweets. After 6 months, J.I. had lost nearly 30 pounds and lowered her cholesterol, and her body mass index (BMI) had dropped from the overweight range to the normal range."[35]

Lessons Learned

SEARHC staff recommend a slow but steady approach to improving heart health. This approach is appealing to the women assisted by the program, and small personal improvements eventually add up to large health gains. Another important lesson is that one program cannot address every issue. Small programs must partner with other programs, and small communities must partner with other communities to foster health in remote villages of Alaska. This strategy encourages individual and community ownership of health programs and increases community participation. Health was a daily process, not a box to check off and forget about. Health programs must set up systems that make it easy for women to make healthy choices each day.

Community-Engaged Heart Health Programs on Moloka'i, Hawai'i[iii]

Description

Moloka'i is one of seven inhabited islands in the Hawaiian archipelago. It is a small island and home to about 8,000 people, and 60% are of NH ancestry. In the mid-1980s, an international research group was funded to conduct the International Cooperative Study on Salt, Other Factors, and Blood Pressure (INTERSALT).[36] Moloka'i was included as a research site because of the large percentage of NH. However, the initially White research group associated with the study make no headway in recruiting community members, as no one from the community knew about the study or had any stake in it. Finally, the Honolulu-based principal investigator approached Dr. Noa Emmett Aluli, a NH family medicine physician practicing on Moloka'i, who agreed to partner in the study to address the lack of data on heart disease among NH, as he was well aware of the burden of heart disease among NH.

Aluli organized a community research "hui" (group) to provide guidance and to support island involvement in the study. The group, all NH, included William "Billy" Akutagawa, Jane Lee, Henry Nalai'elua, Helen O'Connor, Sol Ko'ohalahala, Naomi Brath, Lulu Linker, and Noelani Joy. This hui contributing knowledge in medicine, social work, education, community mobilization, advocacy, and activism.

This group rebranded the study as the Na Pu'uwai Moloka'i Heart Study. Using door-to-door, face-to-face outreach and recruitment, the community research team successfully recruited more than 300 study participants. This began a 35+ year engagement in heart health research and programs that Moloka'i initially participated in and later led, to improve life expectancy and healthy aging on the island. Follow-on studies and programs included (1) the Ho'okē 'Ai Moloka'i Diet Study (1987), (2) cardiovascular risk clinics and programs addressing diabetes management, weight management, and physical exercise through Na Pu'uwai, the Native Hawaiian Health Care System (NHHCS) on Moloka'i (established in 1991), (3) the Native Hawaiian Heart Health Initiative (NHHHI), which supported the statewide sharing of the Moloka'i model of community research and programming for NH heart health (1998–2002), and (4) Hua Kanawao Ka Liko, a generational study of heart health among the Hawaiian people on Moloka'i, funded by the National Institutes of Health (2002–2008). The Moloka'i community research group also advocated for the 1988 passage of the Native Hawaiian Health Care Act

---

iii Funding from NIH NIHLB U01 HL079163 and NIMHD P20 MD00174.

(NHHCA) in the US Congress, which established and funds Papa Ola Lōkahi, the Native Hawaiian Board of Health; NHHCS on five islands, including Molokaʻi; and the Native Hawaiian Health Scholarship Program, which supports the training of NH pursuing degrees in medicine, nursing, psychology, public health, and social work.[37] The NHHCS on Molokaʻi, carrying the name Na Puʻuwai, implemented cardiovascular risk clinics and programs to reduce cardiovascular risk and other chronic diseases. Another offshoot supported by this group was the 1998 establishment of the ʻAhahui o Na Kauka - Native Hawaiian Physicians' Association, which champions superior healthcare for Hawaiians through leadership and advocacy, education (medical, continuing, cultural), and service.

Intervention

The first task of the Na Puʻuwai Molokaʻi Heart Study was to conduct a cardiovascular disease risk factor survey among NH living on Hawaiian homestead lands on Molokaʻi. Hawaiian homestead lands consist of tracts of land allocated by federal law for long-term lease, in individual parcels, to NH with at least 50% Hawaiian ancestry. In addition to the risk assessment questions, the local research team also took blood pressure measures, height and weight, waist and hip circumference, and blood and urine samples for analyses of blood lipids. From these data, they estimated BMI and waist–hip ratio and had cardiovascular risk data (blood lipids) to compare with data from the National Health and Nutrition Examination Survey (NHANES) and the NHIS, both of which published data for the US, but never had a large enough sample of NH to provide estimates for this group.

The survey findings were startling to the community. Approximately 65% of the participants were overweight or obese. About 34% of women and 42% of men said they were current smokers. Although hypertension prevalence was similar to that of the US population (about 25%), greater percentages of NH had hypercholesterolemia and diabetes and low levels of high-density lipoprotein (HDL). The study also found that individuals with significant cardiovascular disease risk were unaware of their risks, were not under treatment, or were not under adequate control.[38]

The Na Puʻuwai community research group had long discussions about what to do with these data. The conversation started with questions like "What happened? How did we get so sick?" as their NH ancestors were a healthy and robust population before Western contact. Incorporating what they learned, Na Puʻuwai agreed to partner with Oregon Health & Sciences University (OHSU) in 1987 on a diet study, which they named Hoʻokē ʻAi Molokaʻi Diet Study. The purpose of the study was to demonstrate the lipid-lowering effects of a high complex carbohydrate diet compared to the standard American diet, which tends to be high in fat (40%), cholesterol (1,016 mg), protein (15%), and salt, and low in fiber.

The Moloka'i team, in consultation with Dr. Kekuni Blaisdell, a NH hematologist and activist who established the Department of Medicine at the University of Hawai'i and instructed and mentored NH physicians for 40 years, and Dr. Claire K. Hughes, the state's first NH registered dietician, insisted that the intervention diet be a traditional Hawaiian, precontact diet, which is composed of 10% fat, 10% protein, and 80% carbohydrates, with 16 grams of fiber and only 2 grams of sodium.[39,40] This diet was based on large amounts of traditional complex carbohydrate foods such as poi (mashed taro), kalo (taro), 'uala (sweet potato), 'uhi (yams), mai'a (banana), and 'ulu (breadfruit). Vegetables included the green leaves of the 'uala and kalo plants, ferns, and a variety of limu (seaweed and algae). Protein sources were primarily fish and other kinds of seafood and occasionally moa (chicken).[41] Ten NH adults with hyperlipidemia participated in the study, consuming the same amount of calories as before, but of only pre-Western-contact foods. The study also included group support and health education sessions by NH healthcare professionals.

After 3 weeks, participants realized significant reductions in cholesterol, triglycerides, and glucose levels (Table 10.1.). Mean blood cholesterol declined from 227 to 206 mg/d and triglyceride from 331 to 174 mg/d. Following three weeks on the Moloka'i diet, participants returned to their Western diets, and their blood lipid values rose to preintervention levels. This study was the first demonstration that NH could reverse their hyperlipidemia by returning to their traditional diet. The research team also observed rapid weight loss among participants at the beginning of the intervention,[42] but controlled for this, as the study was investigating change in blood lipids, not weight. This observation, however, led to subsequent weight-loss programs utilizing the traditional Hawaiian diet.[46]

Community Engagement

Although born and raised on the island of O'ahu, Dr. Aluli chose to practice medicine on the island of Moloka'i after he had spent part of his medical school and residency training there in the early 1970s. The community trusted Dr. Aluli, and many respected him for his leadership and activism in social justice issues to preserve and protect Hawaiian rights to land and water in their homeland.

Based on the trust established by Dr. Aluli and the forming of the community research group, this small island community became fully engaged with the academic partners and worked together to conduct the Na Pu'uwai Moloka'i

Table 10.1. Ka Hoʻoke ʻAi, 1987—Blood Lipids and Blood Pressure

	Baseline Western Diet	After 4 Weeks Molokaʻi Diet	After 3 Weeks Western Diet
Total blood cholesterol	227 mg/dl	206 mg/dl*	234 mg/dl*
HDL	46	42	46
LDL	128	138	154
VLDL	52	32*	40*
Blood triglyceride	331	174*	200
Blood pressure	112/76 mm Hg	109/73 mm Hg	109/71 mm Hg

*$p < 0.05$.

Heart Study in 1985 and the Hoʻokē ʻAi Molokaʻi Diet Study in 1987. Both studies were guided by the community-based research team whose members participated in community networking, wrote letters about the studies to their
neighbors, developed promotional brochures and newspaper publicity, made
telephone contacts, and visited homes to recruit study participants. The project
team successfully recruited over 300 NH participants to the Molokaʻi Heart
Study and 10 to the Molokaʻi Diet Study. In addition to analyzing and disseminating the findings to the community, the community team worked hard to
secure ownership of the data. The team then served as gatekeepers of the data
and pushed to apply findings to support research and healthcare that would
benefit the community. They also insisted that publications be coauthored by
community research members. Data ownership and representation on publications were unprecedented in the mid-1980s, and this group's actions played an
important role as more Hawaiian communities examined equitable rules of
engagement in research, beyond the usual role as "subjects."

The follow-up Hoʻokē ʻAi Native Hawaiian Diet Study was a funded controlled study to test the impact of the traditional diet on BMI and the remedi-
ation of hyperlipidemia. The community research team, with mentor Dr
Kekuni Blaisdell, partnered with researchers from OHSU and maintained a
strong involvement in the control of the study. Program staff, including the
woman who prepared the meals, were all members of the Molokaʻi community. To the extent possible, the foods that comprised the pre-Western diet were
gathered and procured on the island, supporting local fishermen and farmers
and benefiting the island's subsistence lifestyle.[47,48,49]

The group identified Hawaiian cultural values that should be incorporated
into the program, including ʻohana (family), kōkua (cooperation), hoʻomana
(spirituality), aloha ʻāina (honoring the land), and lōkahi (balance between the
environment, God, and humanity). Participants went through the program as

a cohort, convening daily to eat breakfast and dinner together, while learning about the historical, nutritional, and spiritual roles of traditional foods. Education sessions were provided by respected NH health professionals with established relationships in the Moloka'i community. The program had broad appeal because it incorporated NH values and traditions, encouraged the participation of whole families, instilled pride, and built community capacity.

Both studies were examples of community-based research, long before community-based participatory research (CBPR) principles were documented, and long before CBPR was considered by the scientific community as "real science." These studies served as models for future community-driven research and programming in Hawai'i. As required by CBPR principles, both projects provided training and employment opportunities for community members. Without the work of these individuals to explain the potential benefits of research and recruit participants, the studies would have failed.

Outcomes

The Moloka'i-based research group continued to meet over the next three decades, lending support in the development of programs that addressed cardiovascular health and other chronic diseases. The success of the traditional diet program on Moloka'i was soon replicated by other groups, including the Wai'anae Coast Comprehensive Health Center, which serves a large Hawaiian community on the Leeward Coast of O'ahu.[43] In this version, called the Wai'anae Diet, the menu was expanded to include low-fat, high complex carbohydrate meals from other cultures that met the nutrient criteria of the Moloka'i diet. Participants were allowed to eat until full, and all participants lost weight because the lower number of calories per volume of traditional foods naturally caused a reduction in calorie intake and resulted in weight loss.

The program also was replicated by the Department of Health on the island of Kaua'i. As noted in a report on replication efforts on Kaua'i, the program's "unique quality is the strong cultural component that encourages the embracing of spiritual values, ethnic pride, and a sense of familial cohesion. This component appears to be the most enticing element of the program despite the stringent food limitations and the expectations of the program. Participants were willing to commit to a Hawaiian program out of cultural pride and a sense of oneness."[44]

The passage of the Native Hawaiian Health Care Act in 1988 led to the establishment of the NHHCS, agencies on each of five islands to provide health promotion, disease prevention, enabling services (e.g., helping people secure health insurance and get to healthcare appointments, even if that meant arranging transportation and providing childcare), and referrals to needed community and clinical services. By 2000, the five NHHCS were serving 25,000 individuals per year, the majority of whom were NH.

The system on Molokaʻi was named Na Puʻuwai NHHCS, and the members of the Na Puʻuwai research team became founding members of this 501(c)(3). Data then were applied to support the implementation of the Cardiovascular Risk Clinics at Na Puʻuwai NHHCS. At these clinics, islanders received a complete heart health assessment. Information was collected on family history, medical history, and health behaviors, as well as clinical indicators for BMI, cholesterol testing, fasting blood glucose, and blood pressure. Results were shared with the patient's physician, who followed up on abnormal findings and referred them for appropriate services. Many of these services were offered by Na Puʻuwai NHHCS, including nutrition counseling, blood pressure monitoring, and tobacco cessation programs, creating a "revolving door" between screening, treatment, and prevention services. The methodology and success of the Na Puʻuwai cardiovascular risk clinics were shared statewide as the Native Hawaiian Heart Health Initiative (NHHHI). NHHHI events were held on five islands and hosted by NH physicians practicing on their respective islands, reaching 534 community members and involving 60 NH physicians.

In 2006, Molokaʻi General Hospital in partnership with Na Puʻuwai submitted a proposal through the University of Hawaiʻi Medical School to analyze data from the Na Puʻuwai Cardiovascular Risk Clinics. Funding was received from the NIH to find and follow-up on individuals screened between 1992 and 1998. This study was called Hua Kanawao Ka Liko   A Multigenerational Study of Heart Health among the Hawaiian People of Molokaʻi. Of the 855 individuals who had been screened, the research team found that 69 had died. An analysis of their medical records demonstrated that 55% of these deaths were attributed to heart disease. The findings confirmed that cardiovascular disease risk increased with age and that individuals who also had diabetes, hypertension, and/or high low-density lipoprotein cholesterol were more at risk and more likely to die. The community research committee for this study included three of the original Na Puʻuwai study committee members, Dr. Emmett Aluli, Jane Lee, and Lulu Linker, who were joined by other NH members, including Milton Pa, S. Kalani Brady, Barbara Kalipi, JoAnn Tsark, and Dr. Kekuni Blaisdell, and staff, Roy Horner.

Lessons Learned

Several key lessons were learned in this endeavor. First, the initial study to assess heart health on Molokaʻi would have failed without the engagement of the community. There was no trust in outside researchers. Second, when a NH physician leader came forward to support the study, he sought the advice of the community and trusted medical and cultural mentors, and insisted on the engagement and education of community members as coresearchers. This illustrated the critical role of champions of change. Third, the group applied its new learnings to seek benefits for the community, making sure that findings led to programs, that the community retained control over its data, and that community members could coauthor scientific publications. These demands have become commonplace today, but in Hawai'i, this group was the first to question and fight against paternalistic Western research practices. Fourth, the community research team set a precedence for sharing study findings with the community before being reported to funders and published. Fifth, the group had to engage in legislation and secure regular funding for programs to address and reduce heart disease risk on the island. The passage of the Native Hawaiian Health Care Act established and funded these needed heart health services.

Summary

Heart disease is a leading cause of death for Indigenous Peoples. It is caused by many factors, including stress that can stem from the social determinants of health, racism, inadequate income, and limited opportunities for quality education, work, housing, and healthcare. Community-engaged research and interventions, like the ones featured in this chapter, helped Indigenous Peoples gain control over their health. Long-standing engagement of the community in interventions like these also built community capacity to participate in, gain employment from, and lead research. Also important is that community-engaged research and programs led to sustainable healthcare services. This required the use of program and research data in advocacy and policy change.

References

1. Centers for Disease Control and Prevention. Heart disease facts. Accessed February 27, 2021. https://www.cdc.gov/heartdisease/facts.htm#:~:text=Heart%20disease%20is%20 the%20leading,1%20in%20every%204%20deaths.

2. Mayo Clinic. Heart disease. Accessed September 12, 2020. https://www.mayoclinic .org/diseases-conditions/heart-disease/symptoms-causes/syc-20353118

3. Centers for Disease Control and Prevention. Know your risk for heart disease. Accessed May 23, 2021. https://www.cdc.gov/heartdisease/risk_factors.htm.

4. Fryar CD, Chen TC, Li X. Prevalence of uncontrolled risk factors for cardiovascular disease: United States, 1999–2010. NCHS Data Brief. 2012 August;(103):1–8.

5. Jernigan VB, Duran B, Ahn D, et al. Changing patterns in health behaviors and risk factors related to cardiovascular disease among American Indians and Alaska Natives. Am J Public Health. 2010;100(4):677–683.

6. National Congress of American Indians. Housing and infrastructure. Accessed January 1, 2021. https://www.ncai.org/policy-issues/economic-development-commerce /housing-infrastructure.

7. Steptoe A, Kivimäki M. Stress and cardiovascular disease. Nat Rev Cardiol. 2012;9:360–370.

8. Wirtz PH, von Känel R. Psychological stress, inflammation, and coronary heart disease. Curr Cardiol Rep. 2017;19(11):111.

9. Centers for Disease Control and Prevention. *US National Health Interview Survey 2018.* Accessed May 23, 2021. https://www.cdc.gov/nchs/nhis/shs/tables.htm.

10. Hawaiʻi Health Data Warehouse. Hawaiʻi State Department of Health, Behavioral Risk Factor Surveillance System. Coronary heart disease prevalence, for the State of Hawaiʻi, for the years 2011, 2012, 2013, 2014. Accessed September 12, 2020. http://hhdw.org/wp-content/uploads/BRFSS_Heart-Disease_IND_00001_20111.pdf.

11. Juarez DT, Davis JW, Brady SK, *et al.* Prevalence of heart disease and its risk factors related to age in Asians, Pacific Islanders, and Whites in Hawaiʻi. *J Health Care Poor Underserved.* 2012;23(3):1000–1010.

12. US Office of Minority Health. Heart disease and Native Hawaiians/Pacific Islanders. Accessed March 18, 2021. https://minorityhealth.hhs.gov/omh/browse.aspx?lvl=4&lvlid=79.

13. Odani S, Armour BS, Graffunder CM, *et al.* Prevalence and disparities in tobacco product use among American Indians/Alaska Natives - United States, 2010–2015. *MMWR Morb Mortal Wkly Rep.* 2017;66(50):1374–1378.

14. Hawaiʻi Health Data Warehouse. Hawaiʻi State Department of Health, Behavioral Risk Factor Surveillance System. Smoke - current smoker, for the State of Hawaiʻi, for the year 2014. Accessed May 23, 2021. http://hhdw.org/wp-content/uploads/BRFSS_Prevalence_IND_000012_2011.pdf.

15. Benjamin EJ, Muntner P, Alonso A, *et al.* Heart disease and stroke statistics-2019 update: A report from the American Heart Association. *Circulation.* 2019;139(10):e56–528.

16. Hawaiʻi Health Data Warehouse. Hawaiʻi State Department of Health, Behavioral Risk Factor Surveillance System, Weight - overweight or obese, for the State of Hawaiʻi, for the years 2011, 2012, 2013, 2014. Accessed September 12, 2020. http://hhdw.org/wp-content/uploads/BRFSS_Weight-Control_IND_00002_2011-1.pdf.

17. Pan L, Sherry B, Njai R, *et al.* Food insecurity is associated with obesity among US adults in 12 states. *J Acad Nutr Diet.* 2012;112(9):1403–1409.

18. Lee A, Cardel M, Donahoo WT. Social and environmental factors influencing obesity. In: Feingold KR, Anawalt B, Boyce A, *et al.*, eds. *Endotext.* MDText.com, Inc., 2000–2019.

19. Centers for Disease Control and Prevention. *US National Health Interview Survey 2018.* Accessed September 12, 2020. https://www.cdc.gov/nchs/nhis/shs/tables.htm.

20. Hawaiʻi Health Data Warehouse. Hawaiʻi State Department of Health, Behavioral Risk Factor Surveillance System. High blood pressure prevalence, for the State of Hawaiʻi, for the years 2011, 2013. Accessed May 23, 2021. http://hhdw.org/wp-content/uploads /BRFSS_Hypertension-Blood-Cholesterol_IND_00007_2011.pdf.

21. Centers for Disease Control and Prevention. *National diabetes statistics report, 2020.* Accessed September 14, 2020. https://www.cdc.gov/diabetes/pdfs/data/statistics /national-diabetes-statistics-report.pdf.

22. Uchima O, Wu YY, Browne C, *et al.* Diabetes disparities among Native Hawaiians/ Pacific Islanders and Asians who live in Hawaiʻi. *Prev Chronic Dis.* 2019;16:E22.

23. Gone JP, Trimble JE. American Indian and Alaska Native mental health: Diverse perspectives on enduring disparities. *Annu Rev Clin Psychol.* 2012;8:131–160.

24. Bassett D, Buchwald D, Manson S. Posttraumatic stress disorder and symptoms among American Indians and Alaska Natives: A review of the literature. *Soc Psychiatry Psychiatr Epidemiol.* 2014;49(3):417–433.

25. Walls ML, Sittner KJ, Aronson BD, *et al.* Stress exposure and physical, mental, and behavioral health among American Indian adults with type 2 diabetes. *Int J Environ Res Public Health.* 2017;14(9):1074.

26. Elm JHL, Walls ML, Aronson BD. Sources of stress among midwest American Indian adults with type 2 diabetes. *Am Indian Alsk Native Ment Health Res.* 2019;26(1):33–62.

27. Norris FH, Slone LB. The epidemiology of trauma and PTSD. In: Friedman M J, Keane TM, Resick PA, eds. *Handbook of PTSD: Science and practice.* Guilford Press, 2007: 78–98.

28. Kaholokula JK, Grandinetti A, Keller S, *et al.* Association between perceived racism and physiological stress indices in Native Hawaiians. *J Behav Med.* 2012;35(1):27–37.

29. Subica AM, Aitaoto N, Link BG, *et al.* Mental health status, need, and unmet need for mental health services among U.S. Pacific Islanders. *Psychiatr Serv.* 2019;70(7):578–585.

30. Kaholokula JK, Iwane MK, Nacapoy AH. Effects of perceived racism and acculturation on hypertension in Native Hawaiians. *Hawaii J Med Public Health.* 2010;69(5 suppl 2):11.

31. McCubbin LD, Antonio M. Discrimination and obesity among Native Hawaiians. *Hawaii J Med Public Health.* 2012;71(12):346–352.

32. Kuo CC, Howard BV, Umans JG, *et al.* Arsenic exposure, arsenic metabolism, and incident diabetes in the Strong Heart Study. *Diabetes Care.* 2015;38(4):620–627.

33. Muller CJ, Noonan CJ, MacLehose RF, *et al.* Trends in cardiovascular disease morbidity and mortality in American Indians over 25 years: The Strong Heart Study. *J Am Heart Assoc.* 2019;8(21):e012289.

34. Indian Health Service. Special diabetes program for Indians. Accessed January 1, 2021. https://www.ihs.gov/newsroom/factsheets/diabetes/.

35. Centers for Disease Control and Prevention. Southeast Alaska women are changing their lives. Accessed September 12, 2020. https://www.cdc.gov/wisewoman/alaska-searhc.htm.

36. INTERSALT Co-operative Research Group. INTERSALT study an international co-operative study on the relation of blood pressure to electrolyte excretion in populations. I. Design and methods. *J Hypertens.* 1986;4(12):781–787.

37. US Health Resources and Service Administration. Native Hawaiian Health Care Improvement Act (NHHCIA) and Papa Ola Lōkahi. Accessed February 27, 2021. https://bphc.hrsa.gov/program-opportunities/nhhcs.

38. Curb JD, Aluli NE, Kautz JA, *et al.* Cardiovascular risk factor levels in ethnic Hawaiians. *Am J Public Health.* 1991;81(2):164–167.

39. Blaisdell RK. 1995 Update on Kanaka Maoli (indigenous Hawaiian) health. *Asian Am Pac Isl J Health.* 1996;4(1–3):160–165.

40. Aluli NE, Connor WE, Kohn C, *et al.* Effects of pre-Western diet on plasma lipids, lipoproteins and blood pressure in native Hawaiians. Oral presentation at: American College of Physicians, Hawai`i Regional Annual Meeting, March, 1990.

41. Fujita R, Braun KL, Hughes C. The traditional Hawaiian diet: A review of the literature. *Pac Health Dialog.* 2004;11(2):250–259.

42. Aluli NE, Hughes CK, Blaisdell RK, *et al.* Weight control with the traditional Hawaiian diet and cultural education. Oral presentation at 4th National Forum on Minority Health Issues for an Emerging Majority, National Heart Lung and Blood Institute, June, 1992.

43. Shintani T, Beckham S, O'Connor HK, *et al.* The Waianae Diet Program: A culturally sensitive, community-based obesity and clinical intervention program for the Native Hawaiian population. *Hawaii Med J.* 1994;53(5):136–147.

44. Kouchi J, Oana V, Schimmelfennig H. *The Kaua'i Native Hawaiian diet program: A twenty-one day diet intervention valuation.* Kaua'i Community College, 1992.

Contributors

Noa Emmett Aluli, MD (Native Hawaiian) is a leader in research on cardiovascular risk factors among Native Hawaiians. He lives and maintains a family practice clinic on the island of Molokaʻi in the state of Hawaiʻi and also is the Medical Executive Director of Molokaʻi General Hospital. Dr. Aluli founded Na Puʻuwai, Inc., a private nonprofit charitable and educational corporation dedicated to the betterment of health conditions of Native Hawaiians and is the founder and past president of Na Puʻuwai Native Hawaiian Health Care System serving the islands of Molokaʻi and Lānaʻi. He is a founding member of ʻAhahui o Na Kauka, the Native Hawaiian Physicians Association; chairperson of the Kahoʻolawe Island Reserve Commission; founding member of Protect Kahoʻolawe ʻOhana; and cofounder of Pele Defense Fund.

Mapuana C. K. Antonio, MA, DrPH (Native Hawaiian) is a Hawaiian scholar dedicated to advancing the health and well-being of Native Hawaiians and other Indigenous Peoples. She is an Assistant Professor and Head of the Native Hawaiian and Indigenous Health MPH program in the Office of Public Health Studies in the Thompson School of Social Work and Public Health at the University of Hawaiʻi at Mānoa. She holds a joint appointment in the Department of Human Nutrition, Food and Animal Sciences and also is an Adjunct Assistant Professor in the Department of Psychiatry. Her research primarily focuses on community-based participatory research, sociocultural determinants of health, resilience, and general health among Native Hawaiians.

Ken Batai, PhD (Japanese) is a Research Assistant Professor of Urology and Public Health, University of Arizona. He is a cancer health disparities researcher specialized in urologic cancer and men's cancer. His research goals are to understand variation in urologic cancer diagnosis, treatment, and tumor biological characteristics in racial/ethnic minority groups, to identify genetic, biological, and social/behavioral factors affecting cancer health disparities, and to develop programs to reduce cancer burden and improve cancer care in medically underserved populations. He received a PhD in Anthropology from the University of Illinois at Chicago in 2012. He was a postdoctoral research fellow at the Cancer Education and Career Training Program, Institute for Health Research and Policy, University of Illinois at Chicago.

Jessica Blanchard, PhD is an Anthropologist and Research Scientist at the University of Oklahoma's Center for Applied Social Research. Dr. Blanchard's research partnerships address the reduction of health disparities in American Indian, Alaska Native, and other underrepresented communities, with specific attention to cancer care, prevention and delivery, ethical and social implications of genomics research, and community partnerships in health research. At the center of this work is a commitment to ethical community engagement and responsible research practices in communities that have not always been served well by research.

Mark C. Bauer, PhD, is Professor in the School of STEM (Science, Technology, Engineering, and Mathematics) at Diné College, where he has taught courses in math, computer science, and public health since 1980. He integrates the college's Diné education philosophy in designing the curriculum for statistics, research training, and public health planning, implementation, and evaluation, thus making the curriculum more culturally appropriate and tailored to Navajo students. He developed a highly successful Summer Research Enhancement Program to teach public health research methods to undergraduate Navajo and other AI students and support their participation in internships in a variety of programs serving their own communities in various health promotion areas. Since 2000, this program has engaged more than 250 undergraduate AI students in learning and applying quantitative and qualitative research skills.

Kathryn L. Braun, MPH, DrPH is Professor of Public Health and Social Work, and Chair of the PhD in Public Health program at the University of Hawai'i. She also is the Principal Investigator (PI) of Hā Kūpuna National Resource Center for Native Hawaiian Elders. She has codirected several projects funded by the National Institutes of Health (NIH) to train and mentor faculty, students, and community members of Native Hawaiian ancestry and from other underrepresented groups in community-based and translational research methods, including 'Imi Hale—Native Hawaiian Cancer Network. Dr. Braun teaches research methods and is a past winner of a Board of Regents Medal for Excellence in Teaching from the University of Hawai'i.

Linda Burhansstipanov, MSPH, DrPH (Cherokee Nation) has worked in public health since 1971. She taught at universities for 18 years (California State University, Long Beach and University of California, Los Angeles). She was promoted to full professor in 1987 and then developed and implemented the Native American Cancer Research Program at the National Cancer Institute (NCI) from 1989 to 1993. She worked at the Anschutz Medical Center in Denver for 5 years (1993–1998). She is the president of Native American Cancer Initiatives, Inc. (minority woman's for-profit business, 1998) and founded the Native American Cancer Research Corporation (nonprofit) in 1999. She has been the PI or subcontractor for more than 20 NIH grants.

Kevin Darryl Cassel, MPH, DrPH (African American) is Associate Professor (Researcher), Cancer Prevention in the Pacific Program at the University of Hawai'i Cancer Center. He began his career in 1993 in Philadelphia as a cancer prevention and control educator for the NCI, working with underserved communities. After transferring to Hawai'i in 1995, he earned advanced degrees in public health and began conducting community-engaged research in Hawai'i and the Pacific. He has served as PI or Co-PI on numerous projects funded by the NIH, including INdigenous Samoan Partnership to Initiate Research Excellence (INSPIRE), funded by the National Institutes of Minority Health and Health Disparities from 2016 to 2021. INSPIRE provides an example of a project that intertwines academic and Indigenous knowledge to solve problems and build community strengths.

Judith Clark, MPH is the Executive Director of Hawai'i Youth Services Network (HYSN), a statewide coalition of youth-serving organizations and a Pacific Islands training and technical assistance center. HYSN is recognized nationally as a leader in efforts to adapt evidence-based curricula and create culturally relevant educational materials for Pacific Islander and Asian youth. Ms. Clark's areas of expertise include federal grant writing and grants management, designing culturally relevant programs for minority youth, sustainability, and nonprofit management. Judith's awards include Outstanding Advocate for Children and Youth from the Hawai'i State Legislature, the Culture of Respect Award from the National Safe Place Network, and the Weinberg Foundation's AIM for Excellence Award for outstanding nonprofit management.

Jane J. Chung-Do (Korean) is an Associate Professor of Public Health at the University of Hawai'i and a Robert Wood Johnson Foundation Interdisciplinary Research Leaders Fellow. Her research focuses on promoting healthy eating habits through the development and implementation of a family-based backyard aquaponics programming called MALAMA (Mini Ahupua'a for Lifestyle and Mea'ai through Aquaponics) in rural Native Hawaiian communities. Dr. Chung-Do also is cofounder of the Waimānalo Pono Research Hui, a grassroots group promoting community-driven and culturally grounded research, and a director of Ke Kula Nui O Waimānalo. In 2020, she was awarded the Robert Wood Johnson Foundation Health Equity Award as recognition for her work in changing systems and policies at the local level to promote health equity.

May Rose I. Dela Cruz, MPH, DrPH (Filipino) is an Assistant Researcher in the Office of Public Health Studies Program, Thompson School of Social Work and Public Health, University of Hawaiʻi. She formerly worked at ʻImi Hale Native Hawaiian Cancer Network where she aimed to reduce cancer incidence and mortality among Native Hawaiians, Filipinos, and Pacific Islanders through policy, advocacy, programs, and research. Her research projects aim to increase HPV vaccination uptake, decrease minors' access to alcohol, and increase involvement of Filipino communities in health research. Dr. Dela Cruz was born in the Philippines with Filipino indigenous roots in Luzon and the Visayas, and she enjoys creating and testing culturally relevant health education materials for Hawaiʻi residents.

Florence (Tinka) Duran, BS, MPH (Rosebud Sioux Tribe) received her MPH at the University of Nebraska Medical Center in 2018. She serves as the Program Director for Great Plains Prevention Programs of the Great Plain Tribal Chairmen's Health Board. The Great Plains Prevention Programs work on cancer prevention and early detection utilizing evidence-based interventions with the Great Plains Tribes. This includes Tribal Nations in North Dakota, South Dakota, Nebraska, and Iowa.

Leah Frerichs, PhD is a health services researcher in the Department of Health Policy and Management, Gillings School of Global Public Health at the University of North Carolina at Chapel Hill. From 2005 to 2010, she worked for the Great Plains Tribal Chairmen's Health Board, managing their comprehensive cancer control program. She and her collaborators have produced several peer-reviewed manuscripts focused on assessing and documenting American Indian health disparities in a variety of domains including HPV, colorectal cancer, and healthcare access. From 2016 to 2020, she worked with tribes in North Carolina to develop culturally appropriate strategies for colorectal cancer screening.

Francine C. Gachupin, PhD, MPH (Jemez Pueblo tribal member) is an Associate Professor, Department of Family and Community Medicine, College of Medicine, University of Arizona. She received her PhD from the University of New Mexico and her MPH in epidemiology from the University of Washington. She studies primarily chronic diseases and related behavioral risk factors among American Indians. She is the director of the American Indian Youth Wellness Camp. Dr. Gachupin is also currently involved with the University of Arizona Cancer Center (UACC) Partnership for Native American Cancer Prevention (NACP). On the NACP grant, Dr. Gachupin is the UACC PI and NACP Outreach Core PI. The goal of the NACP is to alleviate the unequal burden of cancer among Native Americans of the Southwest through research, training, and community outreach.

Lisa D. Harjo, MEd (Choctaw) is the Executive Director of Native American Cancer Research Corporation (since 2012) and a Senior Researcher for Native American Cancer Initiatives, Inc. Her work in cancer started as a native patient navigator in 2001. She has navigated many American Indian patients to cancer care including quality of life and recovery and has sponsored and facilitated a support group since 2003. She also is faculty for navigator trainings. She has been the project director for multiple federal, state, and foundation grants and has coordinated and supervised multisite, NIH-funded, American Indian research studies and staff locally, regionally, and nationally. She also was Executive Director for the Denver Indian Clinic from the mid-1980s to 2000.

Emily Haozous, PhD, RN, FAAN (Chiricahua Fort Sill Apache) is Research Scientist with the Pacific Institute for Research and Evaluation, Albuquerque office. Dr. Haozous received her BA in music from the University of California, Santa Cruz and her MSN and PhD in nursing from Yale University. Her research is guided by the priorities of her collaborating American Indian partners and collaborators. She has published on cancer pain management, telehealth and video conferencing, elder care, hospice, and palliative care, national trends in premature mortality, and cancer decision-making. She is passionate about policy change that brings equitable healthcare delivery to Indian Country. She is grounded by her family and is most proud of her two teenage sons because they push her to keep asking the hard questions.

Suzanne Held, PhD is a Professor in the Department of Health and Human Development at Montana State University in the area of Community Health. She has worked since 1996 as a non-Indigenous partner with Alma McCormick and other community members from the Apsáalooke (Crow) Nation with the Messengers for Health program in the areas of cancer screening, men's health, cultural competency of healthcare workers, and chronic illness self-management. Her research interests are to work in partnership with communities to establish trust, share power, foster colearning, and examine and address community-identified needs and health issues using strengths-based approaches. She is White, originally from Wisconsin, and understands that health disparities exist because of colonization and current policies that privilege Whites, and she wants to do her part toward a healthier and more equitable future.

Chiu-Hiseh (Paul) Hsu, PhD (Chinese) is a Professor of Biostatistics in the Mel and Enid Zuckerman College of Public Health, University of Arizona. He received his doctorate in biostatistics from the University of Michigan. His research interests include developing statistical methodologies for survival analysis subject to dependent censoring and data subject to the non-ignorable missing mechanism and developing statistical approaches to better analyze biomedical data such as misclassification and variable selection. In addition, he has been working closely with Hopi to evaluate the use of navigators and mobile health to improve cancer screening, particularly for Hopi men, as well as identifying health disparities associated with Americans Indians.

Ilima Ho-Lastimosa (Native Hawaiian) is a cultural practitioner, community leader, and strong proponent of food sovereignty and sustainability. Her life's work is dedicated to promoting traditional growing practices, as well as new technologies, including aquaponics, to give Native Hawaiians the tools, knowledge, and skills to grow and consume healthy foods. Ilima is the Community Coordinator at the Waimānalo Learning Center, working with numerous children in area schools. She also is founder of God's Country Waimānalo, cofounder of the Waimānalo Pono Research Hui, a Director for Ke Kula Nui O Waimānalo, and a Robert Wood Johnson Foundation Interdisciplinary Research Leaders Fellow. In 2020, she was awarded the Robert Wood Johnson Foundation Health Equity Award as recognition for her work to promote health equity.

Christina L. Interpreter, RN, FNP-C (Hopi Tribe and Navajo Nation) is a Family Nurse Practitioner practicing primary care with the Salt River Pima Maricopa Indian Community in Scottsdale, AZ. She attained a BS in health promotion/education and a BS and MS in nursing, and she is a family nurse practitioner. Christina grew up on both Navajo and Hopi reservations. Today, she enjoys spending time with her daughters and grandchildren and resides in Mesa, AZ.

Cornelia "Connie" Jessen, MA oversees the HIV/STD Prevention Program within the Alaska Native Tribal Health Consortium. She also serves as the Program Director for the Native American Research Centers for Health–funded Alaska Indigenous Research Program. Her work experience has given her the opportunity to collaborate with tribal partners and communities on efforts to promote health and wellness among Alaska Natives through community-based and culturally responsive efforts. Ms. Jessen received a bachelor's degree in anthropology and a master's degree in applied anthropology from the University of Alaska, Anchorage.

Jennie R. Joe, PhD, MPH, MA (Navajo Nation) is currently Professor Emerita in the Department of Family and Community Medicine at the University of Arizona. Her joint doctoral degree is from the Universities of California at Berkeley and San Francisco. Her academic studies included disciplines in nursing, public health, anthropology, and medical anthropology. She also was a faculty member at the University of California, Los Angeles, with a joint appointment in American Indian Studies. At the University of Arizona, she directed the Native American Research and Training Center and was an affiliated member in American Indian Studies. Some of her research endeavors gave special attention to the role of culture, environment, and epigenetics as factors impacting chronic diseases, disabilities, and Indigenous health promotion and prevention programs. She continues to focus on various areas of health disparities and their impact on Indigenous populations.

Lloyd Joshweseoma (Hopi Tribe, deceased) worked as the Public Health Compliance technician for the Hopi Department of Health and Human Services. He was involved in several cancer research projects on the Hopi Reservation and most recently served as a native patient navigator in a men's health research initiative for Hopi. Through his work, he collaborated and partnered with Northern Arizona University and the University of Arizona to promote health and wellness among Hopi men.

Lorencita Joshweseoma, MPH (Hopi Tribe) is a facilitator for the Hopi Tutukaihki school on the Hopi Reservation that provides Hopi language immersion through art. She served as the Health Director for the Hopi Tribe for 11 years and served as a Co-PI in projects relating to cancer in Hopi. Her experience as the Hopi Cancer Support Services Administrator has allowed her to assist with research opportunities that led to the overall development of the Hopi Cancer Support Services program. Her overall goal is to work closely with the Hopi community in the area of health and community wellness, to provide opportunities that will enhance services through research initiatives, to ensure that Hopi has a research policy that will protect Hopi people and community, and to provide opportunities for those who are interested in conducting research on Hopi.

Lana Sue I. Kaʻopua, PhD, DCSW, LSW (Native Hawaiian) learned this Hawaiian wisdom early in life: "Mohala i ka wai ka maka o ka pua," which means "unfolded by the water are the faces of the flowers." In plain language, people are like flowers that thrive and bloom when health and well-being are purposely nurtured. This wisdom is a continual reminder to her and motivated her work with Dr. Cassel on the INdigenous Samoan Partnership to Initiate Research Excellence (INSPIRE). Together, they established Le Fale o Soʻofaʻatasiga, a center committed to addressing colorectal cancer and other health disparities. In their chapter, they describe the process of lalaga (weaving) Indigenous and Western knowledge with the cultural strengths of le aiga potopoto (community) of American Samoa.

Keilyn Leinaʻala Kawakami, BA (Native Hawaiian) graduated from the University of Washington with a BA in Global Public Health. She currently is an MPH candidate and a Graduate Research Assistant at the Thompson School of Social Work and Public Health at the University of Hawaiʻi. She has worked on projects through Hā Kūpuna National Resource Center for Native Hawaiian Elders and the University of Hawaiʻi Foundation Barbara Cox Anthony Endowment assisting with community-based participatory research projects to increase health among kūpuna and share Native Hawaiian knowledge with future generations. She was born in Honolulu and is of Hawaiian, Japanese, and Chinese ancestry.

Alma Knows His Gun McCormick, BS (Apsáalooke Crow Indian) has been a leader and community activist for improved health and wellness among the Crow people. Since 2001, she has partnered with the Montana State University, Bozeman and has gained extensive and successful experiences in community-based participatory research in the Crow community, addressing health concerns such as cancer and chronic illness self-care management. She is the Executive Director of Messengers for Health, an Indigenous nonprofit organization in the Crow community. She has multiple publications and has provided presentations nationwide regarding her work. Alma always shares that her passion to help others stems from losing her young daughter to cancer in 1985.

Naomi R. Lee, PhD (Seneca Nation of Indians located in western New York state) is an Assistant Professor in the Department of Chemistry and Biochemistry at Northern Arizona University. She is also an affiliate faculty of the Southwest Health Equity Research Collaborative, the Partnership for Native American Cancer Prevention, and the Center for Materials Interfaces in

Research and Applications. Her research interests are multidisciplinary and focus on novel peptide- and protein-based vaccine development and addressing health disparities in American Indian and Alaska Native communities. Dr. Lee works with various tribal communities across the country, primarily on projects related to sexually transmitted infection prevalence and risk factors.

Pearl A. McElfish, PhD, MBA, MS, PMP serves as Vice Chancellor for the University of Arkansas for Medical Sciences (UAMS), oversees the Office of Community Health and Research, serves as Co-director of the Center for Pacific Islander Health, and holds faculty positions in the UAMS Colleges of Medicine, Nursing, and Public Health. Dr. McElfish's research focuses on reducing health disparities with Pacific Islander and Hispanic communities. She also conducts food systems research and methodological research related to the best methods for conducting community-based participatory research and for disseminating research results to participants and communities. She has published more than 140 peer-reviewed articles based on her community health research in Northwest Arkansas.

Kristen Mitchell-Box, DrPH, MSPH has extensive work experience as a program evaluator and community-based researcher in Hawai'i and Alaska. When she relocated to Alaska in 2011, she first worked as a Research Assistant Professor at the University of Alaska, Anchorage conducting research and providing evaluation services related to suicide prevention programs. She moved to the Alaska Native Tribal Health Consortium in 2015, where she currently serves as a Senior Program Manager at the Alaska Native Epidemiology Center.

Marjoree Neer, FNP joined Toiyabe Indian Health Project in 2011 as the Director of the Toiyabe Public Health Department. She earned baccalaureate degrees from the University of California, Davis and the University of California, Los Angeles and completed her master's in nursing at California State University, Long Beach. She moved to the Eastern Sierra of California in 2000, where she has worked for both the Mono County and Inyo County Health Departments. She is the project director on grants from the Centers for Disease Control and Prevention, e.g., the Special Diabetes Program for Indians and a Public Health Capacity prediabetes grant. She has a great interest in supporting families and assisting them to be healthy and resilient. She believes this support to individuals and communities comes in the form of increasing knowledge, partnerships with families and providers, access to resources and care, and policies and systems that meet the needs of families.

Rachel Novotny, PhD, RDN is Professor and Chair of Graduate Programs in Nutritional Sciences, and Director of the Children's Healthy Living (CHL) Center of Excellence at the University of Hawaiʻi at Mānoa, which focuses on research, training, and outreach in partnership with colleges and Indigenous populations of the US-Affiliated Pacific region. She has worked with diverse populations in the Caribbean, Central and South America, Indonesia, and the Pacific to understand and support ways of life that promote health. She has published more than 150 papers and garnered more than $32 million in federal grants in this work. She has lived and worked in Hawaiʻi for more than 30 years. Her ancestors fled war and persecution in Eastern Europe to the New England area of the US, where she was born and raised.

Marcia O'Leary, BSN is the director of Missouri Breaks Industries Research Inc. (MBIRI), an American Indian–owned research group located on the Cheyenne River Reservation in South Dakota. MBIRI has helped to develop more than 50 projects specific to health in American Indian populations. As a coordinator of the Strong Heart Study, the longest-running study of heart disease in an American Indian population, she has worked to bridge the gap between scientists and communities, to improve capacity and translation of findings, and to narrow time to application of project results. Building capacity and health ownership are key to changing the trajectory of health outcomes, but both must be culturally appropriate and intentional.

Avery Keller Olson, BS is a medical student attending the University of South Dakota Sanford School of Medicine in Vermillion, South Dakota. She received her BS in biomedical science and global environmental sustainability from Colorado State University in 2016 and hopes to continue to pursue a career in medicine with a focus on medically underserved populations. In 2010, she helped to develop and implement a mobile health clinic in the Zumbo district of Mozambique, Care for Zumbo, in coordination with the local department of health. In 2017 she started working with Dr. Daniel Petereit and Walking Forward to address cancer disparities affecting the American Indians living on the Pine Ridge, Rosebud, and Cheyenne River Reservations. As someone born and raised in South Dakota, she plans to return and provide care to American Indian populations after residency.

Donna-Marie Palakiko, PhD, RN, APRN (Native Hawaiian) is a mother, nurse, researcher, and health strategist. Dr. Palakiko has over 20 years of experience as a health strategist with a focus on addressing Native Hawaiian health disparities through community-based participatory research, health promotion and disease prevention programs, and building a Native Hawaiian health workforce. She earned her doctorate from the School of Nursing and Dental Hygiene at the University of Hawai'i, an MS from the University of California, San Francisco with a specialization in community and cross-cultural health, and a BS in nursing from the University of San Francisco. Dr. Palakiko has committed her life's work toward improving the health and well-being of Indigenous Peoples.

Martha Pearson, MA, MPA is Director of Health Promotion for the Southeast Alaska Regional Health Consortium (SEARHC), where she oversees multiple health promotion programs for Indigenous Peoples and rural communities in southeast Alaska. She has worked for over two decades as a health educator and program coordinator for programs in Alaska that address chronic disease prevention, policies, systems, and environmental changes, alcohol and suicide prevention, and home health. Ms. Pearson has lived in Alaska since 1996 and has worked for SEARHC since 2002.

Daniel Petereit, MD is a radiation oncologist in Rapid City, SD, and is the PI of the Walking Forward Cancer Disparity Program, which has been funded by the NCI since 2002. The goal of the program is to lower cancer mortality rates for American Indians through patient navigation, clinical trial access, and identification of barriers to early detection and successful treatment. Published critical outcomes include an establishment of trust within tribal communities, identification of barriers to cancer screenings, creation of research infrastructure, clinical trial enrollment of 4,500 American Indians, and higher treatment compliance and patient satisfaction rates. Walking Forward also has tested multiple interventions for smoking cessation and lung cancer screening.

Erin Peterson, MPH is a Senior Epidemiologist at the Alaska Native Epidemiology Center, Alaska Native Tribal Health Consortium (ANTHC). Ms. Peterson has worked in chronic disease prevention in Alaska since 2002, joining ANTHC in 2015. In her work, she collaborates with tribal health partners to implement policies and practices that increase access to healthy foods and beverages, increase opportunities for physical activity, reduce tobacco use, and enhance chronic disease management. Ms. Peterson holds an MPH from the Rollins School of Public Health at Emory University.

Noel L. Pingatore, MPH is the Director for the Department of Health Education and Chronic Disease at the Inter-Tribal Council of Michigan. She has 25 years' experience working for and with American Indian and Alaska Native populations in Michigan and across the US. Ms. Pingatore utilizes community-based participatory approaches and has worked to improve quality health data and surveillance measures for tribal populations, adapt and implement evidence-based interventions to the unique needs and culture of Native American communities, and facilitate quality improvement processes in tribal health systems, resulting in increased cancer screening rates, improved coordination of care and increased patient satisfaction.

Valerie Rangel (descent of Diné and Oak Springs Apache) is an author, environmental and public health research consultant, and environmental health and justice advocate, as well as being the Fiscal Sponsorship and Outreach Coordinator at the New Mexico Foundation. She earned her master's degree in community regional planning at the University of New Mexico, majoring in Indigenous planning and minoring in public health. She has lectured in earth science, health, and Southwest history courses as a contributing faculty member at the Santa Fe University of Art and Design. In 2018 she presented selections from her book *Environmental Justice in New Mexico: Counting Coup* at the National Environmental Justice conference in Washington, DC. Her book presents stories of strife and struggle in the war to protect the integrity of natural systems, rights to religious freedom, and the continuation of traditional customs.

Noshene Ranjbar, MD originally from Iran, is an Assistant Professor of Psychiatry, Training Director of the Integrative Psychiatry Fellowship, and Medical Director of the Integrative Psychiatry Clinic at the University of Arizona, Tucson. Additionally, she serves as faculty with the Andrew Weil Center for Integrative Medicine and the Center for Mind-Body Medicine. Since 2010, she has been involved in the development of trauma-informed programs using a train-the-trainer model of mind-body medicine in American Indian communities. Using strength-based, culturally sensitive, and community-focused approaches, she leads groups, workshops, and trainings for American Indian youth and adults to address diverse challenges, including the youth suicide epidemic, and to promote resiliency in the face of historical, intergenerational, developmental, and complex trauma.

Diana G. Redwood PhD, MPH is a Senior Epidemiologist at the Alaska Native Epidemiology Center, Alaska Native Tribal Health Consortium. Dr. Redwood has worked in the Alaska Tribal Health System since 2004. Her expertise is in public health and epidemiology, with a focus on cancer screening and prevention. She also researches novel methods of colorectal cancer screening outreach and new screening methods for the Alaska Native population. She is a member of the Indian Health Services Task Force on Colorectal Cancer and has published extensively on her work with Alaska Native people. She consults frequently with states and tribal programs on best practices for colorectal cancer prevention and control and is a passionate advocate for decreasing the burden of cancer among Alaska Native and American Indian people.

Marie Kainoa Fialkowski Revilla, PhD, RDN, LD, IBC (Native Hawaiian) is Associate Professor of Human Nutrition in the Department of Human Nutrition, Food, and Animal Sciences at the University of Hawai'i at Mānoa. Her primary role is to honor her 'ohana (family) through being the best wife, mother, daughter, sister, and niece that she can be. Her secondary role is to honor her community by engaging in work that will raise up the health and well-being of Native Hawaiians and other Indigenous Peoples. She is particularly passionate about promoting the health and well-being of nā pēpē (babies). She hopes to honor all of those who have helped her to get to where she is today by supporting and nurturing the achievement of other Native Hawaiians and Indigenous Peoples in the field of nutrition and dietetics.

Dana Russell, BBA (Navajo Nation) received her Bachelor of Business Administration from Central State University in 1972. She possesses leadership skills in management, training, and the motivation to work with diverse groups and organizations. She has worked extensively with American Indian individuals and entities involving education, entrepreneurship, and nonprofit human services. Her contributions to science include involvement in a 5-year study with the University of Washington to address the incidence of HPV across the life span of Hopi Women. She also served as a Co-PI of a community-based research pilot project with Northern Arizona University and the University of Arizona to determine the efficacy of employing mHealth technology to increase awareness, knowledge, and male cancer screening for Hopi men.

Priscilla R. Sanderson, PhD, MS, CRC (Navajo Nation) knows her maternal clan is Hozii Táchii'nii (Old Orabi Red Running Into the Water People), born for Kinyaa'ánii (Towering House). Her maternal grandfather's clan is Nakaiidini, and paternal grandfather's clan is Bit'ahnii (Leaf). She has been a member of the Northern Arizona University (NAU) Health Sciences faculty since 2009. She was the PI of the Center for American Indian Resilience (CAIR), which partnered with American Indian communities to promote health and resilience. She was PI for the Hopi Men's Pilot Study (2017–2019). She also was PI for an H.pylori study in collaboration with the NAU-University of Arizona

Partnership for Native American Cancer Prevention, and is Co-PI on an NIH H.pylori study. She is a Hampton Faculty Fellow with the Spirit of EAGLES, Mayo Clinic, Rochester, Minnesota.

Ross Shegog, PhD is a Professor of Behavioral Science at the University of Texas School of Public Health and Adjunct Professor with the University of Texas School of Biomedical Informatics. His research focuses on the application of communication technology in health promotion, disease prevention, and disease management to find creative solutions to the challenges of optimally impacting health behavior. His recent projects have focused on the application of computer-based education, decision-support systems, and gaming in the health domains of pediatric asthma management, tobacco cessation and prevention, HIV/STI/pregnancy prevention, violence prevention, physical activity, epilepsy self-management, disaster response worker safety, and HPV vaccination. Dr. Shegog completed his postdoctoral degrees at the University of Sydney and the University of Texas.

Vanessa Simonds, PhD (Crow Tribe and descendant of the Blackfeet Nation) is Associate Professor in Community Health at Montana State University. She earned her graduate degrees from the Harvard School of Public Health. Dr. Simonds uses community-based participatory research approaches to promote health literacy in American Indian communities. She is committed to strength-based, community-centered outreach strategies designed in partnership with Native American communities. For the past 6 years, she has collaborated with tribal partners to implement an environmental health literacy program for youth and their families.

Teshia G. Arambula Solomon, PhD, (Choctaw/Mexican American) is an Associate Professor at the University of Arizona. Dr. Solomon has over 30 years of experience in health research, training, and community engagement with Indigenous populations. Her research has focused on addressing health equity, with emphasis on the preservation and protection of culture. She was lead editor and author of the book *Conducting Health Research with Native American Communities*. Her work guides policy at the national level, including the Cultural Wisdom Declaration published in both the National Tribal Behavioral Health Agenda and the Centers for Disease Control and Prevention Tribal Public Health Agenda. She earned a National Award for Public Health Innovation by the National Indian Health Board in 2018 and was named the University Distinguished Outreach Faculty in 2020.

Christina (Kiki) Stinnett (Chuukese, deceased) was a successful entrepreneur and president of the Chuuk Women's Council (CWC), an umbrella organization in Chuuk State, Federated States of Micronesia (FSM) that collectively promotes women's leadership, education on health and gender issues, environmental conservation, and the preservation of traditional and cultural crafts. She also sat on various boards for both the Chuukese and FSM National Government. Kiki was passionate about women's rights, and CWC is the leading community development and women's rights organization in the FSM. She oversaw many largescale projects as president of CWC, working closely with donors such as the United Nations, the US Agency for International Development, and the Australia Government.

Nicolette I. Teufel-Shone, MA, PhD is the Associate Director of the Center for Health Equity Research and Professor of Health Sciences at Northern Arizona University (NAU). She has formal training in anthropology, nutrition, and community health. She received her masters from NAU and her PhD from the University of Colorado. She has worked with Native Nations since the mid-1980s. She is the Co-PI of the NIH-funded Navajo Nation Native American Research Center for Health Partnership. This initiative is building an educational pathway for Navajo high school, undergraduate, and graduate students to pursue careers in public health and health research. From 2012 to 2017, she coled with Dr. Sanderson the NIH-funded Center of American Indian Resilience, designed to understand and disseminate culturally informed strategies to achieve health equity.

JoAnn 'Umilani Tsark, MPH (Native Hawaiian) is the former Research Director of Papa Ola Lōkahi, a community-based consortium dedicated to increasing the health and wellness of Native Hawaiians, and also served as the Project Director of 'Imi Hale Native Hawaiian Cancer Network from 2000 to 2018. Ms. Tsark brings 30+ years of experience as a public health educator working with groups with low levels of health literacy and with medically underserved communities. She led the 'Imi Hale team to become the leader in supporting emerging Native Hawaiian researchers, providing Hawai'i's only cancer patient navigation training, and developing culturally tailored cancer education materials and tools. She currently serves as a Director for the Community Engaged Core of Ola HAWAII at the University of Hawai'i, John A. Burns School of Medicine.

Jessica Saniguq Ullrich, PhD (Inupiaq) is an Assistant Professor at the University of Alaska Anchorage in the School of Social Work. Jessica has been a scholar with the Native Child Research Exchange program, the Indigenous Wellness Research Institute ISMART program, and Council of Social Work Education Minority Fellowship Program. Jessica's research interests pertain to the promotion of Alaska Native child well-being using an Indigenous Connectedness Framework. This framework highlights the importance of being in right relationship with family, community, the earth, ancestors/future generations, and with spirit. Jessica is currently coauthoring a paper that focuses on the application of Indigenous Connectedness to child welfare, and she will work with Alaska Native youth from three rural communities using digital storytelling to highlight community protective factors.

Index

Understanding and Improving Health for Minority and Disadvantaged Populations

Series Editor: F. Douglas Scutchfield

This series investigates the nature and character of current public health and medical care issues for specific disadvantaged and minority populations in the United States. It also seeks to examine the medical care status and concerns that impact the care these populations receive. Books in this series suggest new approaches based on evidence-driven solutions to the inequities that members of these groups face in health. This series includes coverage of Appalachian, Black, Indigenous, Latinx, and refugee populations, among others, and examines challenges that disproportionately affect these groups. Books in this series describe the notion of socioecological determinants within these populations and examine efforts to mitigate for these determinants. The texts are intended for public health students, educators, and policymakers, as well as the educated lay person with an interest in public health topics and solutions for these marginalized populations.